Nursing Older Adults

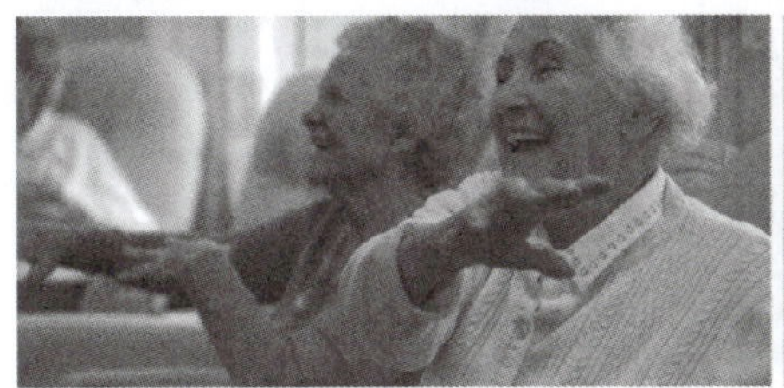
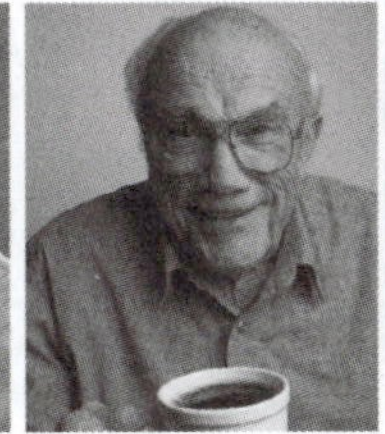
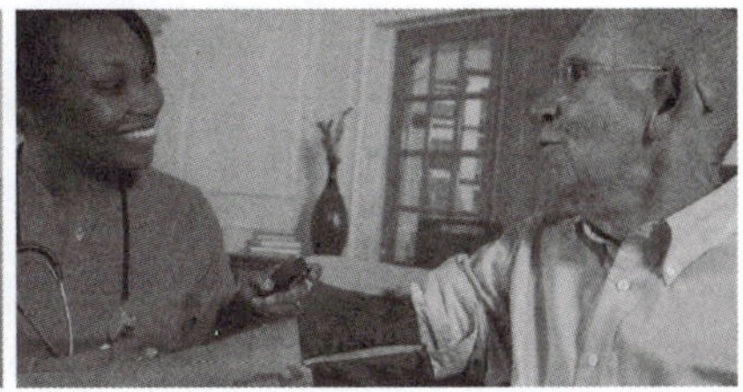

Nursing Older Adults

Edited by Jan Reed, Charlotte L. Clarke, Ann Macfarlane

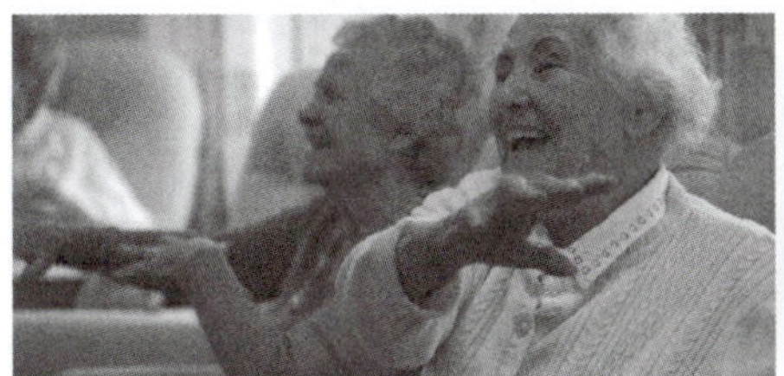

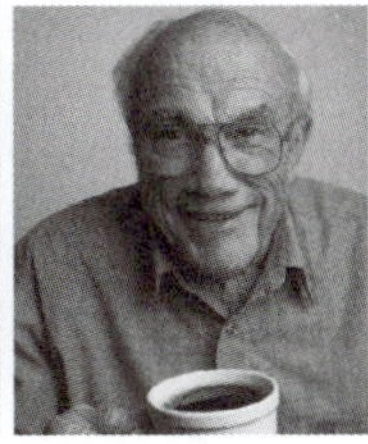

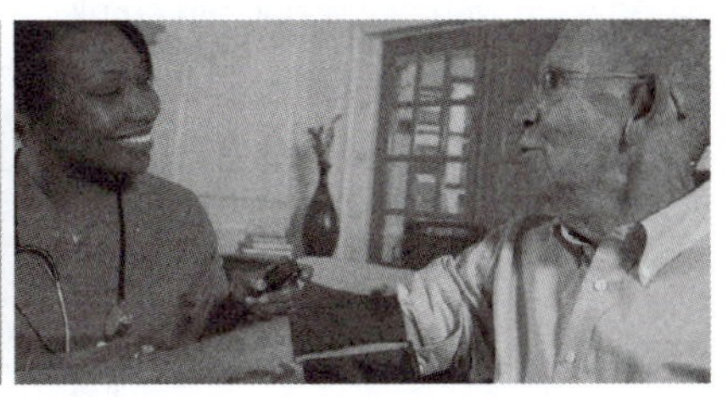

McGraw Hill Open University Press

Open University Press
McGraw-Hill Education
McGraw-Hill House
Shoppenhangers Road
Maidenhead
Berkshire
England
SL6 2QL

email: enquiries@openup.co.uk
world wide web: www.openup.co.uk

and
Two Penn Plaza, New York, NY 10121-2289, USA

First published 2012

A catalogue record of this book is available from the British Library

ISBN-13: 978-0-335-24084-5
ISBN-10: 0-335-24084-4
eISBN: 978-0-335-24085-2

Library of Congress Cataloging-in-Publication Data
CIP data applied for

Typeset by Aptara Inc., India
Printed in the UK by Bell and Bain Ltd, Glasgow.

The McGraw·Hill Companies

Praise for this book

"Never was a book like this more urgently needed. Its combination of authority and experience makes it especially valuable. Its wisdom is based on the knowledge and understanding of how growing frail really afflicts older people. We who have known independence and freedom need to have our lives respected. This book makes a good case for encouraging older people to enjoy as much autonomy as possible and to collaborate with their carers in keeping well. Those who nurse older people will find much sound help within these pages."

Broadcaster and writer Dame Joan Bakewell

"I am delighted to commend this book to you. Putting older people at the centre of their care and support is central in all good nursing care. However, this publication clearly demonstrates the changes to nursing practice that are needed to make this a reality for individual older people. At a time when the number of older people in our society is growing and, when their care is often unfavourable under the spotlight, this publication will provide an invaluable resource for nurses."

Dame Christine Beasley, DBE, Chief Nursing Officer for England

"Nurses have always known the importance of including the consumer's voice into practice; however, this text takes this view to additional heights and incorporates the voice of the older person in true partnership as a book editor. This text makes an extraordinary contribution to scholarship and practice and is sure to be on most undergraduate and postgraduate nursing students 'must have' list of texts."

Wendy Moyle, PhD, RN Director, Research Centre for Community Practice Innovation, Griffith University, Australia

"Nursing Older Adults' edited by Jan Reed, Charlotte Clarke and Ann Macfarlane is a great book: giving a comprehensive insight in the fundamentals of working with older people and key issues in nursing older people. I very much liked the empowering nursing approach, putting the perspectives and resources of older people consequently into the focus of the nursing process. The voice of older people is vividly written in many examples and scenarios given. I recommend this book to nurses, care staff, all who are in the education and qualification sector and other stakeholders in elder care and hope it will be adopted in a broad international context. I enjoyed reading it: very well structured and a work of reference for the issues in nursing older adults."

Professor Dr. Barbara Klein, Fachhochschule Frankfurt am Main – University of Applied Sciences, Germany

Contents

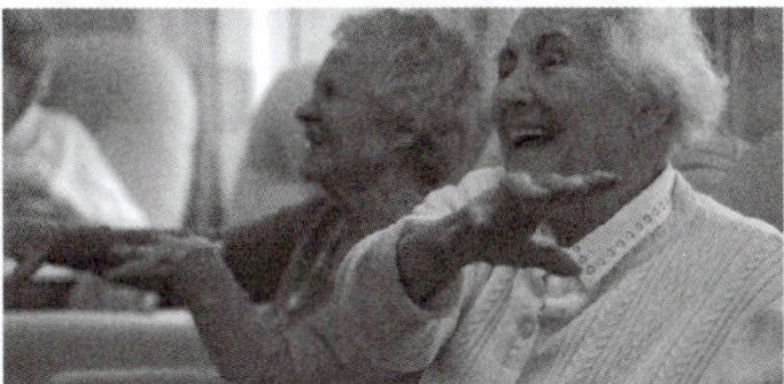 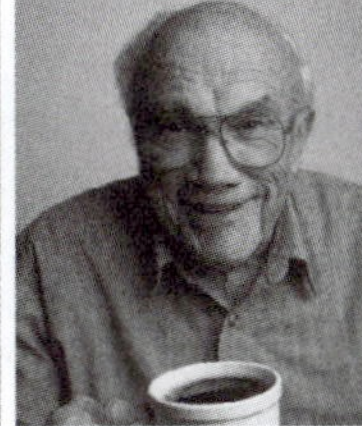 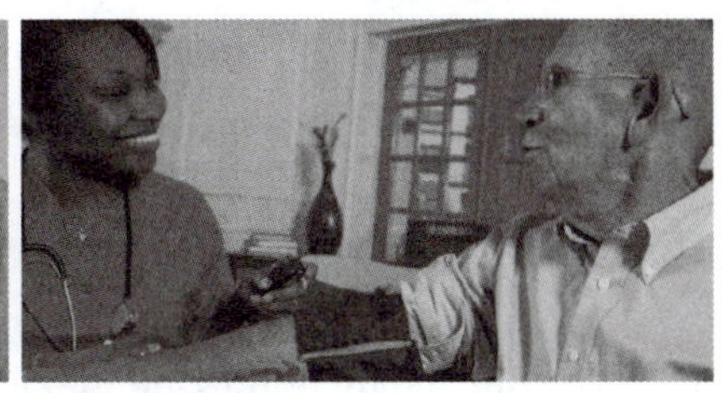

Contributors

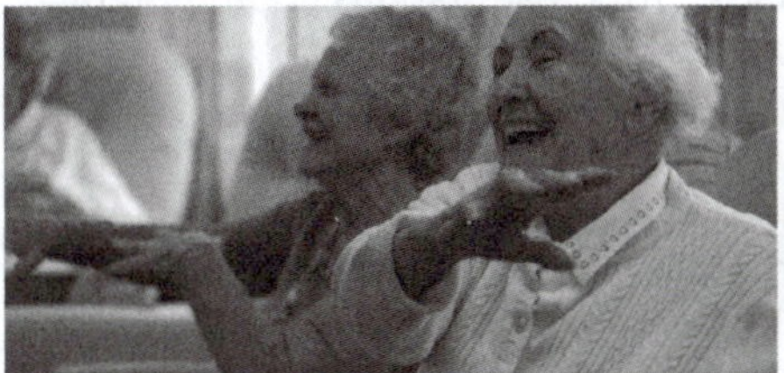
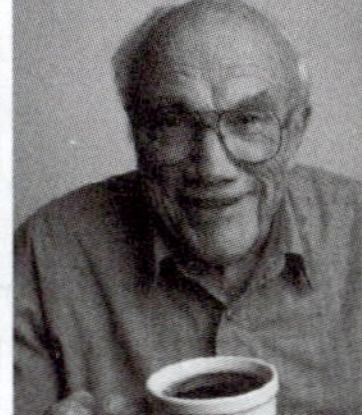
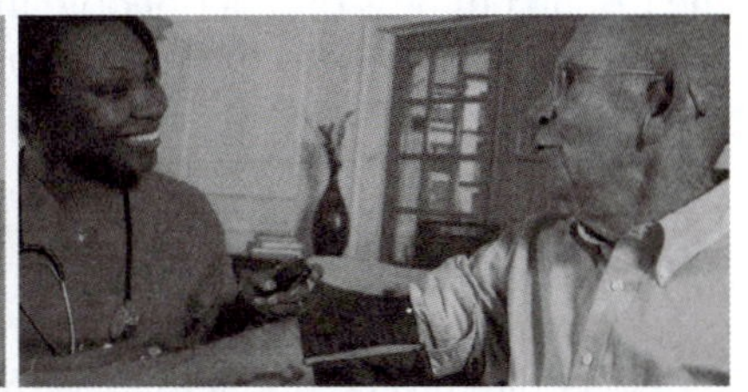

Serena Allan is Head of Care at Braeside House, a Royal Blind care home in Edinburgh, whose purpose is to provide nursing care and support for older adults with visual impairments.

Michael Bauer is a senior research fellow at the Australian Centre for Evidence Based Aged Care at La Trobe University Melbourne, Victoria, Australia where his work is aimed at improving the care of older people. He has a particular research interest in sexuality in long-term care facilities, an area which is still to be acknowledged as a legitimate issue of concern by many aged care service providers. He is a frequent speaker on this topic and has published widely.

Sheena Blair is an occupational therapist by profession and initially her clinical work was in mental health where she specialized in psychodynamic practice, group work and work with older people. She is also Programme Director for Professional Doctorate, School of Health, Glasgow Caledonian University. Her academic interests have also centred upon older people, life transitions especially in later life and the psychodynamics of ageing. She has had a particular research interest in learning in later life and her doctoral thesis was on this topic. Various consultancies have been concerned with helping older people understand the research process and even undertake small research projects themselves. Her career has spanned over 40 years and throughout she has retained a fascination with later life, the dynamics of ageing and the occupational lives of older people and she has contributed to literature in this area.

Jo Booth is a Reader in the School of Health at Glasgow Caledonian University. Her research and practice interests focus on methods of bladder rehabilitation using conservative approaches based on lifestyle and behavioural strategies to promote bladder and bowel continence, particularly in older people and those who have experienced a stroke.

Mima Cattan is a Professor in Public Health at Northumbria University. She has a background in health promotion where she was involved in a range of initiatives relating to mental health promotion and older people. Following on from her PhD on health promotion interventions targeting social isolation and loneliness among older people (University of Newcastle), she has continued to investigate the impact of social support for older people who are isolated and lonely. Her current research focuses on the promotion of mental well-being in older people; for example, transport and older people's mental health, visually impaired frail older people's quality of life, older people's well-being in a multi-ethnic community, the impact of low-level support for isolated and housebound older people, and the resourcefulness of older people in maintaining their well-being. She has co-authored two books: *Mental Health Promotion: A Lifespan Approach* and *Mental Health and Well-being in Later Life*.

Charlotte Clarke is Professor of Health in Social Science and Head of the School of Health in Social Science at the University of Edinburgh. From 1996 to 2011, Charlotte worked at Northumbria University. She has worked in practice, higher education and research with older people throughout her career. She has a particular interest in dementia care and in developing health and social care practice. Her current work includes research into risk management in dementia care, and leading the national evaluation of peer support networks and dementia advisers as part of the implementation of the National Dementia Strategy in England.

Amanda Clarke is a senior lecturer at the Centre of Advanced Nursing Studies, University of Aberdeen. She has extensive experience in both teaching and research. Her research contributes to enhancing understanding of the experiences and perceptions of adults in later life and developing ways to offer individuals education, information and support in the management of health and when thinking about and planning for the end of their lives. This has involved engaging in life story work with older adults and developing more participatory and innovative ways of working with older adults as research participants, service users, co-researchers and peer educators. She is particularly interested in the ways that life story and narrative work may be utilized to gain a more rounded understanding of individuals' experiences and needs from research, policy, educational and practice perspectives. Currently, she is a principal investigator in the Medical Research Council study Engaging with Older People and their Carers to Develop and Deliver Interventions for the Self-management of Chronic Pain which is part of the Lifelong Health and Wellbeing programme.

Christine Brown Wilson is a lecturer in Older People's Nursing at the School of Nursing, Midwifery and Social Work, University of Manchester. Christine promotes evidence-based practice in her work with student nurses with a focus on caring for older people. She achieves this through education and research and is also involved with Local Involvement Networks (Links). Her research focuses on influencing quality improvement in health and social care, particularly in supported living environments. She has published and presented her work on promoting relationship-based approaches to care, valuing the contribution of older people, including those with dementia. Recent projects include improving communication practice with people living with dementia in care homes, and supporting staff attending quality improvement workshops focusing on end of life care.

Angela Dickinson is a senior research fellow at the Centre for Research in Primary and Community Care, University of Hertfordshire. Her work is focused in the area of older people's health and social care and health and well-being with a particular interest in nutrition and working with practitioners to improve clinical practice. Recent work has included work to improve nutritional care of older patients in hospital settings, exploration of community meals for older people, understanding older people's perceptions of fall prevention interventions, and various evaluations of health and social care services for older people, particularly focusing on older people's views and experiences.

Karen S. Dunn is an associate professor in the School of Nursing at Oakland University, located in Rochester Michigan, USA. Karen has published and presented in areas focused on the holistic well-being of older adults, with an increased concentration in spiritual well-being. Other areas included the efficacy of physical restraint use, chronic pain, volunteerism, and predictors of self-rated health in older adults. A recent project compared the use of non-religious and religious music within a multi-sensory environment to prevent agitation in patients with Alzheimer's disease.

Soong-Nang Jang is an assistant professor of public health nursing at Chung-Ang University in Korea. She is a chair of 'Tailored Visiting Health Care Centre' in Hwasung-city. Her current research interest is focused on the psychosocial determinants of older adults' health, including social support, social participation and social capital. She has received a research award about a cross-national comparison of social determinants among older population, and a community-based programme for vulnerable population from the Korean government.

Diana Jones is a Reader in the School of Health, Community and Education Studies at Northumbria University. She is a physiotherapist by profession, currently teaching and researching in relation to the management of long-term neurological conditions, with a particular focus on Parkinson's disease. She has an established interest in the involvement of service users and carers in health care education and research.

Ann MacFarlane a wheelchair user, is a leading Disability Rights and Equalities Consultant, focusing on health and social care. For many years she has been involved in shaping policies in these fields at national and local level. She is an 'Expert by Experience' for the Care Quality Commission, an adviser to the NHS National End of Life Care Programme and is on the Board of the Social Care Institute of Excellence.

Linda McAuliffe is a research officer at the Australian Centre for Evidence Based Aged Care (ACEBAC), a research centre of La Trobe University in Melbourne, Australia. She is also a registered psychologist. Linda has published and presented in the areas of older adults and pain, dementia and sexuality, and is involved in various projects related to aged care and evidence-based practice. Recent projects include staff knowledge and attitudes towards sexuality in aged care; person-centred care; and pain assessment in older adults with dementia.

Brendan McCormack is Director of the Institute of Nursing Research and Head of the Person-centred Practice Research Centre, University of Ulster, Northern Ireland; Adjunct Professor of Nursing, University of Technology, Sydney; Adjunct Professor of Nursing, Faculty of Medicine, Nursing and Health Care, Monash University, Melbourne; Visiting Professor, School of Medicine and Dentistry, University of Aberdeen; and Professor II, Buskerud University College, Drammen, Norway. He collaborates on a number of practice development and research projects in Ireland, the UK, Europe, Canada and Australia that focus on the development of person-centred practice. His writing and research work focuses on gerontological nursing, person-centred nursing and practice development and he serves on a number of editorial boards, policy committees and development groups in these areas. He is the editor of the *International Journal of Older People Nursing*. He has co-authored *Practice Development in Nursing* which has now been translated into two languages and *Practice Development in Nursing: International Perspectives* (published 2008). *Person-centred Nursing*, co-authored with Tanya McCance was published in July 2010. He is President of the All-Ireland Gerontological Nurses Association (AIGNA) and Chairman of the charity 'Age NI'.

Patricia McGeever is Charge Nurse at Roslynlee Hospital, NHS Lothian in Scotland.

Rhonda Nay is Director of the Institute for Social Participation (ISP); Australian Centre for Evidence Based Aged Care (ACEBAC); Australian Institute for Primary Care & Ageing (AIPCA); and is Professor of Interdisciplinary Aged Care at La Trobe University. She is also Director of TIME *for dementia* – the Victorian and Tasmanian Dementia Training Study Centre and a partner in the Dementia Collaborative Research Centre. Her research priority is getting evidence-based, interdisciplinary, person-centred aged care into practice. Specifically, her research focuses on: staff–family relationships; sexual expression and sexuality; person-centred care; and pain assessment and management for people with dementia. She has published and presented extensively on aged care and dementia.

Mike Nolan has been Professor of Gerontological Nursing at the School of Nursing and Midwifery, University of Sheffield and has worked with older people and their family carers in a variety of clinical, educational and research roles for 30 years. He is particularly interested in the interrelationships between older people, family and paid carers. Together with colleagues in the UK, Europe (particularly Sweden), Canada and Australia he has developed a range of assessment approaches in family care and has promoted a relationship centred approach to care using the 'Senses Framework'.

Bhanu Ramaswamy is a physiotherapist by background who has clinically specialized in her practice in the field of rehabilitation of older people and long-term conditions. In addition to clinical practice and post-graduate lecturing, she engages with the voluntary and the social services sectors to promote activity and mobility to people whose medical conditions and frailty put them at risk of developing problems, such as those in care homes, or in the community but with a deteriorating condition. She would like to acknowledge the input of colleagues from AGILE (a Chartered Society of Physiotherapy interest group for physiotherapists working with older people).

Jan Reed is Emeritus Professor of Health Care in Later Life at Northumbria University. She completed her degree in nursing in 1982, and soon after began a doctorate in nursing as a working staff nurse and researcher. This study was about older people and the nursing care they receive. After collecting this data she began work as a lecturer in nursing at Northumbria University. At this university she taught a number of subjects, increasingly focusing on research methods. During this time she was involved in a number of different organizations for older peoople, and was a founding editor of a journal for nursing older people.

Isabell Reid is a team leader for the day services at Midlothian Community Hospital. She leads a small team in providing services for older people with mental health issues to remain living independently, as ability allows, within the community.

Assumpta Ryan is a reader at the School of Nursing and a member of the Institute of Nursing Research at the University of Ulster. She leads the *'Working with Older People'* strand of the Person-Centred Practice Research Centre. Her clinical interest is gerontological nursing and the care of older people. Research interests include the needs and experiences of family carers, community care and the impact of a move to a care home on older people and their families. She has presented papers at a range of national and international conferences and has over sixty publications in peer-reviewed academic journals.

Paula Smith is a senior lecturer in the Department of Psychology and the Centre for Death and Society, University of Bath. She has widespread experience of teaching at undergraduate and postgraduate levels in palliative and end-of-life care. Using a qualitative approach her research focuses on the perceptions and understandings of end of life care for older people, their family carers and the health and social care professionals working with them. She is particularly interested in the psychological adaptation to loss, grief and bereavement of individuals and their families who are living with a chronic illness. Currently, she is working on a number of research projects that combine her interests and expertise in end of life and supportive care for patients and families surviving cancer and stroke.

Alison Steven is a senior lecturer in the School of Health, Community and Education Studies, Northumbria University and is also a staff member of Fuse, the Centre for Translational Research in Public Health – a UKCRC Public Health Research Centre of Excellence. She is a nurse by profession and her main interests lie in the development of professional knowledge and practice, and knowledge translation and exchange via educational initiatives. She has published on patient safety education and safety in health care organizations and has a keen interest in participatory research methods which include the involvement of older people. Her current projects include participatory evaluations of carer health checks and dementia adviser pilots.

Gabriel Telford Steven was brought up from early childhood in India during the days of the Raj. He joined the army as a teenager and fought in Burma during the Second World War. After being demobbed back to Britain, he settled in the Scottish borders and worked for many years as an installation inspector for the South of Scotland Electricity Board until he retired. Over the years he has enjoyed many hobbies and interests including archery, walking, music, books and gardening. He has a passion for wildlife and a long-standing talent for woodworking and woodturning. His perspective on the care of older people, and in particular the concept of risk, is informed by his many and varied life experiences.

Nina Szmaites is the Charge Nurse of an assessment and rehabilitation unit for older people in NHS Lothian, Scotland. The unit's primary role is to prevent hospital admission and to support early discharge from hospital. Her role is to ensure the unit runs ensure the unit runs efficiently providing a rapid and efficient method of assessment by a multiprofessional team. Her primary role is that of a named nurse which gives the client continuity of care from admission to discharge. The unit also sees younger clients whose needs cannot be met by other services.

Debbie Tolson leads the Institute for Applied Health Research, Later Life Research Group at Glasgow Caledonian University. She is a nurse leader with an international reputation for advancing evidence-based care with older people and innovative use of communities of practice to improve quality of interdisciplinary practice within nursing homes, hospitals and community settings. In 2010 her contribution to research with older people was recognized by St Louis University (USA) Medical School through the award of the Jim Flood Memorial Alzheimer Disease Distinguished Lectureship. She is an Honorary Fellow of the Queens Nursing Institute, Scotland. She was the recipient of the Sigma Theta Tau International, 2007 award for the Best of Worldviews on Evidence Based Nursing.

Foreword

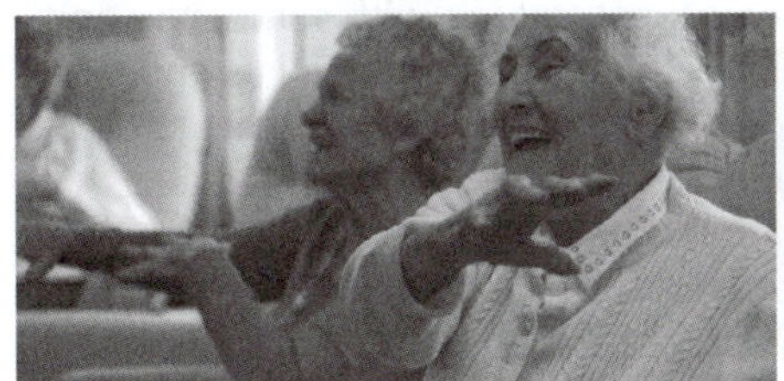
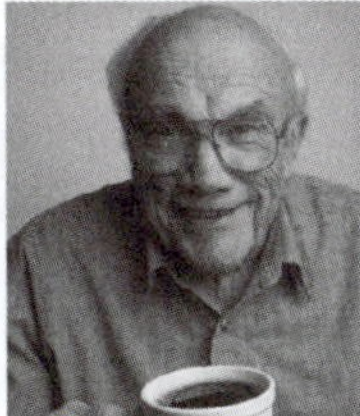
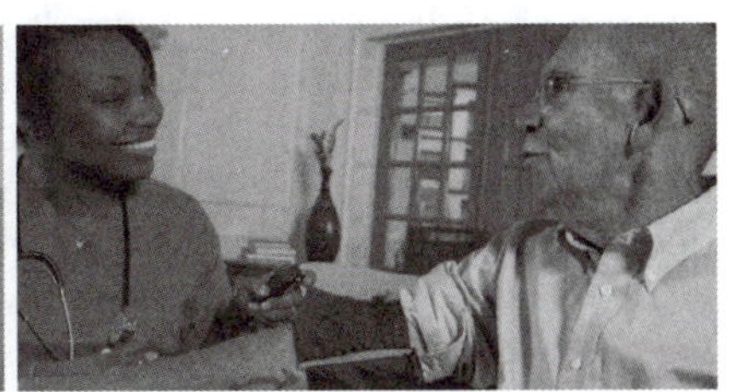

> "No matter what age you are, or what your circumstances might be, you are special, and you still have something unique to offer. Your life, because of who you are, has meaning.
>
> Barbara de Angelis"

Ageism in society means that older people are not always respected for what they have to offer and those looking after them are similarly often disregarded as working within a "Cinderella' or second class service. This book carefully and sensitively challenges the reader to rethink and reframe, placing the older person at the centre by strengthening their 'voice', 'choice' and 'control'; and also helps the reader to appreciate the specialist nature of caring for older people, who often have complex health and social care needs and require highly skilled care.

Given the ageing population, educators need to recognise that nursing older adults is not an optional extra, but rather a core component of health and social care. This book should thus be seen as essential reading, as it revisits the fundamentals of working with older people and, in so doing, captures the most important aspects of the essence of good nursing care in the 21st century.

The dominant feel of the book is that nursing older people is all about listening to and respecting older people and supporting them to determine the support they want to have. The authors practice what they preach by starting every chapter with an older person's views. However, the thing that impressed me most is the fact that one of the co-editors was purposefully selected as an older person and how throughout the book, the voice of older people can be clearly heard.

A systematic review and synthesis of qualitative studies describing older patients' and/or their relatives' experiences of care in acute hospital settings (Bridges et al, 2009) highlights the importance of three paramount themes: "See who I am", "Involve me" and "Connect with me". These themes are also reinforced by older people and their families in long term care settings (NCHR&D 2007). This book keeps these themes central in its writing and highlights the importance of good relationships between older people, their families/friends and staff in delivering person-centred care. The book re-visions nursing as being an interdependent process and thus indirectly challenges much of older people policy which primarily focuses on independence and choice. Further the book's focus on older people's strengths also helps to move away from the current orthodoxy of older people being seen as part of the problem, rather than part of the solution.

The reader may go no further than the index to see the comprehensive nature of this text and the carefully use of language. It covers all expected aspects, along with some new and refreshing topics. In particular, the focus on "spirituality, religious practice, beliefs and values", "sexuality and intimacy" and "risk and safety in nursing older people" makes a welcome addition to usual nursing texts. The attention to detail in use of language also demonstrates a genuine respect for older people that cannot be ignored.

By making clear the expertise of working with older people and addressing this from the perspective of the older person themselves, the authors have produced an invaluable text which should broaden thinking and the hopefully the future engagement of nurses with older people. As well as being valuable for nurses, this text has much to offer all health and social care professionals who are working with older people in a range of settings.

Julienne Meyer
PhD MSc BSc Cert Ed(FE) RN RNT
Professor of Nursing: Care for Older People & Executive Director: *My* Home Life programme, City University

References

Bridges J, Flatley M and Meyer J (2009) *Best practice for older people in acute care settings (BPOP): Guidance for Nurses*. RCN/City University.

NCHR&D (2007) *My Home Life: Quality of life in care homes – Literature review*, London: Help the Aged (www.myhomelife.org.uk)

Acknowledgements

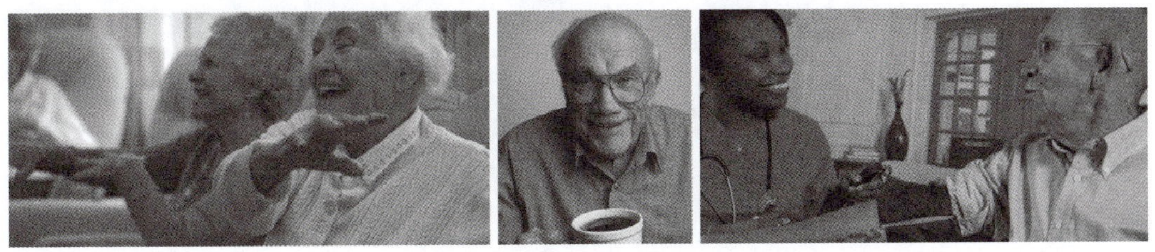

This book is dedicated to all the older people who have taught us so much.

PART 1

The fundamentals of working with older people

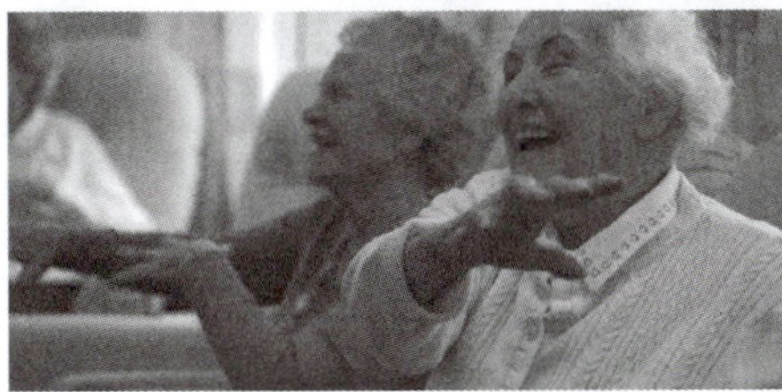
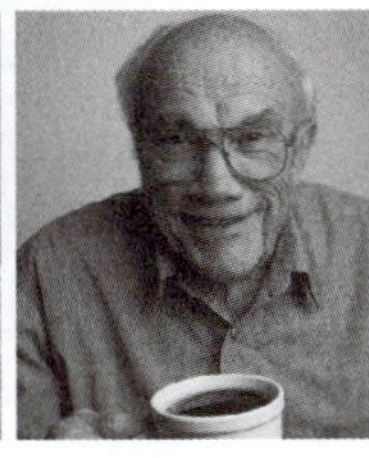
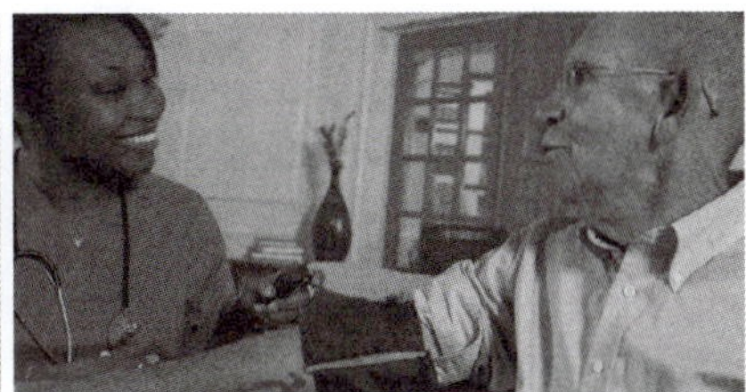

Chapter contents

CHAPTER 1

Introduction to nursing older people

Jan Reed, Charlotte L. Clarke and Ann MacFarlane

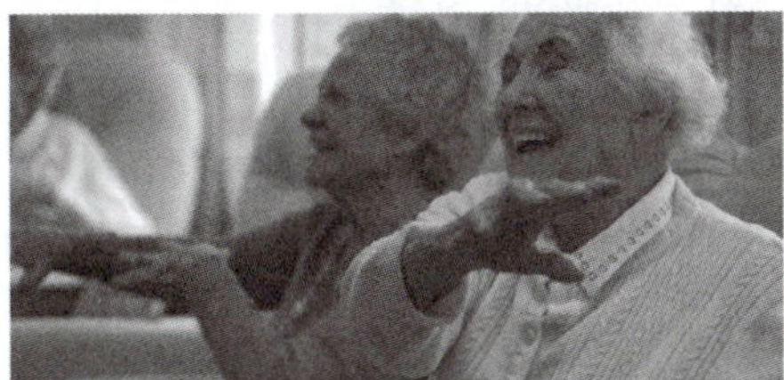
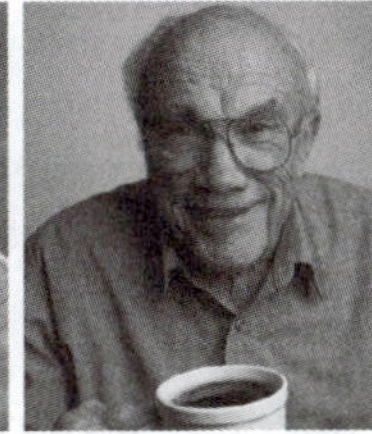
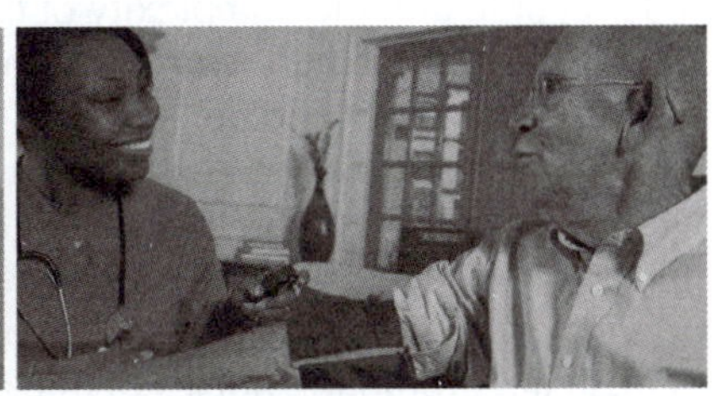

This is the bit that you may be tempted to skip – introductions are quite often dull or unhelpful. We would, however, urge you to read this, because here we set out the way in which this book was developed, some of the ideas and debates that were central to it, and how it fits in with practice. Reading this chapter, then, can place this book in context, and show the ways in which we hope it can be useful to practitioners.

Older people in the book

When we were thinking about and planning this book we wanted to produce something that would help nurses and older people to work together. This means supporting practice which is engaged with the views of older people. One of the features that we insisted on was that each chapter would begin with a comment from an older person. This helps to reinforce the idea that nursing practice is led by the views of older people, and not just by professional interests. This sounds incongruous given the struggle that nursing has had to establish credentials for expertise and knowledge. These can contrast and even conflict with the views of service users. If, as nurses, we feel that we know what is best to do, then it can be tempting to drive this course of action forward, overriding the views of others.

Key point

Nursing practice with older people is led by the views of older people, and not just by professional interests.

This book has, however, been edited by two nurses and an older person, working in partnership, and it is this partnership that we want to emphasize here – it is not a case of nurses and older people working despite each other, but *with* each other. In addition, we want to stress that nurses and older people will also work with other disciplines and professional groups to realize goals, and this will include social care agencies, physical therapists and the voluntary sector, to name but a few of the people who may be called upon in order to develop and meet the aims of care. Each of these agencies will have their own history and reasons for development and this can help explain current practice. Nurses may have more contact, and share more history, with some groups, and older people have more connection to others, but this should not detract from the importance of taking a holistic perspective. In doing so we should appreciate the complexity of the needs and goals of older people and the complexity of the agencies that may contribute to care.

This sounds like hard work, and the effort needed is considerable. In talking to nurses working with older people, however, one thing stands out – their enthusiasm for a field which has, historically, been unpopular. As these nurses show, they value their time spent with older people, a contact which gives them insight into different ways of looking at things, different experiences and different goals and aims. In a world which is often dominated by the priority given to younger people, this contact can offer a welcome breath of fresh air, prompting nurses to think about their work, and their lives, differently.

This enthusiasm has been the basis of the call for specialist nurses to be trained in care for older people. This idea of specialism is quite a new one – earlier notions of older people reflected the idea that there was nothing special about them, and that their health problems were nothing more than the problems everyone else faced. This perhaps often included an added pessimism that these people were dying anyway, so there was not much point in doing more than keeping them comfortable. The idea of expertise in the care of older people was seen as laughable.

More recently, however, the idea of specialist nurses for older people has gained currency in that this field requires an understanding of the issues that older people face, and the way that these issues interact with each other. Trying to maintain a healthy diet, for example, can be shaped by a number of physical, social and economic factors. These factors may gain prominence as we grow older, being unable to get to shops for fresh food for example, so our wish to eat healthy food has to be placed in the context of our ability to achieve this and our wish to do so – we might think that unhealthy food is more fun! Let us take two very practical examples: Jamal is an older person with a deteriorating memory who finds that he is increasingly anxious about leaving the familiarity of his home and so neglects to keep adequate food in stock; Julia has always enjoyed a wide variety of fresh fruit and vegetables in her diet but mobility problems means that she now depends on others to go shopping and they rarely have the time or interest to select good quality foods that are unfamiliar to them.

Balancing all of these factors is where the expertise of specialist nurses lies, and where we hope that this book will be useful, as it sets out key issues and fields which are important when nursing older people. It will also be useful for nurses working in other fields, as they are likely to meet up with older people in their work too. This book will be a useful resource for them, as they try to understand the complexity of the situation of older people.

This work can be diverse, and take place in different settings as older people use a range of different services. What people have found, however, is that access to services can be shaped by age discrimination, in that services can be denied to older people because of their age. This rests on the (ageist) assumptions made about growing older: stereotypes of older people portraying them as having limited contribution to society, limited quality of life and limited life expectancy because of their age.

Talking about older people

Ageism can work both ways – there can be both negative and positive ageism. Negative ageism can assume that older people can be patronized or dismissed, while positive ageism assumes that all older people are wise, good-natured and should be venerated. Both of these ideas lump older people together, and fail to recognize their diversity. Older people are very different, with different values, experiences and views. After all, the category of 'older people' can cover people with 50 years difference in age. If we put other groups in such a broad category, we would think that it was a meaningless process.

This brings us to issues of language. It is critical to the way that we talk about older people. Language can lead us to gloss over diversity, and distances us from the people that we talk about. When we talk about *the* elderly, for example, we indicate their separateness from us. They are a distinct group that we are not members of. Similarly, when we talk about 'geriatrics' we are lumping people together under a heading which is derived from a medical category.

For these reasons, we have thought hard about the language that we use in this book. We use the term 'older people' to signify that we are talking about, and with, people who are older. This emphasizes the idea that these are *people* who are like us, with all the concerns and interests that we can share, and that they are *older*, which means that they may experience some of the social and physical challenges that this may entail.

We have tried to avoid using language that problematizes older people, and that focuses on difficulties rather than achievements. This can be a paradox – nurses can see their role as helping people with problems, and one of our aims in producing this book was to aid nurses in caring for older people who, because they are calling on nurses for help, will be experiencing some difficulties. By using language which reframes problems as challenges then, we are running the risk of hiding difficulties. This is not what we want to do – it would not help anyone if problems were ignored. What we do want to do, however, is move beyond this focus on problems and widen our understanding to encompass the achievements and strategies of older people. In every dimension of living, older people have goals and have thought about ways of reaching them, for example, ways of facilitating mobility. The role of nursing, therefore, might be to support and acknowledge this thinking and action. This approach means that, for example, we have not included a chapter on dementia but throughout the book consider the challenges of memory loss and strategies for living with dementia.

This is why we have tried to use affirmative language; not to hide problems but to help us rethink some of the ideas we have about older people as dependant and passive. We hope that by using this language we will not just see problems but broaden our thinking and our practice to embrace the thinking and activity that older people are engaged in.

Key point

Affirmative language does not hide problems but it can help us rethink some of the ideas we have about older people as dependant and passive.

The structure of the book

Part 1: The fundamentals of working with older people

This thinking about the centrality of older people and the importance of using affirmative language has informed the structure of this book, and the sequence of the chapters. Most chapters begin with a section outlining learning objectives and then have a comment from an older person, anonymous where requested, although this was not always wished, as many older people wanted to have their contributions directly attributed to them. We then follow this with a section on nursing practice. In this we have included some scenarios to illustrate key issues. Some of these are taken directly from specific events in practice, while others draw on a range of experiences. These scenarios can be used by readers to explore practice knowledge and understanding, and to direct reflective exercises in groups or for individuals.

You may also notice that not all of the chapters follow the same structure. This chapter starts the book and also the first section (Chapters 1–5) which give a context for nursing older people. Chapter 6 starts off the next section, on daily activities, and how nurses might support them (Chapters 6–16). Chapter 17 brings the book to a close, with this final word written by a co-editor who is also an older person.

These chapters vary in content, style and structure, both across sections and within them. Some of this is due to the subject matter (e.g. where little research has been done in an area, the relevant chapter may be relatively light on references). Some of this difference may be because of the topic or discipline (there can be different writing traditions in different fields). Some variations may be due to different personal styles. With all these potential factors at play editing has been necessarily light-touch, allowing each author to present what they saw as central, in the way that they thought was most effective. For the reader, editorial work was focused on ensuring that content, style and structure were broadly similar. In calling on experts in different fields we are accessing writers with a substantial grasp of their subject, a significance which makes uniformity unlikely and unwanted.

We start this book with a chapter (Chapter 2) on autonomy; that is the capacity to direct and shape one's affairs and activities. As this chapter discusses, autonomy can be thought of in different ways. We can usually think of autonomy as being an absolute characteristic – we are either completely independent, or completely dependent. It is possible, however, that this view does not acknowledge the complexity of autonomy, and that there are many ways in which it can happen. People may have autonomy in some areas but not others, and at some times but not others. They may also have degrees and different types of autonomy, including the freedom to tell others what to do. This chapter starts with the discussion to prioritize this dimension; a discussion of older people as actively engaged, and the nurse's role as a supporter of this engagement, using the chapter on autonomy and empowerment. This reiterates our views of both older people and nurses as active in choosing and realizing autonomy and empowerment. This chapter then establishes the tone of the whole book, that care for older people is about promoting this engagement.

This promotion can, of course, be insensitive if it is enforced regardless of the goals and wishes of older people. The chapter on autonomy discusses this, but this is also explored in the following chapter, about the goals and aims of nursing care for older people. This focuses not just on actions and behaviours but on feelings and perceptions. The two are connected of course, as actions come from feelings and feelings come from actions. If we have a feeling of safety, for example, we will behave in this context, feeling that we can take more risks. If we take risks in our behaviour, our feelings about safety may change. Nurses can intervene to support not only actions and behaviours, but also feelings and perceptions.

This relationship means that actions are recognized, but there is a focus on people's feelings – importantly, the sense that they have of the goals that they have, or the direction they wish to travel in. These feelings are explored in the next chapter, which talks about the history of nursing older people in acute care settings. This fits goals if a health problem is short term, but does not fit health problems which may have multiple causes or consequences, or are long term or continuous.

This means that the goals of nursing need to change, to centre on feelings. This may mean aiming for something other than physical performance and achievement. Thinking about the personal goals of older people may entail thinking differently, and more holistically, about supportive environments, and ways that nurses can help the reaching of these goals.

All of these models of care have to be developed in the context of changing populations. The third chapter lays out this context by discussing the demographics of current society. Put simply, the population is ageing – older people are living longer and the birth rate is falling. Putting these two changes together, there is the idea that the care needs of the population will increase, and that there will be fewer people to provide it. This idea rests on an assumption that older age will bring care needs, and that younger people will have to provide this. We may need to rethink these assumptions. Perhaps older people will not have increased care needs if we help them to maintain their health. They may, in this situation, be able to self-care to a greater or lesser extent, particularly if they develop the skills and have the equipment to do so.

This brings us to thinking about the resources available to older people, which is where the discussion of policy in Chapter 4 sounds a relevant note. Policy, that is the directions of agencies, directs the resources available and the means of accessing them. Policy, however, is determined by political thinking, and the perceptions of the populace. As a result, a role for nurses might be to be aware of the impact of policy and the ways in which the populace might be made aware of developments and the possibilities for changing policies. This chapter ends the first section of this book, which has set out the context of nursing care for older people. Here we set out some of the key themes and principles which we feel should direct care.

Part 2: Key issues in nursing older people

The second part of the book covers some of the areas where older people may want some nursing support, and it begins with an introduction which explores the fundamentals of care, including the importance of dignity, and revisits the nursing process. Following this, there are chapters outlining issues of mobility, nutrition, continence, mental health, communication, spirituality, sexuality, safety, leisure and dying. These chapters cover issues suggested by older people and nurses, and they follow the principles of models which are organized around activities of daily living.

While this book does not necessarily follow all of the activities found in these models, it follows the ideas of 'activity' and 'daily living'. In other words, it emphasizes the importance of thinking of older people as active, and paying attention to everyday life. We can sometimes think of nursing care as being 'special' care given to passive people. Care might be more constructively thought of as supporting people to achieve a life that is as close to their normal life as possible. This may mean that nurses need to take a back seat – they are supporting, not ordering. The chapters in this book will help in this and many older people have contributed to these chapters.

We finish the book with a reflection from the editor representing older people. Ending with this is one way of emphasizing the collaborative nature of this book, and the importance of the voice of older people. We would urge you to read this, because it covers the experience and insight that many older people can have. Appreciating this can change your practice so it becomes more respectful and collaborative, and we hope these ideas run through this entire book, and will shape your practice.

Learning objectives

At the end of this book, the reader will be able to:

- understand the issues that older people may face and the ways in which these issues interact with each other
- appraise the way that language can be used to describe older people and to use affirmative language to promote the well-being and dignity of older people
- describe a way of nursing older people that emphasizes working in partnership
- identify ways in which nurses may support older people to achieve their goals

CHAPTER 2

Independence and autonomy – the foundation of care

Jan Reed and Brendan McCormack

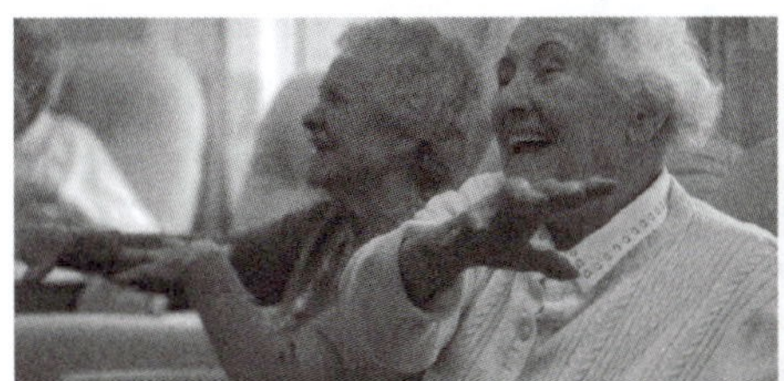
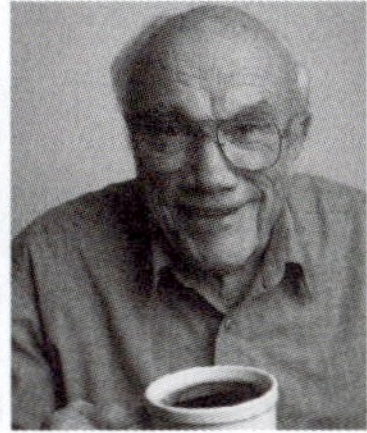
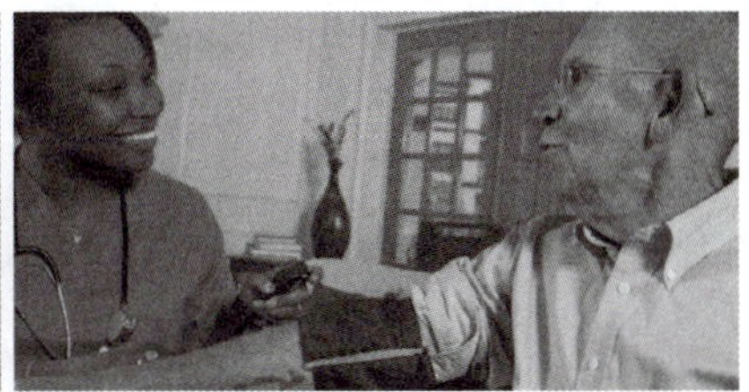

Learning objectives

At the end of this chapter, the reader will be able to:

- understand the complexity of concepts of independence and autonomy
- describe ideas of independence and autonomy for older people
- discuss the significance of assumptions about the passivity of older people
- analyse the challenges faced by health and social care practitioners as a result of needs to empower older people
- discuss the importance of accessing resources for older people at a local and national level

Introduction

Cariad commented:

'I'm used to doing want I want, when I want, and I don't want to lose that. I might need some support or help, but I want to stay in charge.'

The independence and autonomy of an older person are the foundation purposes of nursing care because they help shape and direct practice. Ideas of independence and autonomy can give us a lens to look at the contextual issues of nursing older people. This allows us to explore the impact that nursing care can have in supporting independence and autonomy. The next section of the book deals with some of the aspects of daily living where nursing can play a part, and here again ideas of autonomy shape the ways in which practice is carried out. We can look at processes of assessment and evaluation to see if they affirm and augment independence and autonomy.

Defining independence and autonomy

Independence and autonomy are elusive terms – so what, exactly, do we mean? As Beauchamp and Childress (2001) have discussed, although the idea of autonomy can often be paraphrased, it remains difficult to define. Collopy (1988) has termed this 'conceptual plasticity' (p. 10) and has identified a number of terms that are used interchangeably, or that refer to similar concepts, including liberty, privacy and choice.

Here we use the terms 'independence' and 'autonomy' to refer to the extent to which older people are able to exercise their will, irrespective of the will of others, including carers. As Collopy (1988) says, 'care can slide toward control, not from malevolence but simply from the dynamic of powerful and resourceful professionals interacting with vulnerable and weak clients' (p. 10). This chapter then can act as a cautionary note to nurses and other carers that they should be aware of this driver, and take steps to reflect on and evaluate it.

Scenario 2.1

Mary has dementia and fights to keep her autonomy, something that her partner Peter finds very hard to deal with. In an attempt to keep her safe, he responds by keeping a very close eye on her movements and, in his words, has 'taken over her thinking'. Their community psychiatric nurse is trying to help Peter let Mary retain some choices in her life so that she has some independence and autonomy.

- *What steps could you take to support Mary's wish to be independent?*

Independence and ageing

At first glance the idea of independence and autonomy may feel inappropriate for people who are growing older, as this can be seen as a time of inevitable decline and increasing dependence. These assumptions, however, rest on very simplistic ideas of both independence and growing older. The assumptions that we may have about growing older can be reinforced by the cultural environment in which we live, with images of older people as perhaps figures of fun appearing in the newspapers, advertisements and on TV. Because such images are pervasive and commonplace, their impact can be considerable.

This can have an impact on everyday life – the way that older people can be disregarded in shops, transport or entertainment, for example. This disregard can also affect the way that nurses practise – the way that disregard can permeate the way that we assess for, deliver and evaluate care. We might not do these things because they are thought of as unimportant, but because older people themselves are seen as unimportant. For nursing then there is a challenge to question what we do and the reason we do it. We need to constantly check that we are not enforcing and reflecting stereotypes, particularly those that portray older people as passive and compliant, with little interest in rehabilitation or recovery. As the next chapter argues, the goals of older people can be no different to, and as varied as, anybody else's, and that this should be reflected in our practice. Creating the conditions where an older person can maximize their potential for independence through engagement in autonomous decision-making is a key function of nursing and creating these conditions raises a number of challenges – not least of which is the challenge to the stereotypes we hold about older people and their participation in decision-making.

Key point

Nurses need to constantly check that they are not enforcing and reflecting stereotypes, particularly those that portray older people as passive and compliant, with little interest in rehabilitation or recovery.

These features of the culture in which older people live are pervasive and powerful. Where a culture extols youth and vigour, then older people can be disregarded or devalued. Their experience, knowledge and humanity can be unacknowledged and therefore not considered when care is planned or delivered. Furthermore, the culture in which we live may not encourage, or even discourage, independence – services may be easier to deliver if the people who use them are passive and compliant. The alternative to assumptions of dependence and lack of autonomy can be equally very influential however. An excellent example is in the 2010 Department of Health/Alzheimer Society public awareness campaign for dementia, in which people are encouraged to see the person despite their dementia, using the slogan 'I have dementia, I also have a life'.

An awareness of independence and autonomy is therefore fundamental to the way that we practise – it shapes our goals and the processes of delivering care. This is why we have begun this book with this chapter.

Key point

An awareness of independence and autonomy is fundamental to the way that nurses practise.

Beginning with an exploration of autonomy then sets out one of the key concerns of the book. We hope that the ideas of autonomy will permeate each chapter, and that each will indicate how nurses can promote independence. This is, of course, an ethical question about how we should live, and how we should help others to live. If we stand by the idea that each individual plays a part in shaping the direction of their lives, then as a 'helping profession' we need to find ways of supporting older people to do this.

What this discussion does not do, however, is stick to traditional ideas of autonomy as an 'all or nothing' state where people are completely autonomous or completely dependent. What we argue is that these absolute categories are not useful, and are misleading. No one is completely autonomous. We all depend on others to provide services and goods, and we all have interdependent relationships. The exception would be a self-sufficient hermit, and not many of us fit that description. Similarly, few of us are completely dependant, as we can always find ways of supporting or sabotaging the actions of others. The exception would be if we were very passive to the point of unconsciousness, and few of us fit that description either.

Definitions and dimensions of independence and autonomy

A concept that we take for granted in our everyday lives, such as autonomy, is one that sometimes we struggle to conceptualize in a 'helping' context in settings where older people access health and social care. Originally a term that was used to describe a state's or nation's ability to self-govern, 'autonomy', has over time been adapted to refer to an individual's ability and capacity to make self-determined decisions. Autonomy then refers to a person's capacity for self-determination or self-governance or self-rule; that is, the capacity to make decisions for oneself. However, while on the face of it this is a relatively easy concept to understand, in reality autonomy is complex and gives us much reason for reflection, particularly when linked to the idea of independence. This complexity will also arise and become clear in the final section of this chapter, where the implications for practice are discussed.

If we start by exploring the similarities and differences between 'independence' and 'autonomy' then we can start to see the connections between them.

Independence is a term that points to connection with other people – we are independent *from* something or someone. Autonomy, on the other hand, is a term that refers to a characteristic of a person or an action, which is defined without recourse to anything or anyone else. However, it is difficult to argue the case for independent decision-making without drawing upon the concept of autonomy to justify our right to independence.

Defining our terms

The Cambridge online dictionary, for example, defines independence as:

> *independent (NOT HELPED) not taking help or money from other people:*
>
> e.g. "Grandma's very independent and does all her own shopping and cooking" or "I've always been *financially* independent".

This definition seems very straightforward, but complexities soon arise when we look at definitions of autonomy and autonomous:

> *'autonomy = the right of a group of people to govern itself, or to organize its own activities, e.g. "Demonstrators demanded immediate autonomy for their region" or "The universities are anxious to preserve their autonomy from central government".'*
>
> *autonomous = independent and having the power to make your own decisions: e.g. an autonomous region/province/republic/council*

(Cambridge online dictionary June 2009, dictionary.cambridge.org)

This definition of autonomy brings in a number of other features; namely, power, decision-making and rights, all of which are the subject of much discussion and debate. For the purposes of this chapter we have focused on independence and autonomy, but we should not overlook their connections to empowerment, choice and humanity. These discussions draw on ideas of power, decision-making and rights.

When we think about an individual exercising their autonomy we usually refer to an individual's right to make decisions for themselves. This idea comes from the view that if we are 'free' as people then we have the freedom to make decisions, act on those decisions and reflect on their effectiveness (see Dworkin, 1991). From this perspective, the ability to reflect on our decisions is critical to exercising our autonomy. The autonomous person is one who examines whether or not an independent decision is appropriate and consistent with the values the person holds or not. A person is 'free' when they are able to reflect on the action taken and content that there is consistency between values and action. The approach to self-evaluation needs to be independent in order to constitute personal autonomy. This independence must occur on two fronts – independence from manipulative forces (strong desire for prudence, for example, fostered by a risk averse society) and from the impact of others (e.g. being manipulated into a particular action by another person). When a person acts autonomously, they do not act upon a desire that they reject or would reject, nor do they act vicariously. Instead, the autonomous person identifies with their desires, goals, beliefs and values, and the process of identification must be one that can be defended by the individual and is based on principles that enable the person to see their life as a whole and evaluate a whole way of living their life (critical reflection). In this way the person acts on authentic desires that are truly their own and based on principles that have been critically reflected upon and integrated into their life. It requires the person to distinguish those conditions that restrict and subvert their critical and reflective faculties from those that enhance and improve them. In this sense autonomy is extracted from the narrow view of being free to do what one wants to do at particular points in time to a more global view of life as a whole.

However, when we think about the complexities of health and social care decision-making and the precarious position of many older people in health and social care systems, then exercising autonomy from the position of 'making free decisions' is challenging for many. Consider the following questions:

- How do we find out what older people 'really' think about their future?
- How 'free' (from coercion) are older people in hospital (e.g.) to make independent decisions?

Autonomy is about groups as well as individuals, so as well as the challenges associated with enabling an individual to make authentic decisions we also need to think of social challenges. Although nursing practice places significant emphasis on individualized care and decision-making for individual patients, the notion of groups, however, points us towards thinking at a collective level, about the services and systems that we are all part of and thus how decisions are made that are effective at the group level. If we think at a collective level we may need to reflect on the ways in which services are designed and organized to affect the autonomy of individuals. This can be in the ways that the group can shape services, and the way that services hear and respond to messages. This can be formally organized (e.g. where service user groups are explicitly consulted) or less formal (where comments can be fed into system development). This directs us to thinking about the processes we have to consult service users, and prompts us to be more proactive about this:

- Are there ways to make the views of the group more accessible, and who are 'the group'?
- How can we support people in this process?
- Do we get feedback from a wide range of people?
- How does feedback get responded to? How do we let people know how things are changing?

Supporting autonomy can be particularly demanding when working with older people with altered cognition or who have dementia. There have been several developments recently to support people to express their preferences and choices in life through things like advanced directives which allow people to express their preferences should there be a time when they no longer have capacity to make decisions themselves. Although difficult to broach, nurses can help older people have these conversations which allow them to shape their future and help their family to know what the individual would prefer.

Autonomy and the 'greater good'

It has been argued that 'the greater good' argument (i.e. what is best for a society as a whole, rather than any individual) is more important than a focus on the ability of a person to make decisions and choices for themselves. The arguments from this stance are positioned from the perspective that sometimes decisions have to be made that may violate the autonomy of an individual person but that achieve greater autonomy for a group as a whole. Largely, this requires us to act as moral agents; that is, consider the moral principles upon which we are making decisions and the ethical consequences of our actions. The works of Immanuel Kant (Sullivan, 1990) represent a major influence on understandings of autonomy from this perspective. Moral decision-making is objective and, therefore, overriding. As such, it has rightful priority over all other interests of individuals and groups. The route to deciding on principles for action lies in the central question of Kantian moral deliberation: 'what are the necessary conditions of the moral decisions that we make?' In order to answer this question, Kant focuses on the word 'ought'. Unlike principles that focus on the best option for the individual, autonomous practical reasoning is not based on desire. Therefore reasoning such as, 'I ought not to strike a patient because I might get caught' would not be considered as moral reasoning in the Kantian view as it is based on the selfish desire of not being caught, irrespective of the greater harm caused by the actions. Moral (practical) reasoning concerns what 'ought' to happen and its focus is upon those actions that should be performed and outcomes that would be desired by all persons. Autonomy then is much more than thinking for and about oneself, but requires the person to think from the standpoint of every other person and to think consistently. In the context of older people being consumers of health care, services would not be planned, delivered or developed on the basis of (say) one individual's experience, as such action would be inappropriate unless the choices and decisions made were the same as all similar situations. Conflicts between the rights of the individual and the need for universal principles in health care decision-making are prevalent in debates about state provision of long-term care (Bishop, 1995), rationing of care provision (Aronson, 2002) and reforms to the provision of community care (Glendenning, 2003).

While we can see the importance of a universal position (wanting to do the greater good) in the context of the provision of services, policy and strategy decisions about service design and in care delivery (e.g. in quality improvement programmes or in agreeing generalized standards of practice, e.g. restraint use), it is less easy to see how the principle of 'doing the greatest good' can work in everyday decisions by nurses and care workers with an emphasis on individualized care and person-centred care. Nursing addresses the unique needs of patients as people, and these act as the central ethical concern of nurses. It is this 'everyday' focus of moral decision-making that is central to ethical nursing practice and it is argued that the day-to-day events in this relationship between the nurse and the patient are of greatest ethical concern for nurses (McCormack and McCance, 2010).

Key point

Nursing addresses the unique needs of patients as people, and these act as the central ethical concern of nurses.

Although universal principles can be applied in particular circumstances, it is difficult to see how nurses can do this. For example, how can all patients be expected to participate in their care programmes without considering particular individual circumstances and abilities? How can a nurse treat each patient as an individual under the umbrella of a universal law, without considering the idiosyncrasies of each particular case? Cartwright et al. (1992) argue for an applied ethic, whereby decisions are made according to individual circumstance but based upon a set of well-understood and thought-through generalized moral principles which relate to:

1. preserving the patient's dignity;
2. respecting the patient as a person;
3. allowing the patient access to information;
4. access to appropriate treatments.

Although such principles are all generalizable, at the same time they require knowledge of the individual older person in order for them to be operationalized. However, even such 'obvious' humanistic principles as these are fraught with difficulty in practice and each situation presents a new set of dilemmas for the nurse – dilemmas that Gilligan (1982) suggests can only be addressed through the 'connected' relationship between the nurse and patient and others important to them.

Care and rights

Gilligan argues for an approach to autonomy based on principles of 'care' rather than 'rights'. She argues for a 'responsibility-based' approach as contrasted with an individualistic, rights-based approach. She also suggests that instead of pursuing autonomy from a position where emphasis is placed on the rights of the individual, a position of 'attachment' should be achieved where the emphasis is on an 'ethic of care' (Gilligan, 1982: 164)

> The morality of rights is predicated on equality and centred on the understanding of fairness, while the ethic of responsibility relies on the concept of equity, the recognition of differences in need. While the ethic of right is a manifestation of equal respect, balancing the claims of other and self, the ethic of responsibility rests on an understanding that gives rise to compassion and care.

In the context of a relationship, moral problems arise because of conflicting responsibilities rather than competing rights. Moral problems require an approach to problem-solving that takes into account the context of the problem and the individual's biography; that is, their beliefs and values, rather than the 'formal and abstract' that arises from generalized principles and rules. Gilligan, (1982: 147) views a 'rights-based' approach to moral decision-making (with its emphasis on the protection of individual rights) as a simplistic approach to understanding complex problem-solving, and a failure to recognize the dynamics of relationships: 'Since moral problems arise in situations of conflict where either way I go, something or someone will not be served, their resolution is not just a simple yes or no decision . . .'

Effective decision-making comes from working through everything you think is involved and important in the situation, and taking responsibility for the choice made. This approach by Gilligan requires care workers to engage in active reflection in autonomous decision-making. Here it is also useful to consider the argument put forward by Collopy (1988) about autonomy.

Collopy asserted that autonomy is not, as we said before, a straightforward aspect of care in which someone either does or does not have autonomy. He points to a number of dimensions of autonomy, such as decisions made about long- and short-term issues, or about both mundane and key issues. Importantly, there is a 'continuum of autonomy' where people can have 'decisional autonomy' (i.e. the freedom to make decisions), even if their 'executional autonomy' (the ability to act on these decisions) is compromised (Collopy, 1988: 12).

Scenario 2.2

Fred lives alone since his wife died and he has been recently discharged from hospital having had a stroke. Fred is a great tea-drinker! However, since his stroke he has been unable to make a cup of tea independently. His decisional autonomy to want to drink a cup of tea remains but his executional autonomy to make a cup of tea is now compromised. He is unable to act on his decision to drink tea without support. His district nurse has arranged for someone to go to Fred's house each morning and they make a large flask of tea which Fred keeps beside him and is able to drink whenever he wishes during the day.

- *Are there any older persons who you are working with who have decisional autonomy (they know what they want) but reduced executional autonomy (they are unable to act on their choices)?*

The challenge for nurses and others who provide support to older people then is to support decisional autonomy, and when choices are made ensure that they are carried out. Collopy (1988) terms one dimension of this 'delegated autonomy' as people who are delegated to carry out tasks and, sometimes, decisions. The key to the processes of delegation, however, is that this process is negotiated rather than assumed.

In his model of person-centred care, McCormack (2001) described a form of autonomy that he referred to as 'negotiated autonomy'. By viewing autonomy within an interconnected relationship, an alternative perspective of autonomy can be achieved which is not based on any one person being the 'final arbiter' of decisions, but is instead set within a framework of negotiation based on an individual's values base. The nurse as a facilitator of an older person's autonomy engages in a process of dynamic caring that maintains autonomy at a time when the older person's sense of independence is under greatest threat.

Key point

The nurse engages in a process of dynamic caring that maintains autonomy at a time when the older person's sense of independence is under greatest threat.

When we think about rights, we need to think about both positive and negative rights. 'Positive rights' are the rights to have something; for example, dignity. Negative rights, or the right 'from', are the entitlement to be free from something; for example, freedom from interference or constraint (Reed and Ground, 1997). But where do these rights come from – are they inherent or inborn? Do people have these rights because they are human? If we do decide to accept this inherent nature of rights, we are then in a position where we have to think about how we define humanity.

Humanity and power

Humanity is a more contested issue than we might think, particularly if we define characteristics of humanity as being much like ourselves; that is, aware, articulate and active. This means that the humanity of anyone different to ourselves, such as someone who might have communication or cognitive problems, becomes ambiguous, and we can put respect for rights to the bottom of our priorities. This may make life easier for us, as supporting the rights of people to be autonomous may challenge the way that we (as nurses and services) have organized things. Negating or ignoring rights, however, is also a denial of personhood. If we define humanity and personhood as being like ourselves, then anyone who falls outside this similarity also falls outside this notion of inherent rights.

We need then to challenge this idea of humanity as being similarity, and widen the definition to include people who are different to us; that is, people who think differently or communicate differently. This would include people with dementia, or unconscious people, or people who cannot respond or communicate because of illness. If we broaden our ideas of humanity and personhood, then these people are included, and they have inherent rights, both negative rights to not have harm done to them, and positive rights to have support in their choices.

Power can be something that does not often get discussed – it can be difficult for nurses to acknowledge that, as professionals, they may have more power than service users. Through the knowledge and relationships that professionals have in the environments that they deliver care in, professionals can exert a great deal of influence or power over what happens. This power might be, in part, derived from nurses' status as respected members of a profession regarded as knowledgeable and influential. Conversely, nurses may be regarded as powerless if they are seen to be part of a profession that knows little and has no say in what happens.

These differing views on being power-full or power-less can also be applied to older people. They can be seen as purchasers of health care, and thus able to say what happens and when (as long as they have money – the penniless may also be powerless). On the other hand they may be seen as passive recipients of whatever services are allowed to them. Overarching these differences in purchasing power may also be the shadow of ageism – older people can be discounted because of their age.

Power, then, is a complex phenomenon, and much can depend on the cultural context in which nurses interact with older people. These complexities make an extensive discussion of power inappropriate here, so we are only able to focus on the idea of power sharing between older people and nurses (the reading list at the end of this chapter gives some suggestions for those who wish to explore this issue further).

To increase awareness of power then it would be useful to ask ourselves these questions:

- Who determines what care is given?
- What is the process of consultation?
- Who are the advocates for older people?
- Who is listened to when decisions are being made?

If we ask ourselves these questions then we may come to the conclusion that we have more power than older people. If, for example, we are working in a context where the service has been determined by a body who organizes health services, and who do not consult older people who have no choice or influence on what is provided, then we may conclude that older people may only have the power to refuse care. If even this is constrained by, say, refusal resulting in loss of other benefits, then this power seems hollow.

If, on the other hand, older people determine provision, and in the process of using health services make decisions about the form of care they get, we might think that power is being shared. In both scenarios, however, there may be action that needs to be taken – in the first case to increase the power of older people to determine care and in the second case to maintain it. Perhaps the most difficult scenario, however, is where power imbalances are invisible – where we do not think critically about the ways in which care is shaped. While things may be as they are because of long-standing cultural norms, it is useful to try to explore these and make them visible.

The other element of autonomy that we identified in the dictionary definition was knowledge, the basis of decision-making. Decisions can, of course, be made without knowledge, by instinct or intuition, and even if information is available it may not affect decisions much. At least, however, if information is available, it can be discounted. That is a very different situation to one in which information is not available, and people only have recourse to feelings and ideas to inform decisions.

In order to ensure a wide basis for decision-making then, we need to provide access to information. This may mean thinking through what information is needed and in what form(s):

- Is information needed about health issues?
- Is information needed about services?
- Is information needed about availability of care?

and

- Is information accessible for people with visual difficulties?
- Is information accessible for people with hearing difficulties?
- Is information accessible for people with physical difficulties?
- Is information accessible for people with cognitive difficulties?

These considerations mean that information may need to be about a range of different things, and accessible through different ways. Importantly, it may also need to come from different sources, so that different perspectives are represented. This means that nurses will have to make a considerable effort to make sure that this is all available and that it is offered. This means that we have to do more than keep some leaflets in a cupboard, but we have to think carefully about ways in which this information can be accessed. This may mean using equipment and aides, and, moreover, learning how to use them. It may also mean liaising with other agencies and groups to access different sources of information. Providing information is an important part of some new roles in health and social care, such as health trainers to support older people and dementia advisers who are promoted through one of the key objectives of the National Dementia Strategy (Department of Health (DoH), 2009).

This brief account of some of the dimensions of autonomy point to some of the complexities involved, and readers may well identify more. There are links to concepts such as rights, power and information and each of these needs to be thought through in the context in which we practise and in the context in which an older person lives. As this context is part of the culture in which we live, the danger is that issues of autonomy can become invisible, part of the landscape of our lives.

Alongside this complexity is a growing appreciation that autonomy is not an on/off switch – you do not either have it or not. There are gradations in autonomy, and it needs to be considered from a variety of different angles. The next section explores this complexity further. Furthermore, there are the implications for practice to be thought through, and the final section explores this.

Implications for nursing

All of this makes nursing very complicated – and it makes traditional established notions of professionals being all-knowing and all-powerful untenable! In this model, nurses decide what is best for a patient, and how it can be achieved. The older person would fit into the role of 'patient' as being compliant, grateful and, of course, patient. We can think of this as 'traditional' nursing, whereas what this chapter proposes is a direction for nursing that is empowering in that it focuses on nursing action as designed to work *with* older people to support independence and autonomy. This can be set out as in Table 2.1.

Nursing action	*Traditional nursing*	*Empowering nursing*
Assessment	Nurses decide what should be done, choosing which data to collect and how to collect it. The process of weighing the evidence and coming to conclusion is not disclosed.	This involves the older person as the decider of goals and inputs, and the setting and identification of goals and processes. The nurse supports these decisions after discussion of possibilities with the older person.
Implementation	Nurses do things *to* the patient, who is required to comply and raise no objections.	The older person engages with strategies and changes, developing an understanding of processes and resources.
Evaluation	The outcome of the nursing action is shared with colleagues, not necessarily with the service user.	The older person evaluates the input and its outcome, and modifies it if necessary.

Table 2.1 Nursing action with older people

This table outlines some of the differences between the approaches, but it is not likely that nurses will act according to one column or another, because their practice is likely to be compromised. This might be because of the availability of resources such as time, staff or equipment, or the organizational pressures of targets and procedures. The table then can be used to aid reflection on practice, and how it supports autonomy and independence.

Furthermore, we need to think about ways in which we can support people across different dimensions of autonomy (Collopy, 1988). These dimensions are outlined in Table 2.2.

In all of these dimensions, an older person may need help and support to exercise their capacity for decision-making. This may involve many activities, but will start from a careful and thoughtful discussion with the older person to explore preferences and capacity for decision-making. For example, someone may want to try different medications for a health problem, but will be happy for a doctor, with in-depth knowledge, to identify potential therapies from which to choose.

This type of nursing action may need organizational and practical support; for example, the time to discuss choices, and access to advice and support. If these are not forthcoming, then the nurse's task is more difficult.

What the nurse can hang on to, however, is the idea that older people can exercise independence and autonomy. This idea can clash with images of older people being passive and compliant which are often shown in culture. We have already pointed to some stereotypes of older people, and these can work against non-prejudicial thinking. The nurse then needs to think outside stereotypes and assumptions, and as Collopy (1988) says: 'autonomy can be a source of persistent and serious ethical conflict between the frail elderly and those . . . who provide care to them' (p. 17).

Taking on this conflict is often a brave and controversial course. But we need to remember Collopy's other words 'steering a course through this underlying dilemma is more than a matter of good will' (p. 17). We need then to stop resting on the laurels of benevolence, and enter into a probing discussion with older people about how they wish to exercise their autonomy, and how we can help, now and in the future.

Dimension	*Nursing question*	*Example*
Everyday/ critical	Has this person thought about all aspects of life? Does this cover a range of dimension s from the mundane to the critical?	A person might not be able to get into the kitchen to make a meal– an issue that is not noticed (an everydaymundane issue for staff), whereas issues such as ensuring the older person is given medication are given maximum priority (most critical for staff).
Long term/ short term	What are the immediate issues facing this person and what are the long-term implications?	Access to social events might be considered 'risky' by hospital staff but not by the older person. Not understanding the person's view of acceptable risk (short term) may result in the person losing contact with friends over time (long term).
Decisional/ executional	Does this person want to do things themselves, or simply make decisions about them for others to follow?	A person might choose a style for their clothes (decisional), and ask a friend to buy them(executional).
Direct/ delegated	Does this person want to make the decision themselves, or are they happy to let someone else decide?	A person might directly choose a dish from a menu (direct), but on the basis of the staff knowing the extent of their preferences be happy for their primary nurse to make decisions on occasions when their decision-making ability is reduced (delegated).
Negative/ positive	Does this person want to say no to something or agree to something?	A person might want to not participate in a singing evening but doesn't feel able to be asked to be removed from the communal lounge. However they would agree to a trip to a local library if it were offered to them.
Authentic/ inauthentic	Does this person make decisions that fit with their lifestyle and values?	An older person may go to organised church events but be a declared atheist (inauthentic) as they value the social connection with others and the engagement with families and friends (authentic).

Table 2.2 Dimensions of autonomy (from Collopy 1988)

Conclusion

We have outlined some of the dimensions of autonomy in this chapter, as befits a concept as complex and multilayered as this. In many ways the debates about autonomy chime in with ideas of individualization – one of the basic drivers of nursing practice. When an individual is helped to exercise autonomy then they may differ from the assumed wishes of everyone else, and the services that are established. It is important then for nurses to bear this in mind, and be aware that a difficult time might lie ahead if an older person's wishes are to be supported. However, this is an essential challenge for nurses as it is the way in which we can best support older people to maintain dignity in later life. Crucially, the nurse is in a position to facilitate an older person's autonomy by engaging in a process of dynamic caring that maintains autonomy at a time when the older person's sense of independence is under greatest threat.

References

Aronson, J. (2002) Elderly people's accounts of home care rationing: missing voices in long-term care policy debates, *Ageing and Society*, 22(4): 399–418.

Beauchamp, T.L. and Childress, J.F. (2001) *Principles of Biomedical Ethics*, 5th edn. Oxford: Oxford University Press.

Bishop, C.E. (1995) Sharing the burden: strategies for public and private long-term care insurance, *Journal of Health Politics, Policy and Law*, 20: 811–16.

Cambridge online dictionary, June 2009, dictionary.cambridge.org

Cartwright, T., Davson-Galle, P. and Holden, R.J. (1992) Moral philosophy and nursing curricula: indoctrination of the new breed, *Journal of Nursing Education*, 31(5): 225–28.

Collopy, B.J. (1988) Autonomy and long term care: some crucial distinctions, *Gerontologist*, 28 (Supplement, June): 10–17.

Department of Health (DoH) (2009) *National Dementia Strategy*. The Stationery Office, London: DoH.

Dworkin, G. (1991) *The Theory and Practice of Autonomy*. Cambridge: Cambridge University Press.

Gilligan, C. (1982) *In a Different Voice: Psychological Theory and Women's Development*. Cambridge, MA and London: Harvard University Press.

Glendenning, C. (2003) Breaking down barriers: integrating health and care services for older people in England, *Health Policy*, 65(2): 139–51.

McCormack, B. (2001) Autonomy and the relationship between nurses and older people, *Ageing and Society*, 21: 417–46.

McCormack, B. and McCance, T. (2010) *Person-centred Nursing: Theory, Models and Methods*. Oxford: Blackwell Publishing.

Reed, J. and Ground, I. (1997) *Philosophy for Nursing*. London: Edward Arnold.

Sullivan, R.J. (1990) *Immanuel Kant's Moral Theory*. Cambridge: Cambridge University Press.

CHAPTER 3

The aims and goals of care: a framework promoting partnerships between older people, family carers and nurses

Mike Nolan with scenarios by *Serena Allan, Patricia McGeever, Isabell Reid and Nina Szmaites*

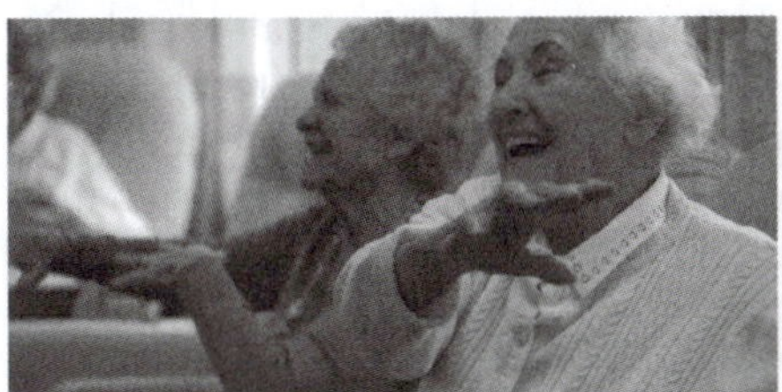
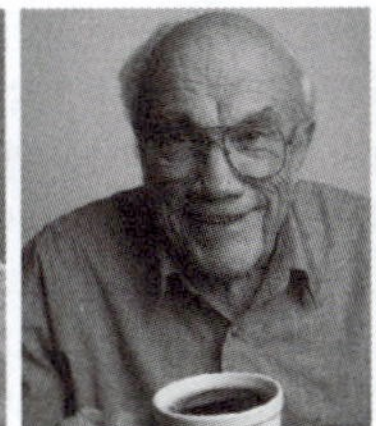
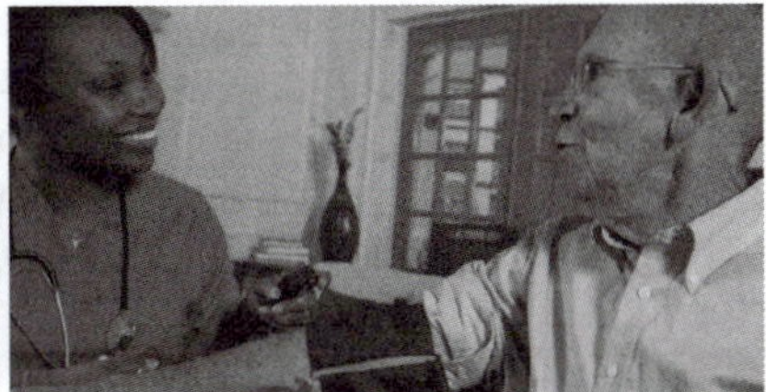

Learning objectives

At the end of this chapter, the reader will be able to:

- discuss the historical and social factors that have shaped the evolution of both health care for older people and gerontological nursing
- identify the limitations of existing practice frameworks/models for work with older people and their families
- understand the principles behind partnership working and a relationship-centred approach to care
- describe the characteristics of an enriched environment of care using the 'Senses Framework'
- provide practical examples of how the 'Senses' may be created for older people, family carers and staff

Freda commented:

'I thought it was lovely how they discussed and told you everything and the consultant drew a diagram to show me exactly what they were trying to do – sat on the end of the bed. Years ago, no-one told you anything.'

Introduction

In the above quotation an older patient describes her positive experiences during a recent admission to an acute hospital. She reflects on how good it felt to be fully involved in her care and to be treated as a 'partner' by her doctor. Working with older people and their families as partners is a central goal of the National Health Service (NHS) in England (Department of Health (DoH), 2008a), and is also promoted in recent standards for the nursing care of older people published by the Nursing and Midwifery Council (NMC, 2009). Promoting such partnerships lies at the heart of this book.

Despite such aspirations concerns over the quality of the care experienced by older people and their families remain. Major advocacy groups such as Age Concern (2006) and Help the Aged (2008) have suggested that standards of care are often 'little short of a national disgrace', and organizations such as the King's Fund argue that the health service has lost its way and no longer routinely provides care and support that ensures respect and treats patients with compassion (Firth-Cozens and Cornwell, 2009). Even the DoH feels the need to re-establish patients' 'Confidence in Care' (DoH, 2008b). It has been suggested that such problems are the result of the current emphasis on cure and the focus on 'technological' solutions to the needs of increasing numbers of frail and vulnerable members of society (Youngson, 2007, 2008). Of course, cure is a most appropriate goal when it is possible and technology will play an increasing role in care delivery. However, many of the problems older people face cannot be cured and the health service tends not to respond so well to the needs of older people with longer-term conditions. In the UK both the Royal College of Nursing (RCN) (2008) and the Nursing and Midwifery Council (NMC) (2009) have expressed concerns about a health service in which success is largely measured by 'targets' and argue that as a result less attention is paid to the overall quality of the experience for older patients and their families. Indeed, it seems that the 'little things' that can make all the difference to the care experienced by older people and their families are seen as increasingly less important (Cass et al., 2009).

This chapter suggests that if the situation is to improve then nurses, and others, working with older people and their carers need a framework for practice that addresses their complex and often subtle needs, while also enhancing the job satisfaction and morale of staff by recognizing the importance of caring relationships and the benefits of working as partners with patients and their families.

It begins with a brief history of nursing older people over the last 100 years or so, and argues that many of the current problems have their roots in a system of care that neither recognizes the needs of very frail older people and their families, nor values those who work with them. This is followed by a short overview of the role played by nursing models and the limitations associated with many existing approaches. The focus then moves to the development of a framework for practice: the Senses Framework, with four scenarios being used to illustrate how this can be applied in practice.

The development of nursing older people

Early pioneers of geriatric (now gerontological) nursing, such as Doreen Norton, writing in the 1950s and 1960s, argued that work with older people who have what we now call 'long-term conditions', represented 'true' nursing and that caring for such individuals was an area of practice in which nurses should excel (Norton, 1965; Norton et al., 1962). However, nursing has never fully realized this potential and, as with medicine, continues to see acute, hi-tech care delivered in hospital settings as being the most skilful and prestigious type of work. Of course, nurses working in acute care play a vital role but to focus on such settings alone neglects the needs of the majority of older people whose problems cannot be cured. Sadly, work with older people has a poor image and gerontological nursing is still the least preferred career option for newly qualified nurses (Nolan et al., 2006). In order to understand why this is the case it is important to look at the way in which both medicine and nursing has developed over time (Evers, 1991).

In their fascinating historical account Wilkin and Hughes (1986) trace how the emergence of modern medicine during the nineteenth century has influenced the way in which health services in general, and those for older people in particular, have developed. During the mid-nineteenth century there were three primary ways of obtaining health care:

- from poor law institutions;
- from voluntary hospitals;
- fee-for-service.

The wealthy paid for their health care privately: fee-for-service. Those with acute illnesses turned to the voluntary hospitals which at that time were emerging as centres for *'scientific medicine'* and the training of doctors. Those individuals who, because of disability or old age, could not be cured (termed the *incurables*) had only one option: the workhouse.

Therefore, from the outset people who were 'incurable' received poorer care and were seen as ever less exciting to work with as advances in medicine gained pace and the prestige and status of the medical profession grew. This remained the case for the next 100 years or so until the pioneers of geriatric medicine such as Marjorie Warren began to demonstrate what could be achieved with the frail older people if they were given the right care. However, despite efforts over the last 60 years, including more recent initiatives such as the National Service Framework (NSF) for older people (DoH, 2001), negative attitudes towards older people remain, as is clear in the language that we use. As the success of the NHS is measured primarily by cure and discharge rates, older people with chronic conditions presented problems from the outset and have increasingly been seen as a drain on resources. Over time the 'incurables' became the 'bed-blockers', and more recently 'frequent flyers'. Indeed, the history of geriatric services is closely linked to the idea of discharge. During the 1950s and 1960s the emerging specialty of geriatric medicine was struggling for recognition and status in the face of stiff opposition from its more prestigious peers, medicine and surgery, who could see no value in 'spending time, money, energy and bed space on redundant senior members of society' (Felstein, 1969). Eventually geriatric medicine was accorded specialty status for largely pragmatic reasons, the desire to free up beds. The existence of geriatric medicine provided medicine and surgery with a way of getting frail older people 'out of their beds' (Wilkin and Hughes, 1986).

Care or cure?

However, as an emergent discipline geriatric medicine was faced with a dilemma: in the absence of cure for many of its patients how could it demonstrate success? According to Wilkin and Hughes (1986) this was achieved by replacing the medical/curative model of health with a functional one in which rehabilitation and the restoration of function became the goals of 'geriatric' care and improved scores on measures such as the Barthel Index became key indicators of success.

The emergence of geriatric medicine, while benefiting those in need of 'rehabilitation', had the effect of further devaluing people with long-term needs who rapidly became an embarrassment to the 'system' and were subject to 'aimless residual care' (Evers, 1991). Essentially, modern medicine has always valued cure more than care (Evers, 1991) and such tensions are still obvious, as evidenced by the need for recent initiatives such as the *Dignity Challenge* (Social Care Institute for Excellence, 2006). Therefore, despite several efforts over the years to promote work with older people as an interesting, challenging and valued area of care, its image remains poor (Nolan et al., 2006). This has not been helped by the way that nursing has developed as a profession.

As the NHS gradually washed its hands of older people in need of long-term care, work with such individuals and their families became more and more unpopular with many nurses. When cure or rehabilitation were not possible, writers such as Reed and Bond (1991) described how nurses focused on 'good geriatric care' in which keeping older people clean and fed provided the measures of success. At this time authors such as Kitson (1987, 1991) were arguing that nurses increasingly viewed the 'technological' aspects of care as more skilful and prestigious but that what the profession lacked was a means of enabling practitioners to 'organize, control and direct' their care. It was here that nursing models were seen to have a key role to play.

Nursing models

During the 1980s and 1990s numerous 'nursing' models emerged, some from the UK, but many from the USA, that seemed to offer the potential to 'organize, control and direct' nursing care. These were adopted enthusiastically, if uncritically, by many nurses and featured prominently in nurse training and in the writing of the time. However, there were also several people who urged caution arguing, for example, that such models, especially those from the USA, were often highly abstract and were both difficult to apply in practice and, because they had an exclusively nursing focus, failed to address the needs of many older people and their families in a holistic fashion (Reed and Robbins, 1991).

In 2003 Wadenstein and Carlsson reviewed the usefulness of 17 nursing models in providing guidance for those working with older people and concluded that none of them was adequate for the task. The highly abstract nature of many models meant that nurses themselves often failed to understand them fully and this was even more difficult for older people and their families. As Clark (2002) notes, many of the ideas that were used were too 'slippery' to be useful in practice. The need to have a framework for practice that is easy to understand and yet can be used in a range of care settings is even more important if older people and their families are to be true partners in their own care. Zgola (1999) has long argued that patients, families and practitioners need to use the same ideas and the same language if they are to communicate effectively, and more recently it has been suggested that ideas underpinning health care need to be expressed in ways that are 'ordinary, accessible, jargon free and commonly understood' (Goodrich and Cornwell, 2008: 24) if they are to be useful for everyone.

It was the desire to provide practitioners with a framework for practice that met the needs of older people, their families and staff working in a range of care settings that was motivation behind the development of the 'Senses Framework', which has emerged over the last 15 years or so. In order to achieve this it was argued that nurses working with older people had to state far more clearly what their goals and priorities of care are (Nolan, 1994). Underpinning the Senses Framework is the belief that, in the past, nurses failed to work in partnership with both older people and their family carers, and often neglected both their wider needs and the expert knowledge that they have (Nolan and Grant, 1989; Nolan et al., 1994). It was suggested that one way of improving the situation was to adopt the model of the 'therapeutic quadrangle' (Rolland, 1988, 1994) as a basis for working more closely with older people and their carers (see Nolan et al., 1994). Rolland (1988, 1994) argued that if services are better to support older people with long-term conditions and their families, there was a need for a new approach. This should reflect the considerable differences in long-term conditions; for example, in terms of their onset, course and duration, and also allow the views of multiple different people to be heard. For instance, following a stroke, which comes on suddenly with very little warning, the needs of an older person and their family are likely to be very different from the needs of a person with dementia, where the condition is gradual in onset and often insidious in the early stages. Rolland (1988) proposed a model called the 'therapeutic quadrangle' which is represented in Figure 3.1.

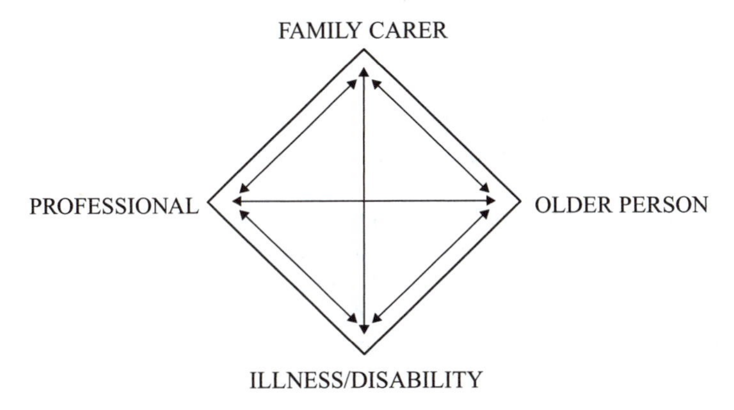

Figure 3.1: The therapeutic quadrangle

Source: Reproduced with permission from Rolland, 1988

Such an approach recognizes that people are often 'interdependent' rather than being independent and that all of us, as human beings, rely on others to have a good quality of life. It is therefore our relationships that largely define who we are in the world. This is especially important for people who need help and support to maintain a good quality of life. This raises questions about the current value placed on autonomy and individuality. For example, from an ethical standpoint MacDonald (2002) contends that the goal of promoting individual autonomy in older people is flawed and that our understanding of autonomy should be underpinned by the belief that humans are 'deeply interrelated and interconnected'. It was from such ideas that the Senses Framework emerged.

Key point

People are often interdependent, rather than being independent, and all of us, as human beings, rely on others to have a good quality of life.

The Senses Framework

The Senses Framework has been applied recently in both acute and community settings, but it was initially developed with care homes in mind. The framework was originally suggested in 1997 (Nolan, 1997), and since then it has been further elaborated upon over a number of years (see Davies et al., 1999; Nolan et al., 2002, 2006; Brown et al., 2007, 2008). The original idea was driven by the belief that staff working in care homes did not receive the recognition that they deserved, and that both academics and policy-makers tended to paint a very negative picture of what it was like to live and work there (Nolan, 1997).

For example, as noted already, studies suggested that care homes provide 'aimless residual care' (Evers, 1981a, 1981b), or at best 'good geriatric care' (Reed and Bond, 1991) where the main goals are simply to ensure that residents are well fed, dressed and kept clean. As important as these activities are, there is more to life than this. It was suggested that nurses, and others, working in care homes had few other therapeutic goals to aim for and that because of this they gained little satisfaction from their work. Indeed, some argued that whereas staff in acute settings suffered 'burnout' because of the highly demanding and rapidly changing nature of their work, staff in care homes were more likely to experience 'rust out' (Pennington and Pierce, 1985) because they experienced so little stimulation.

However, staff working in care homes often have to deal with very complex situations, including increasing numbers of people with considerable physical and cognitive frailty. Based on his experiences as a practitioner and a researcher, Nolan (1997) suggested a framework that would highlight the important role that care homes play, and also provide staff with clear goals to aim for. It was argued that care homes should create an environment in which older people experience six 'Senses'. These are:

- **A sense of security:** to feel safe and secure, not just physically but also psychologically. That is to feel free from threat or harm, and also, for example, to feel free to be able to complain without fear of reprisals.

- **A sense of belonging:** to feel 'part of things', both within the home and the wider community, and to be able to maintain existing relationships and to form new ones.
- **A sense of continuity:** so that people's biography and life history are recognized and valued, and used to plan and deliver care that is consistent with their wishes and preferences.
- **A sense of purpose:** is about having valued goals to aim for, the sort of things that make it worth getting out of bed in the morning and provide a feeling of 'I have a contribution to make'. It is important that older people in care homes have interesting things to pass the time, as many studies suggest that they spend up to 80 per cent of their waking day doing nothing.
- **A sense of achievement**[1]: this is about being able to achieve the above goals and to feel satisfied with your efforts.
- **A sense of significance:** although all the Senses are important, and each one is related to the next – for example, you need a sense of purpose in order to be able to get a sense of achievement – a sense of significance is possibly the most fundamental sense of all. This is about feeling that you 'matter', that your life has importance, and that other people recognize and value who and what you are. As we age our sense of significance is threatened, as we experience multiple losses (of work, of health, of a partner or friends). Entry to a care home also means the loss of your 'home'. Therefore, creating an environment in which older people feel that they really 'matter' is crucial.

Scenario 3.1

Joan had a large family who had moved to live all over the UK and she enjoyed travelling to spend time with them and looking after her grandchildren. When Joan moved into a care home following a fall at home she became very quiet and withdrawn. Her family visited when they could but it was a long journey for them and there was little for Joan's grandchildren to do in the home so they were bored very quickly. The nursing staff in the home recognized that the move into a care home had an enormous impact on Joan's sense of belonging and significance in particular. They worked with a local company to set up a computer in Joan's room with a webcam and now Joan is able to see and talk with her family daily. Through the webcam she is able to stay in touch with changes to her children's homes and her grandchildren can enjoy chatting with her and showing her things that matter to them like a picture they painted at school that day. Importantly, Joan found a new way in which she could feel part of the lives of her family.

- *In what ways are you able to use new communication technologies to support older people to remain in contact with their family and friends?*

However, it was also argued that if staff are to create these Senses for residents then they should experience them too. Therefore, if staff do not experience a sense of security, belonging, continuity and so on in their work, how can they be expected to ensure that residents experience the Senses? This views staff well-being as being essential to residents' quality of life and staff job satisfaction.

---

[1] This was originally termed a 'Sense of fulfilment' but was altered following feedback from older people and staff.

Therefore, staff need to experience a sense of security, not just to be free from physical or verbal abuse, but also to feel confident that they can complain about poor standards, if this is necessary, without risking their jobs. They need to experience a sense of belonging, with there being good teamwork, a happy work atmosphere, and friendly relationships within the home. A sense of continuity is essential, but can be difficult to achieve if there is high staff turnover and extensive use of agency staff. The academic literature suggests that what staff in care homes often lack is a clear sense of purpose – what is their job about, and how do they know that they are doing it well? Creating the Senses for residents helps to provide a sense of purpose for staff, but this requires that all residents' needs are seen as important. Therefore, ensuring that residents are fully occupied and encouraged to form friendships if they wish should be seen as being equally important as meeting their physical needs.

Key point

Nursing staff need to experience a sense of security, not just to be free from physical or verbal abuse, but also to feel confident that they can complain about poor standards.

We all need an occasional 'pat on the back' and to go home at the end of the day feeling, and being told, that we have 'done a good job'. Staff therefore need to experience a sense of achievement, with their efforts being recognized and valued. While the financial rewards in care homes are often limited, the potential for other rewards, for example, ensuring a good quality of life for residents is as great. Indeed, most of the research suggests that staff get their greatest satisfaction from their relationships with residents. This needs to be fully recognized, but so too does the vulnerable position that forming relationships with residents may place staff in. Therefore, the grief that staff often feel when a resident they know well dies must be acknowledged, and there should be support mechanisms in place to help them deal with this grief if they are to feel 'secure' to form close relationships with residents in the future. This demonstrates how each of the Senses influences the others. They are therefore 'interdependent' rather than independent.

Last, and by no means least, staff must also experience a sense of significance. Not only must they feel valued by the organization they work for, but society must also recognize and see the value of the work they do. There is perhaps some way to go before this is achieved but initiatives such as 'My Home Life' (www.myhomelife.org.uk) are leading the way.

Over the years it has been argued (Davies et al., 1999; Nolan et al., 2002, 2006; Brown et al., 2007, 2008) that an 'enriched' environment is one in which both residents and staff experience the Senses. If one group does not, or one of the Senses is missing, then the environment is 'impoverished' to a greater or lesser extent.

An enriched care environment

The Senses Framework has been refined and developed further by working closely with older people, staff and family carers. It very quickly became clear that the needs of a key group, family carers, were missing from the original Framework. It is now recognized that an enriched environment is one in which residents, staff and relatives all experience the Senses.

This is important as there is considerable research evidence to suggest that the best care homes are those in which staff and families work closely together, with each valuing the other's contribution. There is, as Sue Davies has argued, a need to create a 'community' within care homes where it is recognized that residents, staff and relatives all have different but equally important contributions to make in creating an 'enriched' environment (Davies, 2003).

If the argument holds that staff cannot create the Senses for residents unless they experience them too, the same must be true for relatives. Therefore relatives need to feel: safe (to complain if needed for example); that they belong, with it being very important to create a welcoming atmosphere during early meetings, often before admission itself; relatives need to experience continuity and feel that they have a part to play in the life of the home (if they wish, not everyone wants to), and that their efforts are recognized and seen as important, and so on.

Later work showed that if care homes have student nurses, then they need to experience the Senses and to enjoy an 'enriched' learning environment if they are to gain the most from their placement (see Brown 2006; Brown et al., 2007, 2008). Studies have shown that if students experience a positive placement in a care home (they are often expecting it to be a negative experience based on public and media images) then they are far more likely to want to work with older people when they qualify, often in the care home sector. Jayne Brown has described how to create the Senses for students (see Brown, 2006; Brown et al., 2007, 2008) and has recently undertaken work to explore how true partnerships can be forged in all care settings.

An 'enriched' environment of care is one in which all the main groups experience the Senses, as illustrated in Figure 3.2.

Stakeholder / Senses	Older person	Staff	Family carers	Students
Security				
Belonging				
Continuity				
Purpose				
Achievement				
Significance				

Figure 3.2: An enriched environment of care

Since they were originally proposed the Senses have been applied to acute hospital care for older people and have demonstrated how dignified care for older patients can be achieved if the Senses are created (see Davies et al., 1999).

In summary, the Senses seem to work because they 'speak' to people in a language that they understand, probably because they have been developed with the active involvement of older people, staff, family carers and students. They have considerable potential for use in a range of settings. Four 'case' studies are now presented, each of which describes how the Senses have been applied by practitioners working in different care environments. As the Senses were initially developed for use in a care home setting it seems appropriate to start here.

Applying the Senses in practice

We now include several examples of where Senses has been applied in practice, so you can identify and learn from the strengths and experiences of others using Senses framework.

An example from a care home setting

Serena Allan was a charge nurse working in a care home for people with visual impairment when she undertook a leadership training programme aimed at improving the care older people receive by challenging existing models of care and looking for new ways of working. Serena wanted to both change her own style of leadership, which at the time she thought was a little too 'top down', and to challenge some of the current routines within the home that were sometimes more for the benefit of staff rather than residents.

Introducing change is never easy and takes considerable effort, especially when existing ways of working are being challenged. Serena began by reflecting on her own leadership style and realized that by not delegating things as much as she might that she was inadvertently restricting the development opportunities for her staff. She wanted to change this and to offer staff the chance to take on more responsibility themselves. To do this she needed to find out how they viewed their existing work environment.

She therefore adapted a questionnaire called the CARE (Combined Assessment of Residential Environments) Profiles (Faulkner et al., 2006) that was designed to assess the extent to which the Senses are created for staff, residents and relatives in care home settings. At this point Serena focused on staff views as she wanted to capture their feelings about their work.

The results showed that while, overall, staff were generally happy with their work there were areas in which things could be improved. Following the staff survey a series of meetings were held to discuss the way forward and over the next few months a number of changes were introduced, which were initially quite small but became more major as staff gained in confidence. These included:

- Regular monthly meetings so that staff had the opportunity to discuss the way that things were going. These provided a forum where staff were encouraged to challenge the way that care was delivered and to come up with ideas for change.

- In order to 'free up' staff time and enable them to spend more time with residents a review of the pattern of the late shift was undertaken and changes to the hours of working were discussed, agreed and introduced.
- A 'keyworker' system was established in staff who were allocated to work with the same residents. Staff photographs were displayed so that relatives and visitors could identify them more quickly and were encouraged to get to know them better.
- Staff were encouraged to undertake life history work with residents so that they could better understand the influences that had shaped the residents' lives.

All of these changes have helped to create a more enriched environment of care in which the Senses were enhanced for staff, residents and relatives.

The monthly meetings helped to establish a sense of security and continuity. They are well attended and by encouraging staff to talk openly about their views on work and care have created an atmosphere of transparency. The changes to the shift pattern have been valued by both staff and residents and have achieved their goal of giving staff more time to talk to residents. Staff are also clearer about their respective roles and responsibilities.

The photo board and the life story work have helped to create a much stronger sense of belonging for staff, residents and families and a greater sense of teamwork among staff. This has also improved their sense of significance.

Care staff now have more delegated responsibility and can, for example, play a much more active role in planning work rotas, in co-ordinating care and contributing to administrative work if they wish. This, together with the keyworker system, has led to greater clarity about the goals of care and has significantly improved the staff's sense of purpose and achievement.

In reflecting upon what has been achieved Serena has the following to say:

> 'I am pleased with the way that both staff and I have changed. Rather than trying to do everything myself, I now delegate things such as dealing with GP rounds, drug ordering/organization and projects, for example, Life Smile. The change in working hours has been positive for both staff and residents – staff are happy and there has been a benefit to resident care in that there are more staff around at busy times. Staff have moved from being onlookers in the organization of the unit to being working partners. Morale is high and there is excellent teamwork.'

Although on first reading the above changes might seem relatively small, in reality they are highly significant. Introducing change to established practice is notoriously difficult and although successful change is possible this can take months, if not years, to introduce and sustain. Serena's reflections provide a clue as to the roots of her success when she notes that 'Staff have moved from being onlookers in the organisation of the unit to being working partners.' It is the promotion of partnerships that lie at the heart of the Senses Framework and is the key to success.

Having provided an example of how the Senses can be applied in a care home setting, in the next scenario Pat McGeever describes how she transformed the student learning experience on her unit.

An example of creating an enriched learning environment for student nurses

As has already been noted, working with older people is often the least preferred career among newly qualified nurses. Studies have shown that such attitudes are formed during students' training and that it is the nature and quality of their clinical placements that is the most significant influence (Brown 2006; Brown et al., 2007, 2008; Nolan et al., 2006). Placements with older people are often seen as unexciting compared to areas such as A & E or ITU and if students are not stimulated and challenged by their placement with older people then such stereotypes are reinforced.

Pat McGeever, a charge nurse in Roslynlee Hospital, Lothian was concerned that students often felt just like 'another pair of hands' while on her unit and wanted to ensure that they had a more stimulating placement. She therefore introduced the Senses Framework to her ward and encouraged students to use this as a way of both reflecting on their placement and undertaking life story work with patients. To do this she:

- met with the students and introduced them to the Senses on the first day of their placement and discussed how they could be used with patients, relatives and staff;
- asked students to keep a reflective diary focusing on how they felt that the Senses were being met for them;
- devised a questionnaire that students completed about how the Senses were being met on the ward and asked them to identify three things that they thought should be changed or improved on the unit;
- created a new 'buddy' system for students so that they had both a qualified mentor but were also paired with a nursing assistant so that they were always likely to have someone to turn to if they wanted to discuss an issue.

The effect on the unit was dramatic. Students rapidly established a sense of security and belonging so that they felt 'part of the team'. This was helped by having students' names up on the staff board so that relatives knew who they were too. Students had a clear sense of purpose on the unit and worked closely with the occupational therapist in developing the life story work. This also had a very positive impact on patient care as the life stories fed into care planning and ensured that care reflected individual need. Students felt secure to question practice and to raise concerns with Pat. For example, when they noted that the way depot injections were given on the ward differed from how they had been taught in the university this led to a review of practice, so that staff were taught the latest techniques. As a result students' sense of significance was greatly improved. Perhaps most importantly students felt that they had achieved something of value on their placement and reported their very positive experiences (this was something that they had not been expecting) upon their return to the university. However, as Pat's reflections below suggest the benefits of introducing the Senses extend well beyond the student experience:

> 'When I heard about the Senses Framework it just connected with me and the light went on! Taking the Senses forward in my ward has made me feel refreshed and rejuvenated. Spending time with students on the first day setting the scene was the key – spending an hour telling them my story and journey in nursing paid dividends. The other great thing is that all the team wanted to come on board because the Senses remind us of all

> the values we came into nursing for. It was good to see the students leaving happy – one of them is even presenting a paper about her experience on my ward at an RCN National Student Conference!'

Pat's reflection is powerful and attests to what can be achieved if people are open to new ideas. But this takes courage as to openly invite critical comment is a brave thing to do. However, it has clearly paid dividends in this case and has spin-offs for the ward as a whole. Possibly the most important point for Pat and her team is that the Senses 'remind us of all the values we came into nursing for'. It is such values that are under threat in a target driven NHS culture.

The next scenario, Isabell Reid, charge nurse, looks at how the Senses were applied in a day hospital settings, also in Rosslynlee Hospital, Lothian.

An example of rising to the challenge of change

Isabell Reid is a charge nurse working in the day hospital at Rosslynlee Hospital, Lothian. Her staff group have been together for a long time and as she herself said were 'at the mature end of the workforce!'. Isabell was aware that significant changes to the organization of the hospital were being planned and wanted to help her staff to prepare for these changes by introducing reflective practice to the unit. She was aware that this might prove a challenge, for while the staff had a wealth of experience they were also used to a certain pattern of working and may have been reluctant to change. Pat thought that the Senses framework might help the process. She therefore:

- arranged an 'education day' so that the whole team could be introduced to the Senses;
- adapted the CARE profiles questionnaire (as Serena had done in Scenario 3.1) in order to see if staff were currently experiencing the Senses in their day-to-day work. Staff were actively encouraged to provide full and frank answers to the questions;
- asked staff to identify three things that they thought was good about the care they provided and three things that they wanted to change. These were then used as a basis for detailed discussion;
- linked the Senses to the process of staff self-appraisal in order to help them to identify the skills they might need to include as part of their personal development programme.

As a result of this activity a number of things changed. Despite having worked together for a long time staff now felt better able to express their views and felt safe to do so in a supportive environment. As a result communication improved. This helped to foster a greater sense of security and belonging. In order to ensure that good patterns of communication continued a series of two monthly staff meetings have been introduced. The above have enhanced feelings of significance with staff now believing that their opinions really matter. There have also been benefits for day patients and their families. Staff are introducing life story work with patients and using 'question' cards to actively seek the views of patients and relatives about the

(*continued*)

care they receive. This has improved the Senses for users while also adding to the staff's sense of purpose and achievement. Staff are also now spending more time with students and arranging for tutorials with them. A more enriched environment has been created for everyone involved. In reflecting of these changes Isabell notes:

> 'When I first heard about the Senses I was not sure how they would improve what I thought was a good service that we provided. When I found myself enthusing about what I had learned to my staff and seeing my staff listen, I decided to 'give it a try' and see if this would help with the changes that were being implemented. My motivation and that of my team has increased. I am increasingly aware of staffing issues and my awareness of myself has increased allowing me to change. I feel that the changes in myself and the team have improved the client and carer experience. I feel proud of myself and my team for all we have achieved.'

In her reflections Isabell has described changes to the team and benefits for clients and users. But as with Serena perhaps one of the most significant changes has been personal and the Senses have helped both Serena and Isabell to gain new insights into themselves and how the ways in which they work as charge nurses can have a profound impact on the whole environment of care. This is consistent with work on dignified care for older patients in acute settings which has highlighted the key part played by the ward leader in establishing the Senses for everyone else. This key role is further reinforced in the final scenario described by Nina Szmaites.

An example of improving anticipatory care

Nina is a Charge Nurse in an older person's Rehabilitation and Assessment Unit in Edinburgh. At the time she introduced the Senses, the unit was in the early stages of implementing a model of anticipatory care, the aim of which was to take a proactive approach in order to help frail older people remain well, maintain them in the community and to prevent hospital admission. She used the Senses to explore how the current system could be improved and focused in particular on how family carers could be encouraged to play a much more active role. The Senses were used to highlight what the unit currently did well for staff, patients/carers and students. As a result more focus was given to the involvement of family carers, with attention being given to their needs, as well as those of the patient. The staff's roles in the anticipatory care process were clarified and protected learning sessions and regular team meeting were introduced in order to keep everyone up to date. A named co-ordinator was allocated to each patient/carer.

As a result the Senses have been enhanced in the following ways:

- **Security:** Patients and carers are more confident that all their needs have been considered following their comprehensive assessment. This makes them feel safer. Staff are now clear about their role and have well-defined boundaries to work within.
- **Belonging**: Relatives/carers now play a much greater role and are formally involved in care if the patient is happy for this to happen. The regular communication has improved teamworking among staff.

- **Continuity:** The introduction of the named co-ordinator has been positive for everyone and has greatly improved continuity of care, as has the regular input of carers into the work of the unit.
- **Purpose and achievement:** The above changes have resulted in much clearer goals for everyone, with the goals now being reviewed on a more regular basis. Regular feedback from patients and carers ensures that the staff know that their wishes are being met also.
- **Significance:** The increased attention given to patients and carers makes them feel much more significant and recognized as a person of value. The investment in staff training and personal development and the way in which their opinions are actively listened to makes them feel valued and important.

In thinking about what has been achieved Nina notes:

> 'It has been refreshing for the team to celebrate our current practice. This is not about me it is about the team, and the constant effort they put in every day to support the older person through their individual rehabilitation programme. We have had fantastic feedback from patients/carers and outside agencies. We recently offered an assessment to a carer who we were concerned about and he wrote a letter of thanks. When I told him we were just doing our job he said "It's not just what you do, it's the people you are." I can't beat that'.

As Nina notes, one of the real benefits of applying the Senses is that they provide a framework that allows people to reflect upon what they do, to celebrate success and, if needed, to identify areas that can be improved. By focusing on everyone's needs they have the potential to promote an enriched environment for all groups. As they have been developed in close collaboration with staff, students, older people and family carers, they 'speak' to people in a language that they can relate to. Given the diversity of the above settings it also seems that the Senses are relevant in differing care environments. Can they therefore provide a framework for practice with older people with the potential for widespread application?

Relationship-centred care

The Senses reflect important dimensions of caring relationships between older people, family carers and staff across a range of care environments. The framework is essentially about how such relationships can be created and maintained and the role that they play in 'enriching' the environment of care. Many years ago Alison Kitson (1987) suggested that the main goal of nurses working with older people should be to create the right environment for others to grow. However, the Senses is based on the belief that an enriched environment is one in which *everyone* can grow. It has therefore been argued that rather than the current emphasis on person or patient-centred care that the focus should be on relationship-centred care (Nolan et al., 2004). Relationship-centred care was originally suggested as a model for the delivery of health care that was better suited to the needs of people with long-term conditions (see Tresolini and the Pew-Fetzer Task Force, 1994) and the Senses are one way in which such a model can be applied in practice. However, if such a way of working is to be adopted more widely then relationships between staff, patients and families must be valued and seen as an essential aspect of good care, rather than an added extra.

Several writers have recently stressed the need to transform the status of relationships at all levels and between all parties: professionals, patients/residents and families (Baker, 2007; Institute for the Future of Aging Services (IFAS) 2008; Parker, 2008; Szczepura et al., 2008). Baker (2007) contends that there is a need for a new way of thinking about relationships in the context of care, with others arguing that the goal should be to shift the focus away from tasks and towards relationships (Robinson and Gallagher, 2008). This will require a greater recognition and promotion of relational practice (Parker, 2008), which Parker sees as those activities 'necessary to develop and sustain interpersonal relationships' based on an understanding of individual circumstances and their contexts. However, while the new constitution for the NHS explicitly endorses the importance of 'compassion' as a core value for health services, providers are at the same time 'under intense pressure' to shorten, routinize and reduce the interactions that constitute such relationships (Parker, 2008).

'Relational' work appears all the more important in the current acute care-oriented health care environment. Parker (2008) has argued that relational practice requires a number of factors to be in place and comprises several dimensions. She sees these as being:

- accessibility – staff need to be available when they are needed;
- boundary management – staff need to make emotional connections with patients, but also avoid being overloaded;
- connection – the ability to create engagement/empathy and demonstrate emotional authenticity;
- collaboration – all parties need to share information and be involved in relational work;
- continuity – the ability to relate past and present experiences.

However, although such 'relational' practice often occurs between individual patients and staff, Parker (2008) believes that interactions between staff are also critical, and that improving such interactions requires: inter-group support; informal and formal co-ordination systems; the management of membership and boundaries; and a clear understanding of interdisciplinary relationships and status.

Parker (2008) sums her findings up thus:

> “Relational work in caregiving organisations thus depends, not only on the skills of individual practitioners and care workers, but also on the extent to which the workgroup and the organisation are structured and operated in ways that are supportive of relational work behaviours.”

If relational practice is to be at the forefront of care we need to find a new model for health care. The work of the 'Pew-Fetzer' foundation (Tresolini and the Pew-Fetzer Task Force, 1994) that originally coined the term 'relationship-centred' care had just such a goal, arguing that the dominant cure model of Western health care systems was inadequate to address the major health challenges facing modern society. Recently, Youngson (2007, 2008) has advanced a similar set of arguments in promoting compassion as the key to better health services. He argues that there is a need for a move away from a health service based on 'fixing', where the goal is *to provide* a service, to one where the main aim is *to be of* service in order to create a 'healing' environment. Recently, both the Royal College of Nursing (RCN, 2008) and the Nursing and Midwifery Council (NMC, 2009) have produced

RCN 2008	*NMC 2009*
Place – the physical environment and culture of the organization	Place – is care managed and resourced effectively; does the environment encourage an element of calculated risk?
People – attitudes and behaviours of others	People – are they competent, assertive, reliable, empathic and compassionate?
Processes – nature and conduct of care activities	Processes – is there open communication, and partnerships between patients, colleagues and families?

Table 3.1 The three elements of the RCN and NMC models of care

two reports that outline a model of care comprising of three elements, which are again interdependent (Table 3.1).

In a recent analysis of 'interpersonal dignity' in acute care, Baillie (2009) identifies a not dissimilar group of interrelated factors that she asserts either promote or diminish such dignity. These are:

- patient factors – the influence of the patient's own characteristics;
- staff factors – the way that staff interact with patients, families and colleagues;
- hospital environment – the way that the system is structured, especially the culture and leadership that is in operation and the behaviour of other patients in the environment.

The application of the Senses provides a way of addressing such diverse factors and creates an enriched environment of care.

The value of the Senses and relationship-centred care was explicitly reinforced in the latest 'Best Practice Standards' for work with older people in acute care settings (Bridges et al., 2009) that identified three broad areas on which nurses should focus their attention:

- maintaining identity – 'see who I am';
- creating community – 'connect with me';
- sharing decision-making – 'involve me'.

This publication together with others (see Nolan et al., 2006, Davies et al., 2007, www.myhomelife.org.uk) provide numerous practical examples of how an enriched environment can be created in a range of practice settings.

Key point

Nursing staff should focus relationship-centred care on maintaining identify, creating community and involving older people.

Conclusion

This chapter has argued that modern-day health services have evolved into a system that primarily values cure above care and that quality of care is largely focused on meeting 'targets'. Many older people have needs that are not appropriately addressed by such a system. Gerontological nursing has struggled to define its goals of care, especially for people with long-term needs. However, the values of interdependence rather than independence and autonomy should be increasingly promoted, highlighting the importance of relationships and partnerships between older people, their family carers and staff. The Senses Framework provides one way of defining and creating an 'enriched' environment of care in which the needs of all groups are met.

References

Age Concern (2006) *Q is for Quality: The Voices of Older People on the Need for Better Quality Care and Support*. Age Concern. Available online at www.ageconcern.org.uk/AgeConcern/policy-QisforQualityreport.asp; accessed 8 January 2009.

Baker, B. (2007) *Old Age in New Age: The Promise of Transformative Nursing Homes*. Nashville, TN: Vanderbilt University Press.

Baillie, L. (2009) Patient dignity in an acute hospital setting: a case study, *International Journal of Nursing Studies*, 46: 23–37.

Bridges, J., Flatley, M. and Meyer, J. (2009) *Best Practice for Older People in Acute Care Settings (BPOP): Guidance for Nurses*. London: RCN/City University London.

Brown, J. (2006) Student nurses' experience of learning to care for older people in enriched environments: a constructivist inquiry. PhD thesis, University of Sheffield.

Brown, J., Nolan, M. and Davies, S. (2007) Bringing caring and competence into focus in gerontological nursing: a longitudinal, multi-method study, *International Journal of Nursing Studies*, 45(5): 654–67.

Brown, J., Nolan, M., Davies, S., Nolan, J. and Keady, J. (2008) Transforming students' views of gerontological nursing: realising the potential of 'enriched' environments of learning and care: a multi-method longitudinal study, *International Journal of Nursing Studies*, 45(8): 1214–32.

Cass, E., Robbins, D. and Richardson, A. (2009) *Dignity in Care*. London: SCIE. Available online at www.scie.org.uk/publications/guides/guide15/files/guide15.pdf; accessed 12 January 2009.

Clark, P.G. (2002) Values and voices in teaching gerontology and geriatrics, *The Gerontologist*, 42: 297–303.

Davies, S. (2003) Creating community: the basis for caring partnerships in nursing homes, in M.R. Nolan, G. Grant, J. Keady and U. Lundh (eds) *Partnerships in Family Care: Understanding the Caregiving Career*. Maidenhead: Open University Press.

Davies, S., Nolan, M.R., Brown, J. and Wilson, F. (1999) *Dignity on the Ward: Promoting Excellence in the Acute Hospital Care of Older People*. Report for Help the Aged/Order of St John's Trust.

Davies, S., Atkinson, L., Aueyard, B. et al. (2007) Changing the culture within care homes for older people, in M.R. Nolan, E. Hanson, G. Grant et al. (eds) *User Participation in Health and Social Care Research: Voices, Values and Evaluation* (pp. 50–68). Maidenhead: Open University Press.

Department of Health (DoH) (2001) *National Service Framework for Older People*. The Stationery Office, London: DoH.

Department of Health (DoH) (2008a) *Darzi Report: High Quality Care for All: Next Stage Review, Final Report*. The Stationery Office, London: DoH.

Department of Health (DoH) (2008b) *Confidence in Caring: A Framework for Best Practice*. The Stationery Office, London: DoH.

Evers, H.K. (1981a) Tender loving care? Patients and nurses in geriatric wards, in L.A Copp (ed.) *Care of the Elderly*. Edinburgh: Churchill Livingstone.

Evers, H.K. (1981b) Multi-disciplinary teams in geriatric wards: myth or reality, *Journal of Advanced Nursing*, 6: 205–14.

Evers, H.K. (1991) Care of the elderly sick in the UK, in S.J. Redfern (ed.) *Nursing Elderly People*. Edinburgh: Churchill Livingstone.

Faulkner, M., Davies, S., Nolan, M.R. et al. (2006) Development of the combined assessment of residential environments (CARE) profiles, *Journal of Advanced Nursing*, 55(6): 664–77.

Felstein, I. (1969) *Later Life: Geriatrics Today and Tomorrow*. London: Routledge & Kegan Paul.

Firth-Cozens, J. and Cornwell, J. (2009) *The Point of Care: Enabling Compassionate Care in Acute Hospital Settings*. London: The King's Fund. Available online at www.kingsfund.org.uk/research/projects/the-point-of-care-improving-patients-experience/compassion/index.html; accessed 19 May 2009.

Goodrich, J. and Cornwell, J. (2008) *Seeing the Person in the Patient: The Point of Care Review*. London: The King's Fund.

Help the Aged (2008) *On Our Own Terms: The Challenge of Assessing Dignity in Care*. London: Help the Aged, Available online at www.policy.helptheaged.org.uk; accessed 15 May 2009.

Institute for the Future of Aging Services (IFAS) (2008) *State Investment in Culture Change Toolkit*. Washington, DC: IFAS. Available online at www.aahsa.org/uploadedFiles/IFAS/quality_improvement/Culture_Change_Toolkit/Culture%20Change%20Tool%20Kit%204.09Final.pdf; accessed 15 May 2009.

Kitson, A. (1987) Raising standards in clinical practice: the fundamental issue of effective nursing care, *Journal of Advanced Nursing*, 12: 321–29.

Kitson, A. (1991) *Therapeutic Nursing in the Hospitalized Elderly*. London: Scutari Press.

MacDonald, C. (2002) Nursing autonomy as relational, *Nursing Ethics*, 9: 194–202.

Nolan, M.R. (1994) Geriatric nursing: An idea whose time has gone: a polemic, *Journal of Advanced Nursing*, 20, 989–96.

Nolan, M.R. (1997) Health and social care: what the future holds for nursing. Keynote address delivered at the Third Royal College of Nursing Older Person European Conference and Exhibition, Harrogate.

Nolan, M.R. and Grant, G. (1989) Addressing the needs of informal carers: a neglected area of nursing practice, *Journal of Advanced Nursing*, 14: 950–61.

Nolan, M.R., Brown, J., Davies, S., Nolan, J. and Keady, J. (2006) The Senses Framework: improving care for older people through a relationship-centred approach, *Getting Research into Practice (GRIP) Series*, No. 2, University of Sheffield.

Nolan, M.R., Davies, S., Brown, J., Keady, J. and Nolan, J. (2002) *Longitudinal Study of the Effectiveness of Educational Preparation to Meet the Needs of Older People and Carers: The AGEIN Project*. London: English National Board.

Nolan, M.R., Davies, S., Brown, J., Keady, J. and Nolan, J. (2004) Beyond person centred care: a new vision for gerontological nursing, *International Journal of Older People Nursing*, 13(3a): 45–53.

Nolan, M.R., Grant, G., Caldock, K., Keady, J., Iphofen, R. and Jones, B. (1994) *Walk a Mile in My Shoes: A Framework for Assessing the Needs of Family Carers*. Bangor: Rapport Productions, in conjunction with the London Provincial Nursing Services and BASE.

Norton, D. (1965) Nursing in geriatrics, *Gerontologia Clinica*, 7: 57–60.

Norton, D., McLaren, R. and Exton-Smith, A.N. (1962) *An Investigation of Geriatric Nursing Problems in Hospital*. London: Churchill Livingstone.

Nursing and Midwifery Council (NMC) (2009) *Guidance for the Care of Older People*. London: Nursing and Midwifery Council. Available online at www.nmc-uk.org/aDisplayDocument.aspx?DocumentID=5593; accessed 8 January 2009.

Parker, V.A. (2008) Connecting relational work and workgroup context in caregiving organizations, *The Journal of Applied Behavioural Science*, 38(3): 276–97.

Pennington, R.E. and Pierce, W.C. (1985) Observations of empathy of nursing home staff: a predictive study, *International Journal of Ageing and Human Development*, 21(4): 281–90.

Reed, J. and Bond, S. (1991) Nurses assessment of elderly patients in hospital, *International Journal of Nursing Studies*, 28: 55–64.

Reed, J. and Robbins, I. (1991) Models of nursing: their relevance to the care of elderly people, *Journal of Advanced Nursing*, 16: 1350–57.

Robinson, G.E. and Gallagher, A. (2008) Culture change impacts quality of life for nursing home residents, *Topics in Clinical Nutrition*, 23(2): 120–30.

Rolland, J.S. (1988) A conceptual model of chronic and life threatening illness and its impact on families, in C.S. Chilman, E.W. Nunnally and F.M. Cox (eds) *Chronic Illness and Disabilities*. Beverly Hills, CA: Sage Publications.

Rolland, J.S. (1994) *Families, Illness and Disability: An Integrative Treatment Model*. New York: Basic Books.

Royal College of Nursing (RCN) (2008) *Defending Dignity – Challenges and Opportunities for Nursing*. London: RCN.

Social Care Institute for Excellence (2006) *Dignity in Care*. London: SCIE.

Szczepura, A., Clay, D., Hyde, J., Nelson, S. and Wild, D. (2008) *Models for Providing Improved Care in Residential Care Homes: A Thematic Literature Review*. University of the West of England: Joseph Rowntree Foundation.

Tresolini, C.P. and the Pew-Fetzer Task Force (1994) *Health Professions Education and Relationship-Centred Care: A Report of the Pew-Fetzer Task Force on Advancing Psychosocial Education*. San Francisco, CA: Pew Health Professions Commission.

Wilkin, D. and Hughes, B. (1986) The elderly and the health services, in C. Phillipson and A. Walker (eds) *Ageing and Policy: A Critical Assessment* (pp. 163–83). Aldershot: Gower.

www.myhomelife.org.uk

Youngson, R. (2007) People-centred health care. Paper preserved at the International symposium on people-centred health care: Reorientating Health Systems in the 21st Century, Tokyo International Forum, 25 November.

Youngson, R. (2008) *Compassion in Healthcare: The Missing Dimension of Healthcare Reform?* London: NHS Confederation. Available online at www.debatepapers.org.uk; accessed 21 May 2009.

Zgola, J.M. (1999) *Care that Works: A Relationship Approach to Persons with Dementia*. New York: Johns Hopkins University Press.

CHAPTER 4

Demographic change and population ageing

Assumpta Ryan

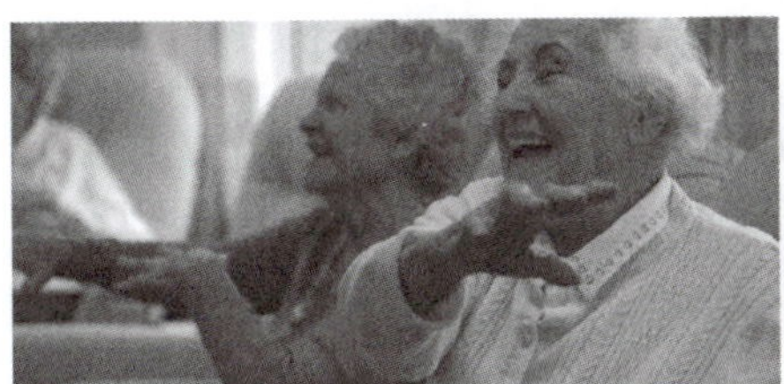
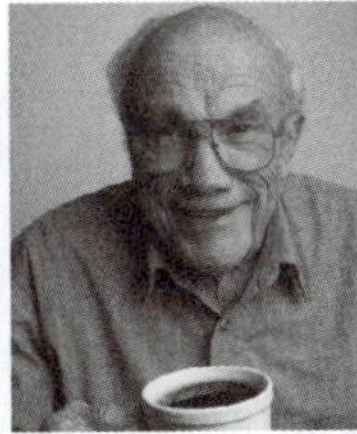
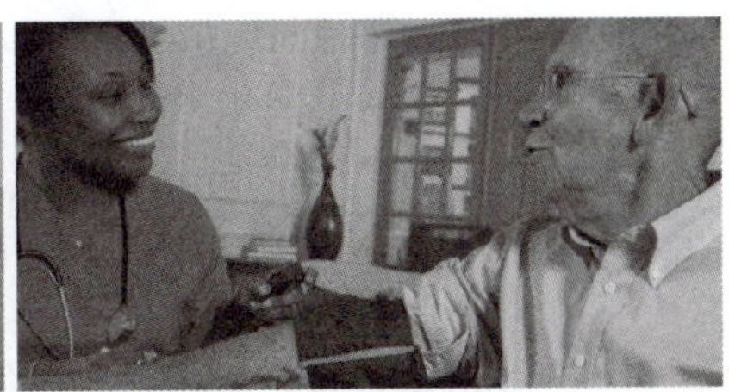

Learning objectives

At the end of this chapter, the reader will be able to:

- understand the causes of global ageing
- describe demographic changes from a national and international perspective
- discuss the significance of changing demographic trends and an ageing population
- analyse the challenges faced by health and social care practitioners as a result of an ageing population
- discuss the importance of ageing in place and social capital for older population groups

Edith commented:

'It's quite nice, being older nowadays – you've got plenty of company, other people going through the same thing. You can share ideas and tricks to get round the system. There's strength in numbers!'

Introduction

This chapter focuses on demographic change and population ageing. It begins with a global perspective on population ageing and moves to a consideration of the European Union (EU) as the region which has the highest proportion of older people. More specific detail is provided on demographic trends in the United Kingdom (UK). The significance of these trends is discussed and the chapter culminates with a discussion of the challenges posed by a rapidly ageing population with a focus on the importance of ageing in place and social capital in the lives of older people.

Background

Demography is the study of the size, growth, age and geographical distribution of human populations, including births, deaths and migrations. The Population Division of the United Nations (UN) has a long tradition of studying population ageing. This includes estimating and projecting the size and characteristics of ageing populations and examining the associated determinants and consequences. The UN has consistently sought to bring population ageing to the attention of governments and the international community (United Nations (UN), 2006) and, in 2007, published a report that highlighted the key indicators and consequences of population ageing. Four major themes emerged:

1 **Population ageing is unprecedented:** Current trends are without parallel in the history of humanity. A population ages when an increase in the proportion of older people (those aged 60 years or over) is accompanied by a reduction in the proportion of children (those under 15 years) and by a decline in the proportion of people of working age (15–59). Worldwide, the number of older people is expected to exceed the number of children for the first time in 2047.
2 **Population ageing is pervasive:** While the focus was originally on ageing in developed regions, population ageing is now almost a worldwide phenomenon. Across the globe, older people are concentrated in rural areas, and such areas are generally characterized by an ageing population (Wenger, 2001). The most significant factors influencing population ageing is a reduction in the fertility rate which has become universal. Because fertility rates are unlikely to rise again to the high levels common in the past, population ageing is irreversible and the young populations that were common until recently are likely to become a rarity over the course of the twenty-first century.
3 **Population ageing is profound:** Population ageing has major consequences for all aspects of human life. From an economic perspective, population ageing will have an impact on economic growth, savings, investment, consumption, labour markets, pensions and taxation. From a social perspective, population ageing influences family composition and living arrangements, housing demands, migration trends, epidemiology and the need for health and social care services. In the political arena, population ageing is likely to influence voting patterns as the 'grey vote' becomes increasing powerful. The impact of mobilizing the 'grey vote' was recently seen in the Republic of Ireland when the government tried to change the automatic entitlement to a state pension in the 2009 budget. The resultant outrage from pensioners and advocacy groups, coupled with street demonstrations and anti-government protests, forced the government to rescind its decision to introduce such a major change.
4 **Population ageing is enduring:** Since 1950, the proportion of older people has been rising steadily, from 8 per cent in 1950 to 11 per cent in 2007 (UN, 2007). It is expected to reach 22 per cent in 2050 (Figure 4.1). As long as old age mortality continues to decline and fertility remains low, the proportion of older people in the population will continue to increase.

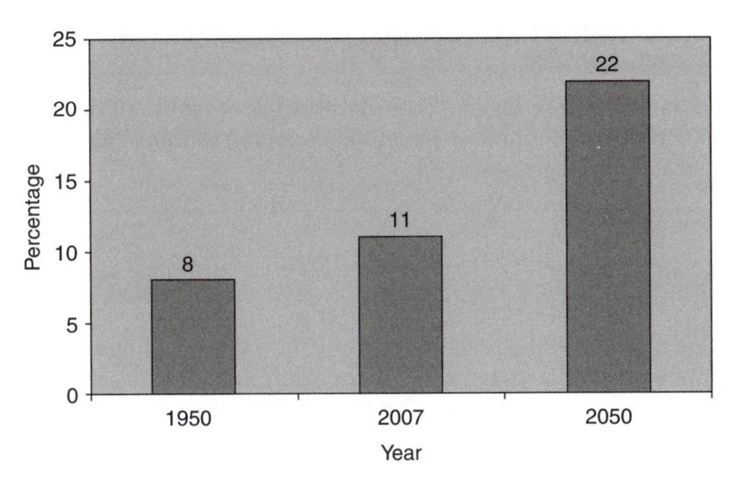

Figure 4.1: Proportion of population 60 years or over: world, 1950–2050
Source: World Population Ageing, United Nations (2007)

Why is the population ageing?

There are two key drivers of population ageing: the decline in fertility rates to below replacement levels and a fall in mortality. The ageing population is also influenced by the approach to retirement of the 'baby boomers' born immediately after the Second World War.

Decline in fertility rates

Fertility decline has been the primary determinant of population ageing. Over the last half century, the total fertility rate decreased globally by almost half, from 5.0 to 2.7 children per woman. Fertility decline in the less-developed regions started later and has progressed faster than in the more developed regions. Over the last 40 years women have been having fewer children; however, in the last decade birth rates have risen slightly. Women in the UK are currently having 1.9 children, the highest figure since 1973, but far lower than 2.93 in 1964.

Rising longevity

As fertility rates move towards lower levels, mortality decline, especially in older ages, assumes an increasingly important role in population ageing. People are living longer through improvements in health, diet, preventative care and technological advances. Not only are more people surviving to old age, but once there, they tend to live longer as the gains in life expectancy are relatively higher at older ages.

The older population is growing at a considerably faster rate than the world's total population. In absolute terms, the number of older people has tripled over the last 50 years and will more than triple again over the next 50 years. The percentage of older people is projected to more than double worldwide over the next half century. Although the highest proportion of older people is found in the more developed regions, this age group is growing considerably more rapidly in the less-developed regions. As a consequence the older population will be increasingly concentrated in less developed regions.

> **Key point**
>
> The older population is growing at a considerably faster rate than the world's total population. The percentage of older people is projected to more than double worldwide over the next half century.

Ageing across Europe

The EU is facing a substantial ageing of its population over coming decades, and demographic ageing is increasingly recognized as an important challenge for policy-makers. In the past, population ageing has often been treated as a 'pensions and care' issue, but there is growing awareness that it is critical for policies related to economic growth, employment and social cohesion.

Fertility has been dropping in the EU for four decades. The total fertility rate for the EU increased from 1.45 children per woman in 1999 to 1.53 in 2000 but still remains low in historical terms (Walker, 2005). At the same time as fertility has declined, life expectancy has increased to about 10 years over the last 50 years.

Europe is currently the world's major area with the highest proportions of older people and it is projected to remain so for at least the next 50 years. Those aged 80 and over currently comprise nearly 4 per cent of the total population of the EU. Over the next 15 years the numbers in this age group will rise by almost 50 per cent (European Commission, 2003). In the four decades since the 1960s, the proportion of people aged 65 and over has risen from 11 per cent to 16 per cent of the EU total population (Walker, 2005). A continuation of this trend is expected and, between 2005 and 2020, the population aged 65 and over will increase by 22 per cent. Growth will be over 30 per cent in Ireland, Luxemburg, the Netherlands and Finland and will be below 20 per cent in Belgium, Spain, Portugal and the UK. Women will continue to outnumber men by a ratio of roughly three to two. Currently, there are fewer than five people in the working ages for every person aged 65 or older in Europe; by 2050 there will be fewer than two.

A UK perspective

Between 2000 and 2020 the relative size of the population aged 65 or older in the UK is projected to increase from 16 per cent to 19.8 per cent. The increase in life expectancy in recent years has been dramatic, particularly for men. Between 1981 and 2002, life expectancy at age 50 increased by four and a half years for men and three years for women. For those aged 65 or older, the extra years of life were three years and two years, respectively. In 2002, women who were aged 65 could expect to live to the age of 84, while men could expect to live to the age of 81. Projections suggest that life expectancies at these older ages will continue to increase in the decades ahead.

In its *Focus on Older People* report, the Office for National Statistics (2005) paints a picture of people aged 50 years and over in the UK today. It includes information on their characteristics, lifestyle and experiences, with particular emphasis on changes associated with age. According to the report, there has been a substantial change in the age composition of older people in the UK over the last 50 years. In 1951, those aged 50–59

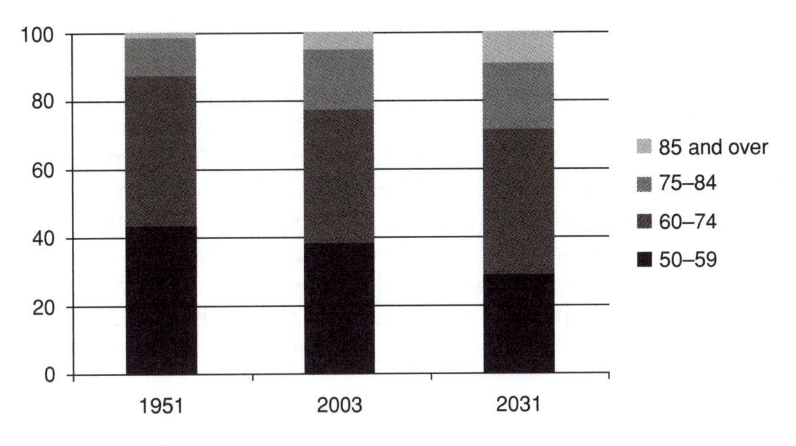

Data for Figure 4.2

	Percentages		
	1951	*2003*	*2031*
50–59	*43.0*	*37.8*	*28.2*
60–74	*44.1*	*39.7*	*43.6*
75–84	*11.2*	*17.0*	*19.1*
85 and over	*1.6*	*5.5*	*9.1*

Figure 4.2: Age composition of the older population (UK) percentages
Source: Office for National Statistics (2005); Government Actuary's Department

represented 43.0 per cent, and those aged 85 and over made up just 1.6 per cent of the 50 and over population. In 2003 the two age groups represented 37.8 per cent and 5.5 per cent, respectively of the older population. Projections indicate these proportions will be respectively 28.2 per cent and 9.1 per cent by 2031 (Figure 4.2).

Older women outnumber older men, as death rates are higher among men than among women. However, the improvement in death rates among older men has led to a narrowing of the gap. There were 77 men in the UK aged 50 and over for every 100 women of the same age group in 1951. The sex ratio increased to 85 men per 100 women in 2003. Projections indicate that the sex ratio will further increase by 2031, when there are expected to be 90 men per 100 women over age 50. The greater number of women than men is most pronounced among the very old, as women tend to live longer than men and as a result of the death of men in World Wars I and II. While in other regions of the world, the difference between the life expectancy of men and women is so great that the concerns of the older population could in fact be viewed primarily as the concerns of *older women*; this does not appear to be the case in the UK.

Living arrangements

Older women are more likely than older men to live alone and the proportion increases with advancing age. Among women aged 75 and over who live in private households in Great Britain, 60 per cent lived alone in 2002 compared with 29 per cent of men of the same age. Widowhood is common among women at older ages: 6 per cent of women aged 50–59 are widowed compared with 79 per cent of those aged 85 and over.

In 2001, 4.5 per cent of people aged 65 and over were resident in communal establishments in Great Britain. This proportion was greatest among people aged 90 years and over. Older women are more likely than older men to live in communal establishments. In 2001, among women aged 75–84, 5.2 per cent were living in communal establishments, compared with 3.2 per cent of men in the same age group. This disparity is a result of gender difference in marital status. Women are more likely than men to be widowed and so be without a spouse to care for them. In addition, at ages over 85, never-married people are even more likely than widowed people to live in a communal establishment. Another important factor is the higher level of disability reported by women than men at any given older age.

Housing

Most older people live in their own homes. However, the proportion of owner-occupied homes decreases with age. Inadequate housing impacts on the quality of life of older people, many of whom are disadvantaged as a result of low income, social isolation, reduced mobility and mental and physical ill health. According to Walker (2005) older people's housing quality is lower in the UK than the European average, especially among the very old, with insufficient heating found in three out of ten older households.

Employment and retirement

Employment is a key determinant of quality of life in old age. It has a direct influence on the amount of pension a person receives and is an important determinant of general economic status. There is no evidence that the absence of employment has a major impact on quality of life in old age, although there is evidence to suggest that compared with other groups in the third age (50–74), those in employment *after* pension age have the highest levels of life satisfaction (Walker, 2005). According to Reichert and Weidekamp-Maicher (2005), the key factors influencing positive well-being in retirement are:

- a positive attitude towards retirement;
- a high degree of satisfaction with achievements in previous employment;
- a transition free from conflicts and entirely voluntary;
- a high level of well-being *before* retirement (optimism, emotional stability and a positive view of old age) which is a predictor of subjective well-being *after* retirement.

According to the Office for National Statistics (2005), over a third of people aged 50–69 in Great Britain who have retired considered that they were forced into retirement. Health problems were the most common reason for those forced to retire before pension age. People in this group were more likely to have no formal qualifications and much less likely to have an income from a private pension, compared with those who retired voluntarily.

Health and well-being

Use of health care services varies, with individuals in older age groups being more likely to seek medical attention. Ill health also rises with age. In 2001, the expected years lived in poor health from age 65 onwards was 4.3 years for men and 5.8 years for women. The proportion of older people with a long-term illness or disability that restricts their daily activities increases with age. Just over a quarter of men and women aged 50–64 in Great Britain reported such a disability compared with two-thirds of men and three-quarters of women aged 85 and over in 2001. The National Dementia Strategy Department of Health (DoH) (2009) reports that around 750 000 people live with a diagnosis of dementia at present, and this is expected to double over the coming 30 years.

Over the last 30 years, there has been a slight rise in the proportion of older people who consulted an NHS GP in the previous two weeks. In 2003, 20 per cent of those aged 65–74 in Great Britain had consulted an NHS GP compared with 14 per cent in 1972. Among those aged 75 and over, the proportion has remained fairly stable at around one in five.

While inequalities in health persist into later life, it is important to note that many people in the older age groups still consider themselves to be in good health, even if they have a long-term illness which restricts their daily activities. In 2001, of all men and women aged 65 and over reporting a limiting long-term illness, just over 10 per cent considered themselves in 'good health' over the year and around 45 per cent reported being in 'fairly good health' (Office for National Statistics, 2005) .

Community care

The majority of older people continue to live in the community well into later life. This has been facilitated by government policy which enables older people to access support services aimed at improving community care provision. Not surprisingly, the volume of home help hours purchased or provided by councils in England has increased significantly over the past two decades. In 1994, 2.2 million hours were provided but this increased to an estimated 3.4 million contact hours in 2004. However, while the overall number of hours has increased, the actual number of households receiving council-funded home care services has fallen, suggesting that councils are providing more intensive services for a smaller number of households.

Family members supply the majority of social care provided in the community. In 2001, over three-quarters (78 per cent) of all older people who reported suffering from mobility problems were helped by their spouse or other household members. As well as receiving informal care, older people are also major providers of care. In 2001, 1.2 million men and 1.6 million women aged 50 and over in England and Wales were providing unpaid care to family members, neighbours or relatives. This represents 16 per cent and 17 per cent of older men and women, respectively.

Family and support networks

It is acknowledged widely that personal relationships are important for well-being and that intergenerational family solidarity is a critical determinant of quality of life in old age (Walker, 2005). There is evidence to suggest that older people living with a partner have better support networks than those who live alone (Victor et al., 2000). On the other hand, older people living alone have more neighbours and friends in their support networks compared to those living with others. Despite the growth of residential separations, research suggests that the levels of social contact between older people and their families remains high (Walker, 1993; Walker and Maltby, 1997).

One of the main themes underpinning a good quality of life as identified by older people themselves is 'having good social relationships with family, friends and neighbours' (Bowling et al., 2002). With greater longevity there is an increasing proportion of families spanning two, three or more generations (Lago, 2000). Nearly everyone in Great Britain has a living parent or child, and many have both. One-third of women born in 1930 still have mothers living when they reach the age of 60. However, major cultural and social changes, especially increased geographical mobility and migration and increased family breakdown mean that intergenerational relationships, roles and expectations are changing. While the role of the family is still central in older people's lives, it differs to that reported in earlier sociological studies (Townsend, 1959).

Scenario 4.1

Elena moved to the UK from Cyprus when she was in her 20s because of the conflict in Cyprus at that time. She and her husband have settled in England but she regards Cyprus as home and returns frequently. Elena's own children live nearby and help her support her husband who has been diagnosed with dementia. However, she misses the support that her sisters would provide. She also finds it hard liaising with services in England as she lacks a lot of confidence in speaking English. The nurse working with Elena and her family has to use a translator to communicate and does not have the same Greek Cypriot background as Elena. Although there is a local Greek Cypriot centre, Elena is embarrassed about her husband's dementia and finds it hard to seek support there.

- *Are there many people in your area who may find it harder to engage with services because of cultural and language differences?*
- *You could find out whether there are any specialist or translator facilities available locally so that you can encourage people to use these.*

Lifestyle

More older people now choose to participate in education and learn new skills including the use of computers and the Internet. In 2002, 51 per cent of those aged 60–69 in England and Wales engaged in some form of learning as opposed to 47 per cent in 1997. In 2002, around three in ten men aged 80 and over and nearly one in five women in England said they owned a mobile phone. Use of mobile phones and the Internet can help older people to remain independent by making it easier for them to communicate with family and friends and to access public and commercial services.

The likelihood of being a member of an organization such as neighbourhood groups falls with age. In 2002, around two-thirds of men and women aged 50–54 in England were a member of an organization, compared with around half of people over 80. Participation in volunteering, cultural and sporting activities also change as people get older. People aged 65–74 have the highest levels of volunteering of all older people. Those in higher age groups are more likely to have health problems or reduced mobility which prevent them from volunteering.

Significance of demographic trends

According to Cowan et al. (2003) current demographic trends raise questions about the future provision of health and social care with a particular focus on reducing morbidity and improving the quality of life and functional independence of older people. Clearly, there is a challenge in identifying *what* type of care provision will be necessary to respond to these demographic changes. Of equal significance are questions pertaining to *who* will provide the care required and moreover *where* this care will be provided.

The ageing population will have major implications for nurses and other health and social care practitioners, the majority of whom currently work with older people. With approximately 50 per cent of hospital beds occupied by older people, hospital-based nurses, with the exception of those specializing in maternity or paediatrics, will invariably find themselves caring for older people. In the community, where over 90 per cent of older people reside, the implications of an increasingly older population will be even greater as nurses and other health and social care practitioners will be providing care for two and perhaps three generations of the same family.

Impact on the family

The health of older people typically deteriorates with increasing age, indicating greater demand for long-term care as the numbers of older people increase. The parent support ratio – that is, the ratio of the population aged 85 or over to that aged 50 to 64 – provides an indication of the level of support families may be able to provide to their older members. Globally, there were fewer than two persons aged 85 or over for every 100 persons aged 50–64 in 1950. Today, the ratio is slightly over 4 per 100 but it is projected to reach 12 per 100 by 2050. That is, persons who are themselves well past middle age will be three times more likely than they are today to be responsible for the care of older relatives. This will have implications for trends in family caregiving as adult children who currently provide care to older relatives will in fact themselves be older and possibly in need of assistance from statutory services.

Older carers

Although caregiving in the main is undertaken by a spouse or adult child, recent research has focused on the needs of older carers (Efraimsson et al., 2001; McGarry and Arthur, 2001). Increasing longevity and demographic changes combined with the emphasis on community care indicate that, in the future, many more older people will be giving and receiving care. Although some older people will be caring for adult siblings, spousal caring is likely to remain the predominant caring relationship. In recognition of the dearth of research in the UK, McGarry and Arthur (2001) carried out a study which examined the experiences of 14 informal carers aged 75 years and over. The results of the study suggested that older carers differed from younger carers in a number of ways. Although they cared for shorter periods of their life, they were more likely to provide care of an intimate nature while having to deal with their own age-related problems. As reported elsewhere, they were also less likely to request or obtain help and perceived caregiving as part of their duty (Brown and Mulley, 1997; Ryan and Scullion, 2000).

There is widespread agreement that family caregiving is primarily a female role (Nolan et al., 1996; Lane et al., 2000; Chambers et al., 2001) and this is equally true for older carers. Twigg and Atkin (1994) described ways in which care provision is modelled on traditional female domestic roles with no comparable provision available to assist with traditional male domestic tasks. From the perspective of older female carers, this deficit can further exacerbate the burden of caring. Additionally, older carers are not perceived as having a social life and consequently receive less support in this area than younger carers (Ryan, 2006). Although the Carers Act (DoH, 1995) gives family carers a right to a separate assessment of their ability to care when a relative's needs are being assessed, this legislation does not appear to have had a major impact on the everyday lives of carers (McGarry and Arthur, 2001).

Loneliness and social isolation

Across the EU, there is a clear trend towards living alone in old age. Older people living alone are at greater risk of experiencing social isolation. A number of factors including demographic variables as well as health, material and social resources are implicated in the loneliness or isolation reported by older people. Vulnerability to loneliness is associated with poor mental health, poor physical health, changes in perceived loneliness compared with the previous decade and time spent alone.

Reduced social contact, being alone, isolation and feelings of loneliness are associated with a reduction in the quality of life of older people (Victor et al., 2000). Increasing numbers of older people, especially older women, now live alone as one partner outlives the other. Living alone, of course, is not synonymous with being lonely, although emerging evidence indicated that there is a clear association (Victor et al., 2000). However, feelings of loneliness can be experienced by those living within larger households such as when a parent moves in with an adult child's family and lives in *their* home or when an older person moves into residential care where any surviving social networks may be disrupted or terminated.

Scenario 4.2

Gladys was widowed 10 years ago and at times likes to be on her own in her own home but at other times she can feel lonely and seeks the company of her children. When Gladys sold her house because she was finding the stairs hard to manage, she moved to live with one of her daughters Mary – an intended temporary stay while she found a more suitable home. Mary's home is very noisy at times, with two young and lively children. Because of her poor hearing, Gladys can find the noise overwhelming at times and increasingly seeks sanctuary in her bedroom and feels rather alone despite being in a busy household. She is in a new part of the country too and has no friends who she can visit easily. For Gladys, it is really hard to find the right balance of being in company and being on her own.

- *How would Gladys be able to find out about social opportunities if she was living in your area?*
- *Are there community-based learning or social groups available?*

Physical and mental health

Future demographic trends suggest that increasing numbers of older people with multiple health needs will place additional demands on health and social care resources (DoH, 2001; Pickering et al., 2001). However, the effects of an ageing population and increasing proportions of older people with complex needs are already evident. There is a well-established association between chronic illness and disability and advanced old age. The most common chronic conditions are lung disease, heart and cardiovascular disease, diabetes, stroke, joint disorders, dementia, depression and impaired vision and hearing. The health complaints that have the strongest impact on daily living, the 'geriatric giants', are mental/cognitive functioning, mobility, balance and stability, vision and hearing and incontinence (Walker, 2005).

Key point

The health complaints that have the strongest impact on daily living are mental/ cognitive functioning, mobility, balance and stability, vision and hearing and incontinence.

Falls are the leading course of injury-related hospitalizations in persons over 65 years and can lead to numerous disabling conditions, extensive hospital stays and death. Approximately 30 per cent of older people experience one or more falls per year and the rate increases with age. Additionally, older people who have suffered a fall are at increased risk of falling again (Lord et al., 2007). Studies on the prevalence of falls have also been conducted in residential facilities, where the reported frequency of falling is considerably higher than among those living in their own homes. A study by Scuffham et al. (2003) found the total cost to the UK government from accidental falls was nearly £1 billion in 1999. The major component was hospital admissions which accounted for nearly half (49.4 per cent) of the total costs. Long-term care costs were the second highest, accounting for 41 per cent primarily in those aged 75 years and over.

The prevalence of dementia increases in old age and places major demands on both paid and unpaid carers, as well as health care systems. For this reason, dementia has been the focus of research and policy initiatives (such as the National Dementia Strategy, DoH 2009). However, it is worth noting that anxiety and depression are also very prevalent in old age and failure to detect and treat both conditions can drastically impact on the quality of life of older persons.

The provision of health and social care services

Older people are the main users of health and social care services and therefore the quality of service provision has a critical bearing on their quality of life. Current UK community care policies focus on supporting individuals who need practical, personal or nursing care so that they may remain in their home environment rather than in hospital or residential settings (Ware et al., 2003). Whereas in the past, older people with such complex needs were cared for in nursing and residential homes, the introduction of the NHS and Community Care Act (DoH, 1990) facilitated such older people to remain at home.

Key point

Older people are the main users of health and social care services and therefore the quality of service provision has a critical bearing on their quality of life.

Changing demographic trends will exert a major influence on the delivery of health and social care to older people in the future. It seems likely that the changes introduced in the Community Care Act (DoH, 1990) will continue to form the basis of future community care provision. However, recent reports about inequalities in resource allocation and the absence of standardized assessment procedures suggest that major changes are required to current service provision (McCann et al., 2005). Despite the limitations of current community care policies, one of the strengths of the present system lies in its recognition of the importance that many older people attach to their homes and communities and the centrality of 'ageing in place' in the lives of these people. Critics may refute these suggestions in their argument that care *in* the community is a contrived policy designed to maximize care *by* the community. While this argument has some support as evidenced by the plethora of studies on family caregiving, it is important that obvious flaws are considered in the context of a policy, which continues to respect the wishes of many older people who want to stay at home.

Although the emphasis on community care is undoubtedly influenced by demographic trends, the extent to which the current model can be maintained is a challenge. This is compounded by factors such as increasing complexity of need, the demand for 24-hour care and recruitment problems in rural areas. Additionally, home help services are easy prey at a time of budgetary problems as cutbacks can often be made in more gradual and less visible ways.

Good community care services are important for older people to be able to live independently in their own homes and prevent deterioration in their quality of life (Walker, 2005). However, The National Service Framework for Older People (DoH, 2001) recognized the lack of consistency in service provision in the UK and the existence of age discrimination in the health and social services. In recent years, social services departments have faced reduced budgets and increasing demands for home care services, resulting in the targeting of services at people with greatest need. An emphasis on meeting high-level need has allowed prevention and rehabilitation work to suffer (Tanner, 2001). However, it is worth noting that older people value the input of low-intensity support services that may enable them to live independently for longer, an option that benefits health and social services as well as older people (Ryan et al., 2009).

Key point

Older people value the input of low-intensity support services that may enable them to live independently for longer.

Domiciliary care provision

Older people have clear opinions on what kind of domiciliary services they need and how these should be delivered to promote quality of life (Raynes et al., 2001). On one hand, they want help with small simple tasks around the home such as replacing light bulbs but they also want rather more fundamental changes at an organizational level. According to Walker (2005), these include: (1) continuity among carers and other services coming into the home to enable them to establish a relationship with service providers; (2) training of care staff to include listening to the older person; (3) adaptations to houses and aids to help promote independence; (4) provision of transport services to facilitate regular contact with friends and relatives and to attend social clubs and other social events; and (5) better health care services.

A recent study by Ryan et al. (2009) revealed that while older people and their families identified areas for improvement, they were generally satisfied with the quality of domiciliary care provision. However, it must be acknowledged that there is considerable research evidence that older people tend not to complain and report high levels of satisfaction with their services (DoH, 2001). The most common difficulties experienced by participants in Ryan et al.'s (2009) study in relation to home care assistants were a lack of continuity and insufficient time.

Ageing in place

'Ageing in place' is a broad term for a policy which recognizes the deep attachments that older people have to their homes. The importance of place has become more recognized with the development of environmental gerontology as a research area. Qualitative studies have investigated the more individual and personal dimensions of place and, in particular, the meaning of home (Reed et al., 1998, 2003). Home, for many older people, is a powerful symbol of autonomy and independence whereas institutions are associated symbolically with the loss of autonomy and independence.

The importance of 'ageing in place' raises concerns about the geographical mobility of older people after their retirement. It is not unusual for retired people, particularly those residing in urban areas, to 'downsize' and move house. Some choose to return to their place of birth, some move closer to adult children and others opt for seaside towns or villages. It would appear that many people make plans for retirement without giving due regard to the consequences of the move should their health fail at some point in the future. The literature on ageing in place appears to question the merits of such decisions. It seems unlikely that older people who are relative newcomers to a community will be in a position to capitalize on the benefits of ageing in place and social capital. While it would be ageist to suggest that older people should not enjoy their lives as they see fit, it is important that such major life decisions are taken with due consideration of all the issues involved.

Andrews et al. (2005) acknowledged that the philosophy of ageing in place recognizes that the movement of older people between care settings and from home to an institutional environment is often to the detriment of their health and against their wishes. However, over half of all the health care beds in the UK are in private nursing homes for older people (Meehan et al., 2002). With demographic trends predicting an increase in the number of older people and a reduction in the number of family carers (Royal Commission on Long Term Care, 1999), it is likely that admission to nursing homes will continue to increase (Ryan, 2003).

Changes in family size and structure and an increasingly migrant population, mean that families often encourage an older relative to relocate close to them so that they can visit on a regular basis. While it is easy to understand why adult children would recommend such a move, it is difficult to reconcile this practice with the importance of ageing in place. While the move may result in closer contact with families, this may be achieved at the expense of contact with friends and neighbours who may not be able to travel to the new location. Geographical distance may not be a concern for car owners but for many older people, visiting a friend or relative outside the locality can be difficult resulting in a loss of contact. This further emphasizes the need for proactive planning and the importance of ensuring that families are fully aware of the literature in this field.

Social capital and older people

The concept of social capital first appeared in 1916 when Lyda Judson Hanifan used the term to describe 'those tangible substances that count for most in the daily lives of people' (1916: 130). Hanifan was concerned particularly with the cultivation of goodwill, fellowship, sympathy and social intercourse among those that 'make up a social unit'. In recent years, the term has been used more widely largely due to the writings of Robert Putnam (2000) in his book *Bowling Alone: The Collapse and Revival of American Community*. Social capital consists of 'the stock of active connections among people: the trust, mutual understanding and shared values and behaviours that bind the members of human networks and communities and make cooperative action possible' (Cohen and Prusak, 2001: 4).

Social capital benefits people by instilling a sense of belonging and establishing relationships of trust and tolerance. No age group relies as much as older people do on the capacity of social connections or community recourse to maintain health and community residence. Gerontological studies of social capital are many and research in gerontology has emphasized the critical importance of network ties and social support in the lives of older people (Kawachi et al., 2008). The informal caregiving literature, for example, has focused on the type; quality and setting of long-term care arrangements, often exploring the impact of kin networks and the implications of gender, age and race for caregiving by adult children.

As older people age in place, they may become more dependent on their community (Kawachi et al., 2008). The type of neighbourhood they live in may influence the extent to which they can take a walk, go shopping or remain engaged in community-based activities. Balfour and Kaplan (2002) found that older adults who lived in neighbourhoods with poorer quality environments (high crime, heavy traffic and excessive noise) experienced a greater risk of functional deterioration. In general, the literature examining the link between individual well-being among people and neighbourhood criminal activity indicated that higher crime rates are associated with community withdrawal, stress and fear of leaving one's home. These conditions may exacerbate an already compromised health state.

Older adults may be more dependent on community level social capital but they may also contribute more to it. Putnam (2000) found that a community with a disproportionate number of older residents was more likely to have an active neighbourhood watch, better social services and, in general, a community more engaged in civic affairs. The literature documenting the positive effects on health of close, personal relationships is extremely convincing with close personal relationships shown to have a positive impact on individual mental health, happiness and physical health (Gold et al., 2002; Halpern, 2008).

The impact of social capital on well-being is indicated by the findings that residential satisfaction is affected more by getting on with your neighbours than by the physical quality of the dwelling (Halpern, 1995). For example, the subjective quality of life of the over 65s has been found to be significantly affected by personal and neighbourhood social capital even after controls have been made for social expectations, personality, health and well-being (Bowling et al., 2002). In contrast socio-economic differences contributed little.

At an individual level, the evidence suggests a strong relationship between social capital and both mental and physical health. In roughly descending order of importance, people who are married, have close friends, go to church or are members of clubs have significantly better health than those who do not. In general, a similar pattern is seen for mental and physical health. Confidence in these results is strengthened by their replication in a large number of longitudinal studies. Individuals with supportive personal relationships are generally less likely to suffer from depression, show less cognitive decline in older age and are several times less likely to die prematurely than the socially isolated.

In principal, the most straightforward way of building up social capital is to go out and invest in it directly. It would seem as if there is nothing to stop us as individuals going out and meeting our neighbours, joining associations, engaging in volunteering and generally being more considerate to one another. However, the evidence on trends suggests that increasingly this is not happening in many countries.

Conclusion

As the twentieth century drew to a close, population ageing and its social and economic consequences were drawing increased attention from policy-makers worldwide. By that time, many countries, especially in the more developed regions, had already achieved population structures older than any ever seen in human history. In most cases, the ageing societies also experienced major economic growth during the second half of the twentieth century. While major shortcomings and unmet needs remained, most developed countries expanded and diversified their systems of social security and health care and, on the whole, the standard of living of older people, as well as the young, improved as populations aged. However, these support systems were strained as the older population increased more rapidly than that of younger adults and as earlier withdrawal for the labour market added to the demands on public pension systems.

The 'maturing' of global societies is a major achievement, with people today living longer and healthier lives than previous generations. This demographic change offers opportunities to harness the experience, expertise and creativity of such a historically large number of older people. There are various options available to both government and private companies to deal with the ageing of Britain's population. The Age and Employment Network (TAEN) argue that the current demographic changes provide great opportunity for businesses. Tapping into a wide pool of talent, experience and skills enables businesses to increase productivity, build competitive advantage and improve the bottom line.

The twenty-first century will witness even more rapid population ageing that we have seen in the past. The challenge for the future is to ensure that people everywhere will be enabled to age with dignity and continue to participate in their societies as citizens with full rights and, moreover, that the reciprocal relationship between generations is nurtured and promoted (UN, 2001).

In summary, this chapter has highlighted that population ageing is unprecedented, pervasive, profound and enduring. This has major consequences for all aspects of human life. Older people are the main users of health and social care services and this trend will increase with rising longevity. However, social capital, if properly harnessed, has the potential to exert a major influence on the mental and physical health of older people. As a result, population ageing is an opportunity for health and social care professionals, particularly nurses, to be at the cutting edge of a demographic change, unparalleled in the history of humanity.

References

Andrews, G.J., Holmes, D., Poland, B., Lehoux, P., Miller, K.L., Pringle, D. and McGilton, K.S. (2005) 'Airplanes are flying nursing homes': geographies in the concepts and locales of gerontological nursing practice, *International Journal of Older People Nursing*, 14(8b): 109–20.

Balfour, J.L. and Kaplan, G.A. (2002) Neighbourhood environment and loss of physical function in older adults: evidence from the Alameda County Study, *American Journal of Epidemiology*, 155: 507–15.

Bowling, A., Gabriel, Z., Banister, D. and Sutton, S. (2002) *Adding Quality to Quantity: Older People's Views on Their Quality of Life and its Enhancement*. Sheffield: Growing Older Programme, University of Sheffield.

Brown, A.R. and Mulley, G.P. (1997) Injuries sustained by caregivers of disabled elderly people, *Age and Ageing*, 26: 21–23.

Chambers, M., Ryan, A.A. and Connor, S.L. (2001) Exploring the emotional support needs and coping strategies of family carers, *Journal of Psychiatric and Metal Health Nursing*, 8(2): 99–106.

Cohen, D. and Prusak, L. (2001) *In Good Company: How Social Capital Makes Organizations Work* (pp. xiii, 214). Boston, MA: Harvard Business School Press.

Cowan, D.T., Fitzpatrick, J.M., Roberts, J.D., While, A.E. and Baldwin, J. (2003) The assessment and management of pain among older people in care homes: current status and future directions, *International Journal of Nursing Studies*, 40: 291–8.

Department of Health (DoH) (1990) *The NHS and Community Care Act*. London: Her Majesty's Stationery Office (HMSO).

Department of Health (DoH) (1995) *Carers' (Recognition and Services) Act*. London: HMSO.

Department of Health (DoH) (2001) *The National Service Framework for Older People*. London: HMSO.

Department of Health (DoH) (2009) *National Dementia Strategy*. London: HMSO.

Efraimsson, E., Hoglund, I. and Sandman, P. (2001) The everlasting trial of strength and patience: transitions in home care nursing as narrated by patients and family members, *Journal of Clinical Nursing*, 10: 813–19.

European Commission (2003) *The Social Situation in the European Union*. Luxembourg: Office for Official Publications of the European Communities.

Gold, R., Kennedy, B., Connell, F. and Kawachi, I. (2002) Teen births, income inequality and social capital: developing an understanding of the causal pathway, *Health and Place*, 8(2): 77–83.

Halpern, D. (2008) *Social Capital*. Cambridge: Polity Press.

Halpern, D.S. (1995) *Mental Health and the Built Environment: More than Bricks and Mortar?* London: Taylor & Francis.

Hanifan, L.J. (1916) The rural school community centre, *Annals of the American Academy of Political and Social Science*, 67: 130–8.

Kawachi, I., Subramanian, S.V. and Kim, D. (2008) *Social Capital and Health*. New York: Springer.

Lago, D. (2000) *Older Women: Key Intergenerational Figures*. Available online at www.agexted.cas.psu.edu/docs/21600477.html (accessed 15 June 2010).

Lane, P., McKenna, H.P., Ryan, A. and Fleming, P. (2000) *Listening to the Voice off Carers. An Exploration of the Health and Social Care Needs and Experiences of Informal Carers of Older People*. Republic of Ireland: South Eastern Health Board.

Lord, S.R., Sherrington, C., Menz, H.B. and Close, J. (2007) *Falls in Older People: Risk Factors and Strategies for Prevention*. Cambridge: University Press.

McCann, S., Ryan, A. and McKenna, H. (2005) The challenges associated with providing community care for people with complex needs in rural areas: a qualitative investigation, *Health and Social Care in the Community*, 13(5): 462–69.

McGarry, J. and Arthur, A. (2001) Informal caring in later life: a qualitative study of the experiences of older carers, *Journal of Advanced Nursing*, 33(2): 182–89.

Meehan, L., Meyer, J. and Winter, J. (2002) Partnership with care homes: a new approach to collaborative working, *NT Research*, 7(5): 348–59.

Nolan, M., Grant, G. and Keady, J. (1996) *Understanding Family Care: A Multidimensional Model of Caring and Coping*. Maidenhead: Open University Press.

Office for National Statistics (2005) *Focus on Older People*. Newport: ONS.

Pickering, G., Deteix, A., Eschalier, A. and Dubray, C. (2001) Impact of pain on recreational activities of nursing home residents, *Aging*, 13(1): 44–48.

Putnam, R.D. (2000) *Bowing Alone: The Collapse and Revival of American Community*. New York: Simon & Schuster.

Raynes, N., Temple, B., Clenister, C. and Coukthard, L. (2001) *Getting Older People's Views on Quality Home Care Services*. York: Joseph Rowntree Foundation.

Reed, J., Payton, V.R. and Bond, S. (1998) The importance of place for older people moving into care homes, *Social Science and Medicine*, 46(7): 859–67.

Reed, J., Cook, G., Sullivan, A. and Burridge, C. (2003) Making a move: care-home residents' experience of relocation, *Ageing and Society*, 23: 225–41.

Reichert, M. and Weidekamp-Maicher, M. (2005) Germany: quality of life in old age, in A. Walker (ed.) *Growing Older in Europe*. (pp. 159–78). Maidenhead: Open University Press.

Royal Commission on Long Term Care (1999) *With Respect to Old age: Long Term Care – Rights and Responsibilities*. London: The Stationery Office.

Ryan, A.A. (2003) Rights, risks and autonomy: a new interpretation of falls in nursing homes, *Quality and Safety in Health Care*, 12: 1–2.

Ryan, A.A. and Scullion, H. (2000) Nursing home placement: an exploration of the experiences of family carers, *Journal of Advanced Nursing*, 32(5): 1187–95.

Ryan, A.A. (2006) *Rural Family Carers' Experiences of the Nursing Home Placement of an Older Relative: A Grounded Theory Approach*. Unpublished PhD thesis, University of Ulster, Faculty of Life and Health Sciences.

Ryan, A.A., McCann, S. and McKenna, H. (2009) Users' perspectives o the impact of community care in enabling older people with complex needs to remain at home, *International Journal of Older People Nursing*, 4: 22–32.

Scuffham, P., Chaplin, S. and Legood, R. (2003) Incidence and costs of unintentional falls in older people in the United Kingdom, *Journal of Epidemiology and Community Health*, 57: 740–4.

Tanner, D. (2001) Sustaining the self in later life: supporting older people in the community, *Ageing and Society*, 21: 255–78.

Townsend, P. (1959) *The Family Life of Old People*. Harmondsworth: Penguin Books.

Twigg, J. and Atkin, K. (1994) *Carers Perceived: Policy and Practice in Informal Care*. Maidenhead: Open University Press.

United Nations (2001) International Strategy for Action on Ageing 2002. Draft text proposed by the Chairman of the Commission for Social Development acting as the preparatory committee for the Second World Assembly in Ageing at its resumed first session, New York, 10–14 December. E/CH.5/2001/PC/Lq. Available online at www.un.org/esa/socdev/ageing/waa/isaale.htm; accessed 18 October 2010.

United Nations (2006) *Population Ageing 2006*. New York: Department of Economic and Social Affairs, Population Division.
United Nations (2007) *World Population Ageing 2007*. New York: Department of Economic and Social Affairs, Population Division.
Victor, C., Scambler, S., Bond, J. and Bowling, A. (2000) Being alone in later life: loneliness, social isolation and living alone, *Reviews in Clinical Gerontology*, 10: 407–17.
Walker, A. (1993) *Age and Attitudes*. Brussels: European Commission.
Walker, A. (ed.) (2005) *Growing Older in Europe*. Maidenhead: Open University Press.
Walker, A. and Maltby, T. (1997) *Ageing Europe*. Maidenhead: Open University Press.
Ware, T., Matosevic, T., Hardy, B., Knapp, M., Kendall, J. and Forder, J. (2003) Commissioning care services for older people in England: the view from care managers, users and carers, *Ageing & Society*, 23: 411–28
Wenger, C.G. (2001) Myths and realities of ageing in rural Britain, *Ageing and Society*, 21: 117–30.

CHAPTER 5

Working together: participation with older people

Christine Brown Wilson

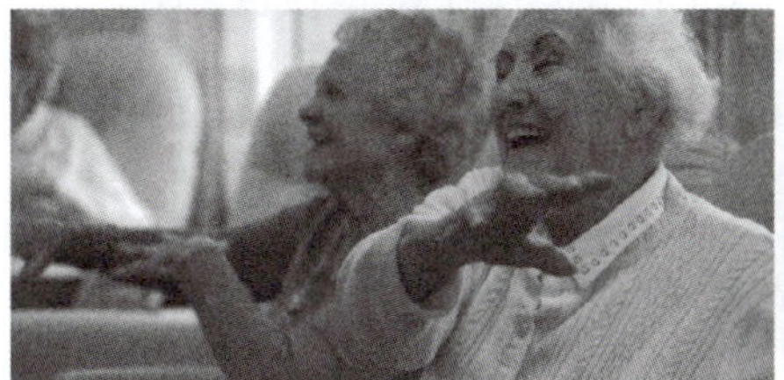 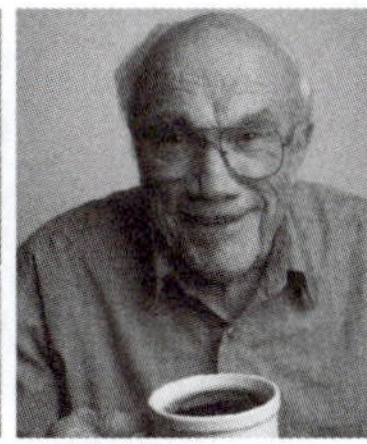 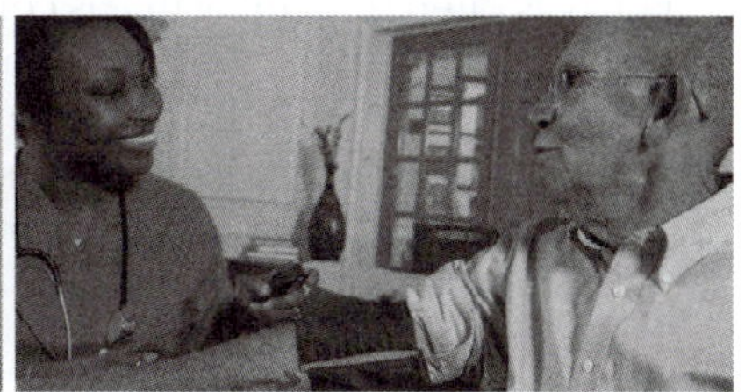

Learning objectives

At the end of this chapter, the reader will be able to:

- explore the implications of health policy in different economic, social and cultural contexts
- discuss the participation of older people in the development of policy and services from the perspective of the older person
- critically examine the practical implications of participation of older people for nursing practice

Making a difference – Commentary by Ros Nesbitt:

'I like to keep active and be involved. I am on the [service user] board for physical disability and learning disability, as I have a disabled daughter. I am not frightened to speak out especially if it is something I feel positive about. They [the local authority representative] are pleased I am not afraid to speak. I must be doing something right as they keep asking me back: now I am on the board for long term conditions.

If we work together, yes we can make a difference and that's what it's all about, making that difference. I can't do it on my own, nobody can but as part of a team, maybe we can make things better for people living here – that's what it's all about.'

Introduction

This chapter explores the goals identified in policies relevant to older people using the framework of Active Ageing. It will consider how nurses might enact the goals identified within polices to promote the health and well-being of older people through the assessment and care process. Strategies for promoting participation by engaging older people in decision-making are presented within a framework that incorporates the perspective of older people, their families and staff. A range of scenarios are explored that provide practical strategies supporting nurses in aligning quality criteria with a more person-centred focus, reflecting the goals of many policies that shape the delivery of health and social care. The chapter concludes with how an older person is participating in the process of health and social care policy to create more responsive services that meet the needs of the community.

Policy is often something that is considered to be distant from the workings of everyday life; something that is enacted by others and not really affecting day-to-day decisions. However, policy decisions intimately influence every aspect of life as they regulate the amount of tax paid and the services received in return. In this way, policy impacts particularly on the quality of life of older people, determining their finances and making decisions that influences their access to health and social care. For example, the type of services provided in a locality and how they are configured often depends on the policy direction. The opening years of the twenty-first century have seen many different types of services developed to support a health and social care system that will meet the demands of a growing older population. The role played by nurses has changed with these services and will continue to do so as the policy direction changes with different political administrations who direct resources for service provision which, in turn, influences decisions made by service providers. Financial constraints have meant that local and central governments often look for services that can be provided at the lowest cost. Working to such financial constraints within health and social care might be interpreted as a competing priority to the provision of quality care.

With a greater focus on the accountability of public services, older people are involved in shaping, assessing and monitoring public services at a local level. As we saw from the opening commentary, older people are also being enabled to work within the policy processes. This process provides opportunities for older people to contribute to their community, making a difference to the lives of others. As older people are the greatest users of health and social services, it makes sense that policy and its implementation are shaped by their perspective. A further impact of health and social care policy is on the quality of the service provided. While this is to be welcomed, there is growing concern that nurses are spending less time involved in direct care as they complete paperwork demonstrating that they meet quality criteria. This has left nurses feeling the tension between two competing priorities; providing care and demonstrating that care has been delivered. This perpetuates the perception that policy is removed from day-to-day practice. Strategies that seek to address this tension are explored throughout this chapter.

Key point

Older people are the greatest users of health and social services so it is important that policy and its implementation are shaped by their perspective.

Background

The number of persons aged 60 rose to 737 million in 2009 (United Nations (UN), 2010), with 35.6 million people living with dementia worldwide (Wimo and Prince, 2010). Over the next decades, the rate of increase for older people, particularly in the older age groups, will be four times faster than the younger population (UN, 2010) with the amount of people living with dementia increasing to 65.7 million by 2030 (Wimo and Prince, 2010). As many countries have invested in health to reduce mortality rates, this now means a high proportion of people are living longer – requiring care and support as they age. The reduced birth rate in many countries also means that there are fewer young people working and paying taxes. This raises concerns as to how services for this growing population of older people will be funded in the future. An additional issue is the feminization of ageing, as older women are living longer than their male counterparts. Few societies recognize the unpaid work of women as carers within family structures, leaving many older women without financial resources in later life. Older women in particular may need additional resources to maintain independence when confronted with ill health and/or disability as they age. Box 5.1 identifies strategies being adopted by different countries to address these issues. There is currently a system in place in the UK where health care is free at point of delivery but social care requires a level of payment. As with all countries, UK policy-makers are now considering issues of long-term economic sustainability in the provision of health and social care for older people.

Box 5.1 Funding principles in different countries

In Europe, health care is provided and resourced according to political principles. For example, Sweden's long-term care system is founded on social democrat principles where care is heavily subsidized and eligibility is judged against an inability to meet needs through social support. Contrastingly, in Asia a co-payment principle exists with health care being paid partly by the individual and their family alongside government subsidy (Chan, 2006). For example, in China a rural co-operative medical scheme is financed jointly between regional government, local government and individuals (Xu et al., 2009).

Key point

Few societies recognize the unpaid work of women as carers within family structures, leaving many older women without financial resources in later life.

Policy is concerned with how the citizens of a country are enabled to live safe, healthy lives and how they are enabled to fulfil what they wish to achieve. It is concerned with the social relations on which well-being is founded and what is required to live a good life. Defining what is meant by a good life will be different across countries and is often influenced by the culture of a country, socially determined and guided by the political values of those who make decisions. The political framework of a country generates policies that promote these values but may also be influenced by pressure groups, both nationally and internationally. From this brief overview of what policy is, we might conclude that it is beneficial to consider policy as a conceptual framework with a specific goal which will be influenced by the cultural context in which people live. This suggests that policies that apply to older people will reflect how ageing is valued within society. Given the increasing numbers of older people, globally, the World Health Organization (WHO) suggests Active Ageing as a means of framing policy within a life course perspective. Active Ageing is an example of a conceptual framework with the goal of promoting health, participation and security for older people globally (WHO, 2002).

Promoting good health through effective policies

When considering the range of demographic data about the health of older people, it can be difficult to make international comparisons. For example, if we compare healthy life expectancy between countries (Box 5.2) we need to interpret figures with caution as data is collected differently around the world. Healthy life expectancy is defined as years spent in good health before death. This suggests that the longer someone remains in good health, the less time they will require supportive services. We can see from Box 5.2 that although people in many countries are living longer, they are living their later years with disabling conditions. This means that many older people will need some level of care and support as they age. As we are seeing higher prevalence rates of chronic conditions in both developing and industrialized countries, policies and resources will need to be deployed differently to meet the health needs of communities. This will have implications for how services are configured and the role nurses play within them.

Box 5.2 Healthy life expectancy between countries from WHO (2009)

There will be key differences between countries, even when on similar continents such as Asia. In India for example, a woman can expect to live to 65 and a man expect to live to 63. However, their healthy life expectancy might only be 56 years. Contrast this to Japan where life expectancy is 79 for men, 86 for woman with 76 years expected to be lived in good health (WHO, 2009). Key differences also exist between and within developed countries such as the United States, Europe and Scandinavian countries, with policies needing to be viewed in the political, social and economic context of each country (Howse, 2007). For example life expectancy in the UK is 81 years for women and 76.6 for men (Office for National Statistics (ONS), 2008). However, after 65 years, women are expected to live for 14.5 years in good health and men for 12.5 years, which means that older people, on average, are living for over 4 years in poor health (ONS, 2008).

Older people have been at the forefront of policy initiatives since the turn of this century. Policies in themselves develop and change according to political priorities and available resources. In considering the breadth of policy initiatives within the UK, three goals appear to underpin the provision of health and social care services for older people:

1 Providing a service that meets the needs of older people, promoting their dignity, independence and choice.

2 Ensuring a quality service that uses standards or benchmarks to protect the public.
3 Developing an efficient and accountable service.

> **Key point**
>
> Older people have been at the forefront of policy initiatives since the turn of this century.

While these goals are clearly relevant to policy, they seem quite removed from practice-based goals of person-centred or relationship-centred care. Research relating to the care of older people often describes the importance of relationships in the delivery of health and social care. This important aspect of practice does not initially appear to fit into the three goals stated above. The difference between practice-based goals and policy-based goals might account for the dissonance some nurses feel between the expectations placed on them in delivering person-centred care and the type of paperwork being asked of them to fulfil quality requirements.

Understanding how relationships influence care

We know from successive policy documents and consultations across the UK that older people wish to remain in their own homes, have choices in their care provision and be treated with dignity and respect. Although older people speak about 'independence' in these documents, they also refer to the importance of reciprocity and mutual exchange in social relationships, specifically with any help received being negotiated to maintain their role as both givers and receivers of care (Godfrey et al., 2004). Older people also have parallel networks of support provided by families, friends and neighbours and these social relationships and networks are integral to their well-being. Social networks also play a crucial role in supporting people with dementia to remain active within their community. Understanding how these relationships might be disrupted or threatened by life changes and the subsequent impact on health and well-being is a crucial aspect when supporting older people.

Older people wish to be involved in different types of social and leisure activities that connect them to people and places with whom they have shared interests (Godfrey et al., 2004). Changes in health can threaten this involvement by creating difficulty in accessing opportunities in the community resulting in loneliness or social isolation (Allen, 2008). People living with dementia are at particular risk of social isolation and need the opportunity to join in with others, but also to be able to meet together with others who also live with the condition. In an attempt to address these needs, peer support networks have been promoted for people with dementia and their supporters. Such networks may take the form of Dementia cafés for example, where people can come together with shared experiences and in the knowledge that the environment is appropriate for people with dementia. We know that a range of factors may adversely influence an older person's mental health and well-being but the importance of relationships and social networks are not always addressed by nurses whose focus may be on physical conditions. Older people often reveal significant information about their lives through stories they share and nurses need to be alert to these clues, as illustrated in Scenario 5.1.

Key point

Older people often reveal significant information about their lives through stories they share and nurses need to be alert to these clues.

Scenario 5.1

One gentleman who had restricted mobility shared stories about his past role as a coach for the local football team. The nurse who heard this story referred this gentleman to the community services, who were able to provide a volunteer to take him to the local club where he was able to get involved in coaching again. Nurses visiting people at home are in a unique position to identify when other services might be approached. On this occasion, a community-based service was able to support this person in maintaining a valued activity within the wider community.

- *How do you learn about the past lives of the older people you are working with?*
- *How could you use this information to enhance their lives now?*

Due to increasing frailty or deterioration of health, there will be a proportion of older people for whom living in the community will no longer be possible. The concept of 'home' is a powerful symbol of autonomy and independence, with care homes often representing a loss of these attributes (Wiles, 2005). In the UK, 4.1 per cent of people aged 75–84 in 2006 lived in a care home, rising to 17.1 per cent for people aged over 85 and we know that nearly one-third of those living with dementia live in residential environments (Department of Health (DoH), 2009). This suggests that older people entering care homes are more likely to have an increasing level of physical and cognitive frailty. Although the frailty of older people in long-term care creates challenges, older people entering care homes actively reconstruct their lives to provide meaning in their new environment, with many actively creating new relationships (Brown Wilson et al., 2009; Cook and Stanley, 2009). Older people and their families in care homes often communicate what is important to them through stories about their lives (Brown Wilson et al., 2009). This information can be used to support older people, including those with dementia to remain part of the community, enjoying activities they have always been involved in. One research study demonstrated how the stories shared by older people and their families could be also be used to continue significant care routines providing a positive experience for the older person, their family and staff (Brown Wilson and Davies, 2009). Therefore, to facilitate the quality of life for older people in care homes, nurses working in these environments must consider how the biography of older people, including those with dementia, might be integrated into personalized routines and meaningful activity.

Acknowledging that older people live active lives, engaging in decision-making that enables them to do so, even in poor health, is the first step for nurses to move from a dependency model to one where older people are active partners in formulating goals of care.

Using relationships to promote shared decision-making

The assessment process undertaken by nurses is a key area where an older person could be involved in decisions that will impact on their quality of life by shaping future care needs. Many environments caring for older people use models based on Activities of Daily Living, each of which are dealt with later in this book. This section provides practical strategies in how these models might be adapted using a biographical approach. A biographical approach to care planning acknowledges that older people have aspirations and goals influenced by their past experiences, relationships and values which can be accommodated within their ongoing care (Clarke et al., 2003). A similar concept is described as person-centred planning, which aims to sustain those activities that are valued, substituting those that can no longer be accomplished (Godfrey et al., 2004).

For older people to be more active in health care decisions, they need information that they are able to interpret that also takes into account their needs and preferences. Nurses are often in a unique relationship with an older person, often hearing stories about their lives and experiences. These stories may reflect goals and aspirations, values and important relationships in the life of the older person. Understanding the relevance of these stories has the potential to support nurses in shaping information that will enable older people to participate more effectively in the decision-making process.

Key point

For older people to be more active in health care decisions, they need information that they are able to interpret that also takes into account their needs and preferences.

A further challenge for nurses lies in finding ways of recording and reporting what might be considered to be anecdotal information to influence the care planning process. For example, when an older person's mobility alters, knowing that gardening was an important feature in their lives would enable rehabilitation to be focused on how this significant activity might be continued or modified. Stories that would enable nurses to shape care in this way are often shared during periods of intimate care, and may be considered 'too insignificant' to report. However, adopting a biographical approach to care planning might support the involvement of older people in decisions, using the stories they share to shape their care. Therefore, nurses have a role in ensuring that all staff recognize the value of these stories, incorporating this anecdotal information into systems of record keeping.

Developing a relationship based approach to quality care

The previous section demonstrated how nurses are involved in the first goal of policy: enabling a service to meet the needs and aspirations of older people. While many nurses might involve older people in developing goals of care in this way, it is often difficult for nurses to describe how this approach to assessment contributes to the second goal of policy: a quality service. This section focuses on a quality framework that enables nurses to articulate how these strategies promote quality of care.

It is outside the scope of this chapter to critique models of quality, but it is probably fair to say that most quality models relevant to older people focus on the measurement of clinical indicators related to activities of daily living. While these clinical quality indicators are necessary to ensure benchmarks are reached, they may also perpetuate a task-focused approach to care, whereas alternate policy drivers appear to direct staff to a person-centred approach. This creates a dilemma in practice environments as quality criteria appear to reward a task-focused approach, with no apparent mechanism to reward a person-centred approach. The previous section outlined the importance of relationships in involving older people in decisions relating to their care. This section proposes a quality improvement model based on relationships developed through the caregiving process.

Promoting relationships in care environments: the PRICE model

The model presented in this section is derived from a secondary analysis of data that explored relationships in care homes (Brown Wilson, 2007). This research captured the views of older people, families and staff and suggested that relationships promoted positive experiences for everyone involved. The type of relationships that could be developed were often dependent upon the approach staff adopted in their care, described as individualized task-centred, person- and relationship-centred. Older people, families and staff often described their experiences and relationships in relation to the caregiving tasks being undertaken. It was these items of data that were mapped to the structure, process and outcome model of quality (Donabedian, 1986) and analysed for statements that described satisfaction with the care being given or received. Initial findings suggest that older people, families and staff are more likely to describe a positive experience of care when they are involved in person- or relationship-centred care, with a less positive experience being expressed when there was a focus on the task. This led to the development of the PRiCE (Promoting Relationships in Care) model (Figure 5.1).

Individualized task-centred care

The PRiCE model (Figure 5.1) suggests that individualized task-centred care is the minimum standard, concerned with meeting care goals in a way that is individual to the resident. Staff adopting this approach described how focusing on a task, such as personal hygiene, enabled them to make sure everything was done and so provide good care. While some staff routinely focused on the task, others described how organizational constraints, such as lack of staff, meant they sometimes adopted this approach. Families and older people shared their experiences of individualized task-centred care, describing this as 'the bottom line'. Families described clinical care being delivered to a minimum standard but raised concerns that their family member might not always receive the care that was required (Scenario 5.2). Older people described the discomfort of having to wait to go to the toilet or the boredom of sitting at the table long before the meal was ready. These examples suggested that individualized task-centred care provided the least positive experience for older people and families. Staff who did not routinely focus on the task also described a poor experience of the day, when organizational constraints meant there was little choice but to adopt this approach.

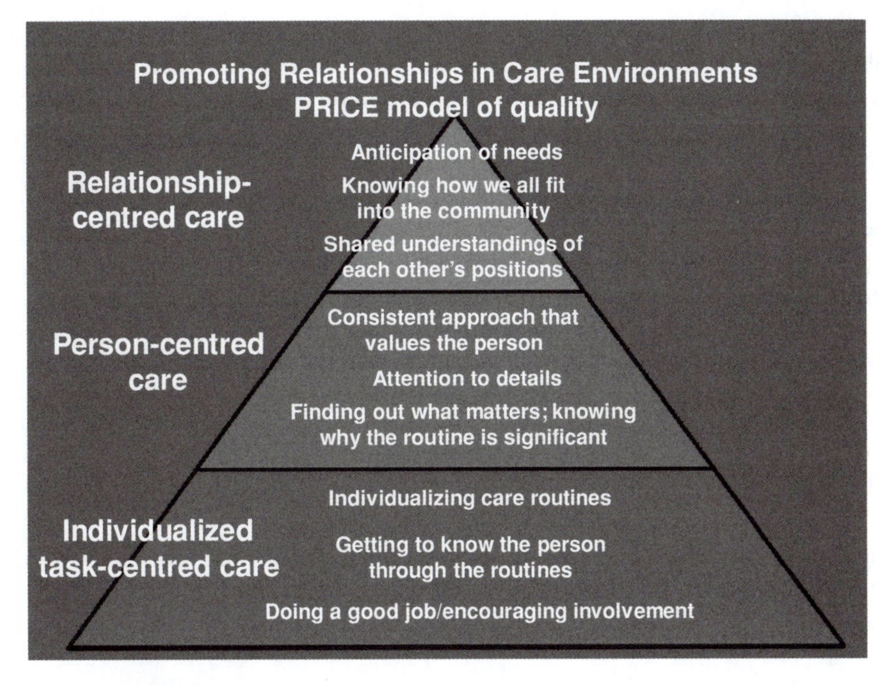

Figure 5.1: The PRiCE Model
Source: Adapted from Brown Wilson (2007)

Scenario 5.2 – the family perspective

One family member asked staff what her husband had eaten as he was unable to recall this information. The staff member replied she had been too busy to notice. When older people are unable to remember what they might have had for dinner or even if they have eaten, families feel concerned that they might not be receiving the care they need. When staff are so busy with ensuring that everybody has eaten, they may be unable to recall specific details when questioned by families. Families then feel they need to come in and check themselves that this care is being delivered.

- *What could the nurse in this situation do in the future to ensure that staff know what an older person has eaten – is it enough and who knows about it?*

Person-centred care

In this approach, the focus was on the person rather than the task. This was achieved by using the stories shared by older people and their families to shape personal care routines. This information was collected through a biographical approach to care planning. Staff would establish the small but significant details that improve a person's care, ensuring the older person and their families felt that staff understood the person and what was important to them. Overall, person-centred care provided a good experience for older people, families and staff. However, the needs of families or staff were not always recognized. Person-centred care sometimes depended on 'who' was on duty and the approach they adopted. While staff were able to adopt a consistent approach to care, when different staff members adopted different approaches, there might not have been the same consistency (as in Scenario 5.3).

Scenario 5.3 – the older person's perspective

Significant details impact on an older person's experience of the day. One lady who lived in residential long-term care believed she lived in a flat and that she was going 'out' to the communal areas. For this reason, it was important that she had her make-up on before she left her room. One day when this make-up had not been applied, she was withdrawn and did not engage in her usual way with others in the community. Two care workers sat beside her and asked if she would like help with her make-up. They helped her apply this and as they left, this lady had been transformed into her usual chatty, engaging self. When I asked the care workers why they did this, they told me how important it was for this older woman to have her make-up on before she came out of her room – without it she had a poor experience of the day.

- *Make a list of all the things that you like to have done each morning before you meet someone. Would an older person feel any differently?*

Relationship-centred care

Staff who adopted a relationship-centred approach acknowledged that everyone (older people, families and other staff) had a contribution to make within the wider community. This meant that the needs of everyone involved in the relationship of care were taken into account. A key aspect of a relationship-centred approach was how care was organized to take into account the needs of each person in context to others who might have competing needs. Not only were the needs of older people taken into account, but also the needs of staff and families. Decisions often took into account the significant details for each older person and what was most important to each individual. As far as possible, care was then directed to attend to each older person in a person-centred way (Scenario 5.4). When this was not possible, staff would involve the older people in the decision-making process according to their abilities. In this way, a decision was reached in how to manage care in the best way for everyone. Staff also considered who might be the 'right' member of staff to support people who might not understand changes to their care routine. This meant that staff needed to be able to work flexibly as a team, supporting each other as well as the people they were caring for. The most positive experiences described by older people, families and staff were from those who experienced or adopted this approach to care.

Scenario 5.4 – the staff perspective

A senior care worker described how he would organize care while considering the significant details for all the older people in the residential environment. For one lady, retaining her continence was exceptionally important and so staff organized their assignments to enable three people to be in the right place at the right time to take this lady to the toilet. Times were negotiated with this resident according to the needs of others in the environment. When staff anticipated her needs and let her know that they knew what was important to her, she was able to relax, knowing that someone would come when they were needed. Staff were able to balance other assignments and families felt secure that staff were working to meet her physical needs but also understood what was important to her as a person, who wished to retain her dignity.

- *Think of someone who you are working with – what do you do to make sure their dignity is maintained?*

In considering these approaches, many nurses will be able to identify how they adopt a person-centred approach. Adopting a person-centred approach is often possible in one-to-one interactions with individual staff choosing to work in this way. The dilemma for quality improvement is how this approach is maintained across all shifts with all staff rather than it being dependent on the person or team on duty at the time. To achieve this, relationship-centred care is necessary where all contributions are valued and care is organized in a way where everyone has their significant details attended to in their care routines. This suggests that person-centred care is also necessary if relationship-centred care is to be delivered. There may be times when person-centred care is preferable; for example, when supporting a person experiencing dementia in a communal environment when they are unable to understand the environmental context in which they find themselves. Person- and relationship-centred care therefore might be considered as aspects of a continuum of care. For example, when staff adopted a relationship-centred approach, they spoke about organizing care in relation to the significant details for individual residents. What made this different from person-centred care was that they were able to see these individual person-centred needs in the context of other residents within the community. Relationship-centred care, therefore, moves beyond the focus of the individual person to consider the needs of everyone within the community. Staff who adopted a relationship-centred approach were more aware of the contribution older people wished to make in the wider community. These members of staff were aware of relationships between residents and how older people liked to spend their time. Often older people require support from staff to enact their contribution or make choices and staff who adopted a relationship-centred approach recognized this. This meant residents were supported in undertaking everyday activities such as visiting people who were unwell, sitting beside friends, giving out mail or folding linen. This enabled reciprocal relationships between older people, families and staff to be developed (Brown Wilson et al., 2009). Considering how to create person- and relationship-centred care routines provides staff with a starting point in how to achieve relationship-centred care and so improve the experience of older people and their families.

Documenting relationship-based approaches to care

For nurses, the next systematic step in the quality process lies in capturing information that can describe how care is delivered. The examples provided for each approach to care reflect what is generally regarded as everyday interaction, or described as 'the way we do things'. For example, in considering meal times from an individualized task-focused approach, we might document that a person ate well and if they enjoyed their meal; that they liked certain foods and disliked others. If we wanted to document a more person-centred approach, we might document if it was important for someone to eat a certain way, or that they were used to eating certain foods in their lives and how this influenced how they approached their meals now. It would also include how their current health status was impacting on their intake and what was being done to address this (Scenario 5.5). To document a relationship-centred approach, we might include how assistance for each meal was negotiated and the impact this style of eating had on not only the physical intake of the person but also the social interaction with fellow diners and staff. Documenting the support for both the older person and other diners in this situation would be important. Documentation might also include discussions with families.

Scenario 5.5

Jack is a fiercely independent man and does not like to wear a clothing protector during meals – when staff put this on, he often removes it before his meal arrives. He often likes to feed himself but his manual dexterity has been affected by his stroke. Staff keep an eye on Jack to see how he is managing each meal and then offer to help. He will either accept or decline this offer. When he completes his meal independently, he requires a change of clothing which staff attend to after they have supported some of the more frail older people back to bed for an afternoon rest.

- *Can you identify a situation in your area where different staff have different views on how to manage a situation?*
- *How do you try to resolve these differences?*
- *How to you decide on care that respects an older person's wishes even when not all staff are in agreement?*

This section provides a starting point for nurses to think about how they might use the quality models they work with to demonstrate a relationship-centred approach when supporting older people. This approach supports older people in becoming involved in decisions that affect their day-to-day care even when they require support to enact these decisions. The following section considers the third goal of policy: creating an efficient and accountable service. The focus in the following section considers how older people might participate in shaping services to meet the needs of the wider community.

Shaping policy: the older person's perspective

A common thread throughout this chapter has been the involvement of older people in shaping their care. Older people who experience ill health or disability with health conditions describe themselves as working at staying well, with many seeking to adapt their lives in ways that could bring them continued meaning and pleasure (Allen, 2008; Godfrey et al., 2004). This means that older people may perceive health and social care services as a means of supporting these goals and aspirations. Unfortunately, for many older people, services do not always meet these aspirations, focusing on a professional definition of needs. To address this, there is now a requirement for local authorities to involve service users at all levels of decision-making in the policy process. This concluding section presents the experience of an older person in this process and suggests strategies that enable older people to shape the policies affecting their care.

> **Key point**
>
> Older people who experience ill health or disability with health conditions describe themselves as working at staying well, with many seeking to adapt their lives in ways that could bring them continued meaning and pleasure.

Successive older generations will have differing expectations of services, be better informed about potential health interventions and more inclined to demand their rights. This is particularly relevant in Western administrations where the ageing 'baby boomer' generation present a very different lifestyle to previous generations asking new and different questions of policy-makers. Politicians and clinicians recognize that although they are developing new policies for their ageing populations, current policies should only be considered a stopgap (Phillips and Chan, 2002). The concept of active ageing implies that older people continue to be active throughout their lives, making decisions as they age in how to adapt, grow and develop even in the face of concomitant losses. This section draws on the experience of one older person, Ros, who experiences a number of health challenges resulting in restricted mobility and periods of being acutely unwell. However, Ros maintains her involvement in a number of local user groups and it is this experience which is drawn on for this final section.

Public participation has been developed within the UK to ensure improved quality of services while devolving responsibility for their provision to local government bodies. One way successive governments have sought to achieve this is by public consultation; asking those who use the services (in this case, older people) what they feel should be part of the services being provided. In responding to these exercises, there are underpinning themes of independence, dignity and choice in current UK policy. This approach could be described as a consumerist approach – asking older people's views on a service as consumers. While consultation is an important part of the policy process, this approach alone does not enable older people to influence decision-making (Carter and Beresford, 2000). Ros describes her experience of this approach:

> “ a group of us were asked to go the new hospital. I was there to look at mobility issues, there was also a woman who was blind. They took us around and the corridors were so narrow. It is a long way for people to walk and there are no chairs if people get part way and need a rest. I can't see how they will have the space to do that, but that's what they need. It will cost too much for them to change it now. They took me in a wheelchair they had to pull and I was going backwards, you can only see where you need to go once you've passed it. It lacks dignity. ”

In this situation, service users were asked for their opinions after the event, rather than shaping the process. This raises the question of whether the consultation is effective or if, in Ros's words, it is simply a 'tick-box exercise'. In situations such as this, Ros feels that services 'are not listening', which can be frustrating. This is in contrast to the experience Ros has had on a local authority user group board where she is able to address disability issues with those who run the services. On this board, she has requested that information on accessible transport be made available to people with disabilities coming into the city:

> “I asked her [the service provider] what she has done about it since the last meeting and she hadn't done anything. It is quite simple to do. I let it go this time, but I told her that I expected something to be done by the next meeting and I will make sure it is.”

This is an example of a democratic approach (Carter and Beresford, 2000) addressing issues of power by enabling older people to bring services to account for their actions. Older people have often been marginalized from this process due to issues of age, disability, gender or the demands of the political system (Barnes, 2005). Ros describes herself as 'feisty' and not intimidated by people in positions of power, putting this down to her experience as a nurse. However, there may be people who require support to develop personal confidence or assertiveness. This suggests that not only do older people need a forum giving them the power to make decisions but also support that enables them to act effectively within that forum.

Enabling participation

Older people need support to become involved in areas described by Ros. This includes physical access to the environment, access into organizations responsible for policy and practice and support to be able to influence their decisions. Social and psychological factors are often influenced by an older person's life experiences and these need to be taken into account if older people are to be supported to have meaningful roles. Ros became involved in influencing policy following a meeting with her care manager, where she shared stories about what she had done with her life. These stories demonstrated that Ros was an active person and this conversation led the case manager to ensure Ros was invited to a public meeting to become involved as a service user representative. As a retired nurse Ros retained an interest in health issues and has been invited to work on the long-term care physical disabilities board. As part of her involvement she has been asked to give an opening address at a local involvement network meeting for service professionals and volunteers. She found this very daunting but this showed her how she had developed her skills through her involvement in these activities.

Policies and programmes for involvement of older people need to be respectful of their views and aspirations (Barnes, 2005). Ros described factors she feels are necessary in the day-to-day work of service user groups:

- Group cohesion – having a common goal to work towards.
- Supportive and enabling leaders that provide a conduit between the group and the more formal policy mechanisms.
- Working as a team – local authority responsiveness to the concerns raised by the group.

Crucial too is that older people receive feedback on their suggestions and a report of actions taken in the light of their comments.

Ageing has historically been considered as a period of decline, with biological, social and psychological models of ageing presenting either a fatalistic view of decline or an overly optimistic view of positive ageing. While there is evidence to suggest that many people are living longer and in better health than previous generations, older people still tend to have more disabling conditions due to either co-morbidities or increasing frailty. Older people such as Ros often refute the perception of ageing as a period of decline, seeing opportunities for further growth and development. While Ros recognizes that she has a disabling chronic condition, she also sees herself in good health, able to manage all her activities that give her life meaning. This might not be the case for all older people but there is growing evidence to suggest that how older people perceive their health might be influenced by how they have approached their life previously (Godfrey et al., 2004). Therefore, understanding how people have grown and developed throughout their lives is becoming increasingly important if we are to support older people in maintaining their health, supporting them to fulfil their aspirations and goals in life.

Conclusion

A key driver within polices has been to provide person-centred services that meet the needs and aspirations of older people. This chapter began by describing the goals underpinning policies relating to the care and support of older people. The goals of efficiency and quality may at times focus on the task of care, which is in direct contrast to a person-centred approach. This situation can create dissonance for nurses as they strive to meet what may be perceived as competing priorities. This chapter has presented strategies to support nurses in articulating how they address each policy priority through day-to-day care practice. Strategies such as listening and responding to the stories older people and their families share provide a starting point for nurses to support older people in decision-making. This strategy supports a biographical approach to assessment and care planning, which enables nurses to share this information in more formal settings such as multidisciplinary team meetings. Sharing the views of older people and their families with other professionals will ensure that the needs and aspirations of the older person are met. Working in this way supports the positive experience of older people, families and staff contributing towards quality care. Using the quality framework described within this chapter will support nurses in articulating their practice to demonstrate the quality of care they deliver.

Acknowledgement

I wish to extend my thanks to Ros Nesbitt who took time out from her other activities to share her story. She has asked that we use her real name.

References

Allen, J. (2008) *Older People and Well Being*, Institute for Public Policy Research. Available online at www.ippr.org.uk/publicationsandreports/publication.asp?id=620; accessed 8 April 2009.

Barnes, M. (2005) The same old process? Older people, participation and deliberation, *Ageing and Society*, 25: 245–59.

Brown Wilson, C.R. (2007) Exploring relationships in care homes: a constructivist inquiry. Unpublished PhD dissertation, University of Sheffield.

Brown Wilson, C. and Davies, S. (2009) Using relationships in care homes to develop relationship centred care – the contribution of staff, *Journal of Clinical Nursing*, 18: 1746–55.

Brown Wilson, C., Davies, S. and Nolan, M.R. (2009) Developing relationships in care homes – the contribution of staff, residents and families, *Ageing and Society*, 29: 1–23.

Carter, T. and Beresford, P. (2000) *Age and Change: Models of Involvement for Older People*. Joseph Rowntree Foundation (JRF). Available online at www.jrf.org.uk/sites/files/jrf/1859353215.pdf; accessed 10 January 2010.

Chan, A. (2006) Ageing in Southeast and East Asia: issues and policy directions, *Journal of Cross-cultural Gerontology*, 20: 269–84.

Clarke, A., Hanson, E.J. and Ross, H. (2003) Seeing the person behind the patient: enhancing the care of older people using a biographical approach, *Journal of Clinical Nursing*, 12: 697–706.

Cook, G. and Stanley, D. (2009) Quality of life in care homes: messages from the voices of older people, *Journal of Care Services Management*, 3(4): 1–23.

Department of Health (DoH) (2009) *Living Well with Dementia: National Dementia Strategy*. London: DoH.

Donabedian, A. (1986) Criteria and standards for quality assessment and monitoring, *Quality Review Bulletin*, 12: 99–108.

Godfrey, M., Townsend, J. and Denby, T. (2004) *Building a Good Life for Older People in Local Communities: The Experience of Ageing in Time and Place*. Joseph Rowntree Foundation. Available online at www.jrf.org.uk/bookshop/; accessed 21 May 2006.

Howse, K. (2007) Long term care policy: the difficulties of taking a global view, *Ageing Hoizons*, 6: 1–11. Available online at www.ageing.ox.ac.uk/system/files/Ageing%20Horizons%206%20Howse.pdf; accessed 29 January 11.

Office for National Statistics (ONS) (2008) *Social Trends* (No. 38). Basingstoke: Palgrave Macmillan.

Phillips, D.R. and Chan A.C.M. (2002) (eds) National policies on ageing and long-term care in the Asia-Pacific issues and challenge in Ageing and Long-term Care (ch. 1). National Policies in the Asia-Pacific. Available online at www.idrc.ca/fr/ev-28466-201-1-DO_TOPIC.html; accessed 20 June 2009.

United Nations (UN) (2010) *Department of Economic and Social Affairs: World Population Ageing*. Available online at www.un.org/esa/population/publications/WPA2009/WPA2009-report.pdf; accessed 21 January 2011.

Wiles, J. (2005) Conceptualising place in the care of older people: the contribution of geographical gerontology, *International Journal of Older People Nursing,* in association with *Journal of Clinical Nursing*, 14(8b): 100–108.

Wimo, A. and Prince, M. (2010) *Alzheimer's Disease International World Alzheimer Report 2010: The Global Economic Impact of Dementia*. Available online at www.alz.co.uk/research/worldreport/; accessed 30 September 2010.

World Health Organization (WHO) (2002) *Active Ageing: a Policy Framework*. Available online at www.whqlibdoc.who.int/hq/2002/WHO_NMH_NPH_02.8.pdf; accessed 23 June 2009.

World Health Organization (WHO) (2009) *World Health Statistics 2009*. Available online at www.who.int/whosis/whostat/EN_WHS09_Full.pdf; accessed 21 June 2009.

Xu, K., Saksena, P., Huang Fu, X., Lei, H., Chen., N., and Carrin, G. (2009) *Health Care Financing in Rural China: New Rural Cooperative Medical Scheme* (No. 3). Technical briefs for policy-makers. Available online at www.who.int/health_financing/documents/pb_e_09_03-china_nrcms.pdf; accessed 10 January 2010.

PART 2

Key issues in nursing older people

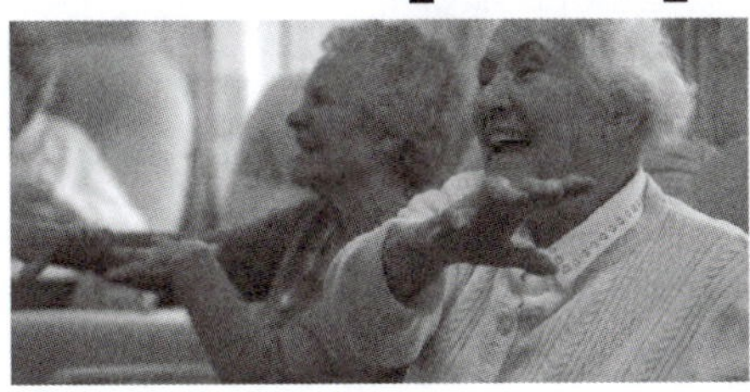
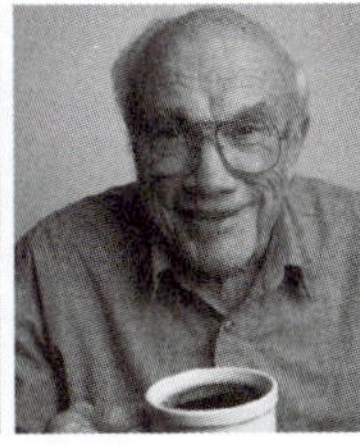
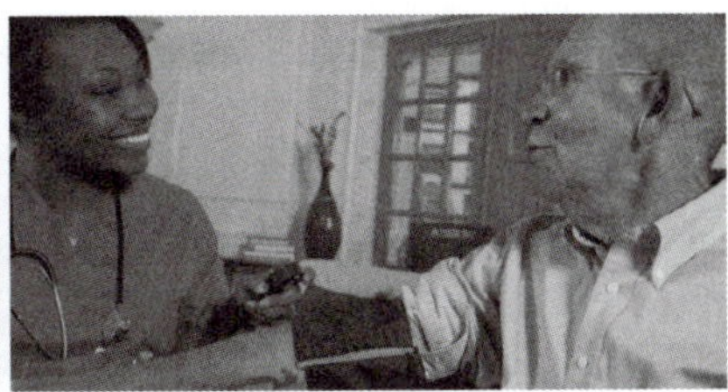

Chapter contents

CHAPTER 6

Fundamentals of nursing

Charlotte L. Clarke

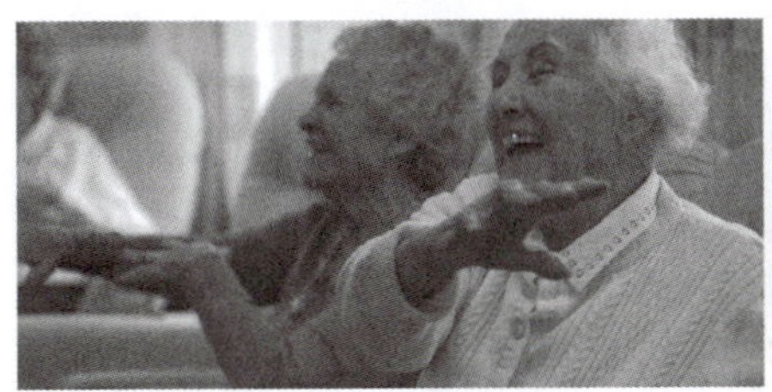 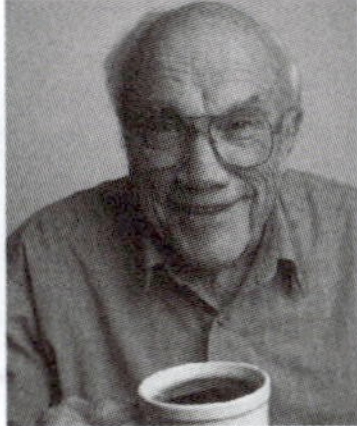 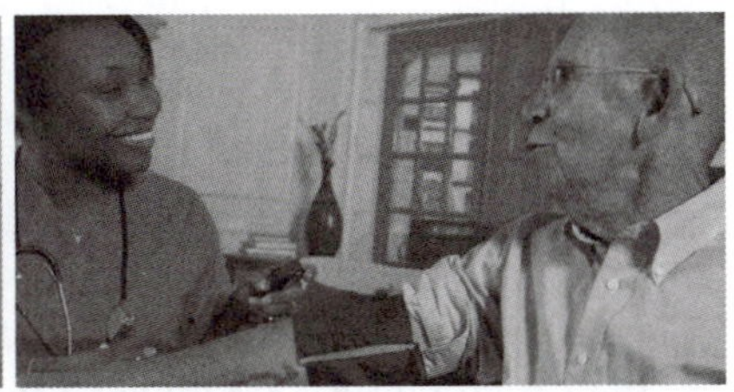

Learning objectives

At the end of this chapter, the reader will be able to:

- describe the holistic nature of nursing practice for older people, with attention required to the full social context and strategies for maintaining well-being
- identify the importance of sustaining the independence of older people and augmenting existing strategies of self-management
- critique the subtle but essential ways in which care is provided for older people in maintaining choice and dignity
- identify the role of nurses in assessing, planning, intervening and evaluating in partnership with an older person

Jack lives with dementia and in conversation with a researcher reflected on the way staff relate to him:

'They're inclined to be a little bit fussy in the centre that I go to. If somebody doesn't stick to the path sort of thing. I mean with the best of intentions, they are anxious that you don't do anything by which you'll injure yourself. When I first went there I was a bit piqued because I didn't think I was that bad... – So what kind of things do they discourage you from doing there? – Well stepping out of the building. I wanted to get some fresh air. Anyway, they found somewhere I could sit, which solved that problem. ... oh they're very exact about the way I walk, the way I use my walker because I'm inclined to cross my hands or something silly like that or just put it one-handed and they stop me doing that but they do it in the best, in a good humoured way.'

Introduction

This chapter seeks to bring together some of the many issues raised in this first section of the book and explore the ways in which nurses can plan and implement care. Fundamental to this process of nursing is that there is an effective identification of the needs of the older person which is conducted in partnership with them so that goals of care are mutually agreed.

Background

The Nursing and Midwifery Council in the UK (NMC, 2009) state that there are three main elements to providing care to older people:

- **People** – requiring nurses who are efficient and able to deliver safe, effective, quality care. This requires nurses to be competent, assertive, reliable and dependable, empathetic, compassionate and kind.
- **Processes** – delivering quality care which promotes dignity by nurturing the older person's self-respect and self-worth. This is achieved through communicating with older people and listening to what they say, assessment of need, respect for privacy and dignity, partnership working with older people, families and colleagues.
- **Place** – attending to the diverse environments in which older people receive nursing care (be it in the community or hospital) and ensuring a commitment to equality and diversity, that it is appropriate, adequately resourced and effectively managed.

Achieving these elements is underpinned by an approach to people that conveys 'care', and that means being able to communicate effectively. I am struck, and moved, by the notion that nurses can 'do' things but may do so with or without 'care'. For example, words spoken without care fail to communicate and indeed may even be harmful. Does this notion of 'with' or 'without' care apply to all of the other areas of practice? Would continence management be compromised if it was 'without care'? How do older people experience 'care' and what effect is there if they receive interventions and words 'without care'?

We can 'do' nursing by identifying deficits as peoples' needs. However, perhaps we should instead be providing care by identifying peoples' strengths and unmet needs, in a way that offers a more genuine approach to caring. Spilsbury and Meyer (2001) argue that it may never be possible to define the contribution of nursing to patient care since it is ever changing. However, perhaps this notion of 'care' seems to be something that adds value to the actions and words that form the behaviours of practice.

Nursing 'with' care is very much more demanding than 'without' care – involving an emotional labour of care. But this is where the nursing of older people can be such a great privilege. To be working with people who have such a lifetime of knowledge and experiences, and who are now perhaps at their most vulnerable in their adult lives, is both rewarding and challenging. So long as we allow ourselves to get to know people.

Key point

Nursing 'with' care is very much more demanding than 'without' care – involving an emotional labour of care.

The need for an intimate knowledge of the person's life story is being increasingly recognized as necessary in providing effective support for older people (Crisp, 1999; Keady and Gilleard, 1999). This is the personal knowledge, known by family carers and older people themselves, but which is of limited availability to professional carers (Clarke and Heyman, 1998). Without access to this knowledge, our awareness of the older person is restricted and our ability to allow their biography to inform present intervention and future planning is consequently limited. So it is important to make the time to get to know the older people who you are nursing – this is not an 'added extra' to nursing work but is fundamental to ensuring that good quality care is provided that respects the individual person and their strengths.

Needs, resource and nursing processes

Some of the essential issues concerning the nursing care of older people have been mapped out in the previous chapters of this book. Largely, these are based on the following three goals:

- Autonomy in which older people are enabled to be able to make decisions and manage their own life, albeit with the assistance of others at times.
- Choice and personalization in which there is an emphasis on people being able to co-ordinate their own support to be able to live independently and to continue to be active participants in their community.
- Dignity in which staff, families and others demonstrate a person's self-worth by showing respect, maintaining privacy and promoting autonomy.

In the following section, the ways in which these principles underpin nursing practice are explored in relation to various aspects of caring for older people – mobility, elimination, sexuality, and so on. The need for attention to nursing practice cannot be underestimated. Here are some key facts drawn from chapters in this section:

- 71 per cent of people aged 65 and over have a longstanding illness, mostly musculoskeletal problems, heart and circulatory diseases diabetes, arthritis and emotional/anxiety related problems (English Longitudinal Study of Ageing (ELSA), 2002; Health Survey for England (HSE), 2004, 2005).
- 42 per cent of men and 46 per cent of women report that their illness limits their activities in some way (ELSA, 2002; HSE, 2004, 2005).
- More than three million people in the UK are malnourished or at risk of malnutrition (BAPEN, 2009).

So there are some very real problems that people face as they age and for which they may turn to nurses for care and advice about. Miller (2004) emphasizes that typically an older person has a combination of chronic conditions and that the manifestations of ill health in older people are likely to be more subtle and less predictable than in younger adults (an acute infection is more likely to cause an acute confusional state in older adults for example). Moreover, the consequences of ill health are likely to have a greater impact on older people, with a longer period of recovery and possible longer-term legacies such as an ongoing fear of falling following a fall and fracture which limits the extent to which the older person wishes to leave their own home. All of these factors make nursing older people both very challenging and rewarding. Miller (2004) describes assessment processes as needing to be 'detective-like' and addressing the full complexity of an older person's situation.

But there are also some more 'iatrogenic' problems that older people have to navigate – problems that come about as a consequence of the attitudes and beliefs of society, members of the public and health and social care staff such as nurses. The effects of dynamics and prejudices such as ageism, explored in the earlier section of this book, have a very significant effect on older people, and Steven et al., Chapter 13 (p. 206) write that:

> “ The notion that risks and safety issues escalate in later life permeates most of lay and professional thinking. This may be compounded by frequent reports in the press which relate to elder abuse or the poor care of older people with an underlying ageist ethos. The majority of older people negotiate later life uneventfully and take a measured approach to their own management of risk and safety awareness. ”

As Steven and Steven say, most older people take into their later years a lifetime of learning about themselves, their strengths and weaknesses and the strategies they use for getting through life. It is foolish for us as nurses to underestimate this, and certainly detrimental to the welfare of older people. We should not judge people's needs, their risks and safety on the fact that they are of a certain age alone.

A nursing process with older people

As nurses, we need to assess what older people's actual needs are and what their resources are for managing this themselves, identify any shortfall of resource and then plan and evaluate how these needs may be met. In nursing, we go through a process of decision-making and action which assesses need, plans and implements actions and may (or may not) undertake an evaluation (see Figure 6.1).

What we need to do more explicitly is assess the resources of older people themselves and jointly plan care (as in Figure 6.2). As a result, we may make an assumption that they need to hand over their care to staff rather than retain as much self-management (and so dignity) as they choose.

We must not underestimate the resource base that older people have. This will have many aspects to it: financial, social (family and community), psychological coping strategies, and so on. It is also a part of people's lives that can have an enormous impact on their well-being. There is now a growing recognition of the importance of social participation, social networks and social support and their role is vital for successful ageing and active ageing. Indeed, there is an increasing recognition that social factors such as these are

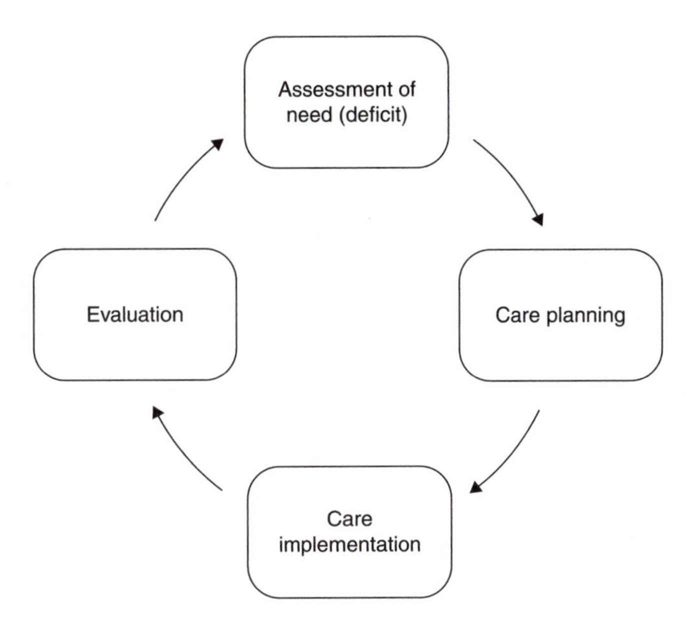

Figure 6.1: Traditional view of the nursing process – emphasizing need (deficit), care and dependency

important in the development of issues such as physical disability, cognitive function, depression and chronic disease including cardiovascular disease in the older population. For example, the National Dementia Strategy (DoH, 2009) promotes the use of peer support networks. As such, social factors may have a large protective influence on the course of ill-health for an older person – and if we weaken such factors through our care then we may exacerbate someone's ill-health.

Key point

Nurses must not underestimate the resource base that older people have.

In considering the resources that an older person has, and the strategies used to allow these resources to influence their health and well-being, it may be useful to draw on the work of Baltes and Baltes (1990). They propose a resource model with three aspects:

1 **Selection** – an older person will actively or passively reduce the number of goals and activities they engage with in order to focus on those that are most meaningful to them.
2 **Compensation** – an older person will develop new or alternative ways of achieving goals and activities when functional changes mean these cannot be achieved by the former ways.
3 **Optimization** – an older person will enhance and refine the means of maximizing resources (perhaps disinvesting time and energy on things that can be functionally achieved but which detract from having time and energy to do the activities selected as being most important).

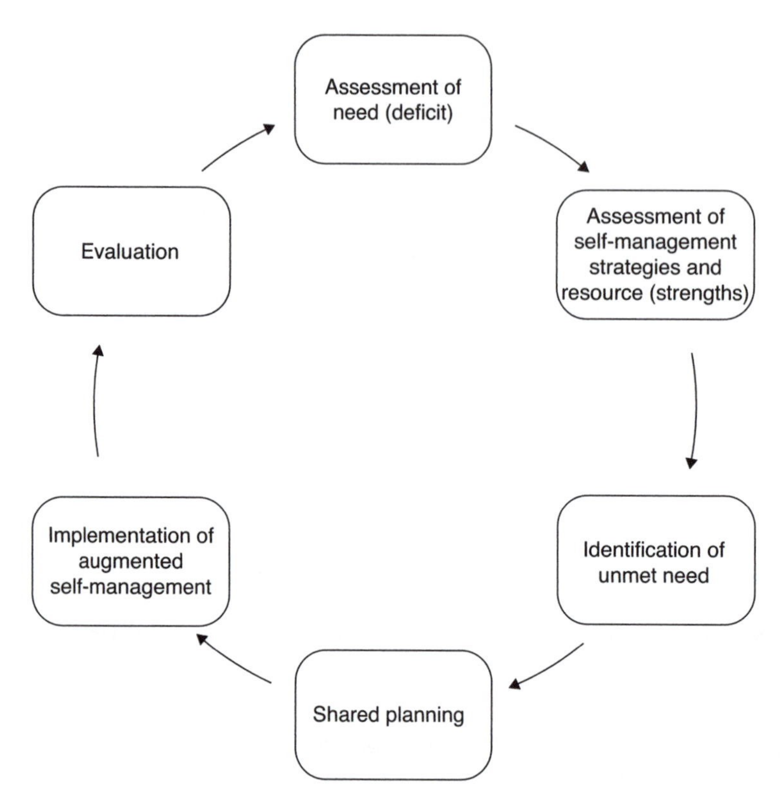

Figure 6.2: Strengths-Based Approach to the nursing process – emphasizing need (deficit), resource (strengths), shared planning and augmented self-management

Lang et al., (2002) found that for those older people with a limited resource base (defined in this study as sensorimotor, cognitive, personality and social resources), the use of the strategies of selection, compensation and optimization increased the likelihood of survival over a four-year period.

Exploring ability and disability of older people

Getting to know people, their strengths and abilities as well as needs, is a key challenge in nursing practice. It is why the process of assessment is central to subsequent planning and care actions. Our understanding of what we view an individual's health needs to be is shaped by many dynamics. Some of these are more value-laden than may be acknowledged and it is important to expose the assumptions underpinning care practices that purport to meet health needs. Some of these assumptions concern age, biography, focus of care and, very importantly, dependence.

Looking at just dependence, for example, Hill (1999) argues that the distinction between dependent and independent is too simplistic and that interdependency between people needs to be more fully recognized. Such approaches to the complexity of dependency and independence have informed in part the emergence of relationship-centred care in the nursing of people with dementia (e.g. Clarke, 1997; Nolan et al., 2004). Swain et al. (2003) also seek to disentangle what is meant by the concept of dependency, identifying the word 'independence' as having two meanings: to need other people's help, and to be free from control in judgement and action.

This latter meaning, being free from control in judgement and action, is of particular concern to nursing older people. If we are to support independence for older people, then it is necessary for us to understand that this means freedom from the control of others over their decisions and action. It does not just mean ability to manage without the help of others. Indeed, the help of others may allow the older person to have control over their decisions and actions (the use of advocates for people with dementia for example). Contrast this with a study that interviewed 20 nurses and found that 'for patients, dependency on care is a miserable loss of self-determination and self-worth' (Strandberg and Jansson, 2003: 84). So it is crucial that if older people become dependent, they retain control over their own decisions even if they are dependent on the help of others to execute those decisions, needing help for example to dress in the clothes of their choice.

Key point

Getting to know people, their strengths and abilities as well as needs, is a key challenge in nursing practice.

It is in this context that a range of frameworks of assessment and intervention are now emerging such as relationship-centred care (Nolan et al., 2002; Nolan et al., 2004). There is a need to focus on the interpersonal dimensions of families and care (Clarke, 1997). These approaches recognize that older people exist and function as part of wider family networks and the whole of their social relationships needs to be taken into account when assessing and planning care – they do not exist in a social vacuum.

Defining need

Another key influence on health care need is the process by which professionals and services define need. There are marked differences between the dominant knowledge of professional and lay carers (e.g. Clarke and Heyman, 1998). The older person and their family have a knowledge of that person that is normally denied to practitioners and that is inevitably drawn from a domain of personal values and meanings (Clarke, 1999a; Nolan and Keady, 2001). Practitioners, however, have a knowledge base that arises from their past knowledge and experiences of caring for older people. The care provided by practitioners is determined by a knowledge of the 'right' way of caring. This assumes, potentially, that there is single evidence base and may lack acknowledgement of the values and meanings associated with the knowledge domains of the older person and their family. Indeed, it may result in care which undermines the goals of older people themselves, as illustrated in Scenario 6.1.

Scenario 6.1

Mabel was a former teacher who was in hospital following an acute illness which meant that her pre-existing poor mobility from her arthritis worsened and she could no longer get around her home. To Mable's distress, discussions were taking place to find a suitable care home for Mable to live in. However, Mable then improved considerably and she needed fewer and fewer analgesics to control her arthritis-related pain. As a result, it was agreed that Mable could return to her own home and she was delighted.

The day after Mable was discharged she was readmitted. But now she was much more content though clearly in considerable pain. Evidently she had purposefully refused analgesia in the preceding week because she wanted to persuade the staff that she was much better and able to return home. Why? 'I just needed one last night in my house before I see out my days in a home'. But why had none of the staff recognized this need? Why had she felt unable to express this and instead deprived herself of much-needed analgesia? Mable had taken what action she felt was in her control and it is us as nursing staff who need to answer some questions about why she felt it had to be done this way.

- *Can you identify an older person who is distressed by what is taking place in their lives?*
- *How can you support them to share their concerns?*

In this scenario, Mable felt excluded from the decision-making process and took matters into her own hands as best she could. Had she been enabled to share decision-making, she might have been able to express her wish to say goodbye to her own home and been supported to allow that last night there to happen in a way that did not harm her.

In a similar way, in a study into the construction and management of risk in dementia care, Clarke et al. (2004) argue that risk assessment and management are processes that have the potential to marginalize and exclude people from social participation. This results from professionals having a knowledge base that is perceived to be more influential than older people's (derived from research evidence rather than lived experience) and a greater ability to make things happen (older people, and people with dementia in particular, being relatively 'powerless'). Bond et al. (2002) argue that a diagnosis of dementia can lead to professional judgements about lack of insight that result in depersonalization and loss of independence, and in this way removal from the probabilities of risk.

Needs and services

The previous sections have argued that there is a difference between health need and service provision to meet that need and that this difference sometimes leads to a gap in meeting the needs of older people themselves. This arises for three reasons (Clarke, 1999b):

1 There are considerable differences between lay and professional conceptions of health and pathology.
2 There is philosophical diversity in professional practice ranging from pathophysiological models through to interactionalist, social constructionist and socio-critical models, each

bringing its own set of assumptions about needs, assessment, intervention, role of the family and relationship between professionals and client.

3 These conflicting knowledge domains generate ethical dilemmas in clinical decision-making.

Health care itself has a set of needs that are influenced by its own organizational biography, and often it is these needs that preside over the needs of individual clients and families. In a soft systems methodology evaluation of a Health Action Zone (Carr et al., 2006), focusing on partnership working and community development, the dynamics of engagement and entrenchment were identified which shape the needs of any health provider organization. Patterns of entrenchment were those in which decisions and actions reinforce historical patterns of service delivery, health was clinically (ill health) defined, power continued to be distributed according to traditional hierarchies, and change upheld disease-oriented individualistic definitions of health and the historical distribution of power. On the other hand, patterns of engagement were those in which decisions and actions focused on meeting population health need regardless of traditional boundaries of service delivery. Health was defined as a universal attribute possessed by all, available to all, and the responsibility of all. Change challenged traditional power hierarchies and promoted partnership working across professions, organizations and statutory and voluntary care sectors.

Underpinning several issues here is the way in which knowledge is created, communicated and used in services and in a way that seeks to minimize the loss of knowledge to the system. In a study of adult mental health services that developed a new pattern of service delivery (involving a higher proportion of non-professionally qualified staff; shared health and social care staff offices and high level of joint-disciplinary activity between Community Mental Health Nurses (CMHNs) and social workers) (Cook et al., 2001; Gibb et al., 2002) it was possible to identify ways in which the service had developed so positively. These included: feeding service user knowledge into the care system; minimizing information transaction time (especially between the social workers and the CMHN); creating an early warning system; interdisciplinary knowledge exchange; and an increased capacity for receptivity and critical analysis of knowledge. Similarly, Garvin (1993) emphasizes the importance of quick and efficient transmission of knowledge through an organization in order to enhance decision-making, inform new policy and practice and provide the capacity for effective action (Senge, 1990). As such, it is imperative that the evaluation of assessment and interventions are not overlooked. Evaluation will not only ensure that the care plan for an individual older person is continuing to meet their otherwise unmet needs, but will inform the development of the service and ensure its continuing ability to meet the needs of older people.

Scenario 6.2

Raaj has experienced several admissions to hospital, normally over the winter when his breathing deteriorates as a result of an exacerbation of his chronic obstructive pulmonary disease (COPD). This gets him down and he dreads the winter approaching. He has been receiving regular visits to check his diabetes and blood sugar levels as these have been rather poorly controlled recently and as a result he has

(*continued*)

got to know Mary, the community nurse, quite well. Mary has been encouraging Raaj to lose some weight and do some gentle exercises to improve his diabetic management but also to improve his breathing which Raaj has benefited from.

One day Mary notices that Raaj takes longer to answer the door than usual and is looking a bit different to usual; his colour is rather grey and his lips and fingertips are much bluer than usual. Mary is able to get the GP in to check Raaj's condition and together they are able to intervene at a much earlier stage than in previous occasions to avoid his COPD deteriorating further and manage to avoid Raaj being admitted to hospital.

In this situation, Mary draws on her knowledge of physiology to recognize the signs of Raaj's COPD deteriorating, but can only do so because she has got to know him quite well and what he is normally like. She is able to work with Raaj to get some additional medical support and together they were able to achieve the mutual goal of avoiding a hospital admission.

- *Think of a situation in which you have been nursing an older person whose condition has been deteriorating – how have you known this?*
- *What knowledge have you drawn on?*

Types of knowledge

These threads of knowledge which underpin nursing are described very lucidly and thoroughly in work by Liaschenko and Fisher (1999). They describe three types of knowledge for nursing:

- **Case knowledge** – of anatomy, physiology, pharmacology, clinical procedures for example.
- **Patient knowledge** – of how the individual is identified as a patient, of individual's response to intervention, knowing how to get things done and of other providers.
- **Person knowledge** – of the individual patient's personal biography.

Key to Lianschenko and Fisher's model is that each of these types of knowledge are linked by 'social knowledge'. The social knowledge that links case and patient knowledge concerns knowing the skills and working patterns of others involved in the patient's care (e.g. social workers, medical staff) so that the nurse is able to co-ordinate care and ensure that the correct expertise is available for the patient. The social knowledge that links patient knowledge and person knowledge requires an understanding of the patient's world beyond receiving health care – for example, the social context of their life, the impact of any disease on their independence and ability to self-manage their care, the stigma that may be present, and 'the degree to which the individual takes up the dominant cultural discourse about their particular disease and impairment. For older people, there are contradictions and paradoxes inherent in living as an older person in a disabling society, which has the potential to accelerate the restriction of choice and decision-making (Swain et al., 2003). There is interplay between self and society, and a relationship between the potential difficulties accompanying growing older and the context in which it takes place (Clarke, 2008).

Conclusion

This chapter acts as a bridge between the first section of the book and the second section, which explores in some detail many aspects of nursing practice with older people. As the first section highlights, nursing practice is coloured by society's attitudes, national policies, professional guidance and local practices and contexts. Older people, in turn, bring to their later years a lifetime of experiences, learnt strategies for managing problems and a resource base which needs to be deployed appropriately to help them achieve their full potential in later life. To achieve this, the nurse needs to assess not only the deficits and needs of the individual, but also their resources and self-management strategies. This requires an approach to nursing older people which requires partnership with older people and their families and is a key way in which nurses demonstrate their care.

In summary, 'care' is fundamental to good quality nursing intervention, and adds essential value to the acts and words used when working with older people. The essential goals in working with older people are independence, choice and personalization, and dignity. The issues faced by older people arise not only from their own age-related changes (such as poorer mobility) but from the attitudes of other people (who may feel that older people with memory problems are unable to make their own decisions for example). Care planning for older people needs to include an assessment of their strengths and approaches to self-management, and to involve them in joint planning decisions. However, there are factors built into professional practice and into service delivery that can make it harder to assess and plan care jointly with an older person.

References

Baltes, P.B. and Baltes, M.M. (1990) Psychological perspectives on successful aging: the model of selective optimization with compensation, in P.B. Baltes and M.M. Baltes (eds) *Successful Aging: Perspectives from the Behavioural Sciences* (pp. 1–34). New York: Cambridge University Press.

BAPEN (2009) *Combating Malnutrition: Recommendations For Action: Report From The Advisory Group On Malnutrition*. Redditch: BAPEN.

Bond, J., Corner, L., Lilley, A. and Ellwood, C. (2002) Medicalization of insight and care-givers' responses to risk in dementia, *Dementia*, 1(3): 313–28.

Carr, S., Clarke, C.L., Molyneux, J. and Jones, D. (2006) Facilitating participation: a Health Action Zone experience, *Primary Health Care Research & Development*, 7: 147–56.

Clarke, C.L. (1997) In sickness and in health: remembering the relationship in family caregiving for people with dementia, in M. Marshall (ed.) *The State of the Art in Dementia Care*. London: Centre for Policy on Ageing.

Clarke, C.L. (1999a) Family caregiving for people with dementia: some implications for policy and professional practice, *Journal of Advanced Nursing*, 29(3): 712–20.

Clarke, C.L. (1999b) Dementia care partnerships: knowledge and ownership, in T. Adams and C.L. Clark (eds) *Dementia Care: Developing Partnership in Practice*. London: Ballière Tindall.

Clarke, C.L. (2008) Editorial – risk and long-term conditions: the global challenge, *Journal of Nursing and Healthcare of Chronic Illness*, 17(5a): 1–3.

Clarke, C.L. and Heyman, B. (1998) Risk management for people with dementia, in B. Heyman (ed.) *Risk, Health and Healthcare: A Qualitative Approach*. London: Chapman & Hall.

Clarke, C., Luce, A., Gibb, C., Williams, L., Keady, J., Cook, A. and Wilkinson, H. (2004) Contemporary risk management in dementia: an organisational survey of practices and inclusion of people with dementia, *Signpost*, 9(1): 27–31.

Cook, G., Gerrish, K. and Clarke, C.L. (2001) Decision making in teams: issues arising from two evaluations, *Journal of Interprofessional Care*, 15(2): 141–51.

Crisp, J. (1999) Towards a partnership in maintaining personhood, in T. Adams and C.L. Clarke (eds) *Dementia Care: Developing Partnerships in Practice*. London: Ballière Tindall.

Department of Health (DoH) (2009) *National Dementia Strategy*. London: Her Majesty's Stationary Office (HMSO).

English Longitudinal Study of Ageing (ELSA) (2002) Available online at www.ifs.org.uk/elsa/; accessed 30 May 2009.

Garvin, D.A. (1993) Building a learning organisation, *Harvard Business Review*, 71(4): 78–92.

Gibb, C.E., Morrow, M., Clarke, C.L., Cook, G., Gertig, P. and Ramprogus, V. (2002) Transdisciplinary working: evaluating the development of health and social care provision in mental health, *Journal of Mental Health*, 11(3): 339–50.

Health Survey for England (HSE) Available online at www.dh.gov.uk/en/Publicationsandstatistics/PublishedSurvey/HealthSurveyForEngland/index.htm; accessed 30 May 2009, utilizing data mainly from the Reports of 2004 and 2005.

Hill, T.M. (1999) Western medicine and dementia: a deconstruction, in T. Adams and C.L. Clarke (eds) *Dementia Care: Developing Partnerships in Practice*. London: Ballière Tindall.

Keady, J. and Gilleard, J. (1999) The early experience of Alzheimer's disease: implications for partnership and practice, in T. Adams and C.L. Clarke (eds) *Dementia Care: Developing Partnerships in Practice*. London: Ballière Tindall.

Lang, F.R., Rieckmann, N. and Baltes, M.M. (2002) Adapting to aging losses: do resources facilitate strategies of selection, compensation, and optimization in everyday functioning? *Journal of Gerontology*, 57B(6): 501–9.

Liaschenko, J. and Fisher, A. (1999) Theorizing the knowledge that nurses use in the conduct of their work, *Scholarly Inquiry for Nursing Practice: An International Journal*, 13(1): 29–41.

Miller, C. (2004) *Nursing for Wellness in Older Adults*. Philadelphia, PA: Lippincott, Williams & Wilkins.

NMC (2009) *Guidance for the Care of Older People*. London: NMC.

Nolan, M. and Keady, J. (2001) Working with carers, in C. Cantley (ed.) *A Handbook of Dementia Care*. Maidenhead: Open University Press.

Nolan, M., Davies, S., Brown, J., Keady, J. and Nolan, J. (2004) Beyond 'person-centred' care: a new vision for gerontological nursing, *International Journal of Older People Nursing*, 13(3A): 45–53.

Nolan, M., Ryan, T., Enderby, P. and Reid, D. (2002) Towards a more inclusive vision of dementia care practice and research, *Dementia*, 1(2): 193–211.

Senge, P. (1990) *The Fifth Discipline: The Art and Practice of the Learning Organisation*. London: Doubleday/Century Business.

Spilsbury, K. and Meyer, J. (2001) Defining the nursing contribution to patient outcome: lessons from a review of the literature examining nursing outcomes, skills mix and changing roles, *Journal of Clinical Nursing*, 10: 3–14.

Strandberg, G. and Jansson, L. (2003) Meaning of dependency on care as narrated by nurses, *Scandinavian Journal of Caring Sciences*, 17(1): 84–91.

Swain, J., French, S. and Cameron, C. (2003) *Controversial Issues in a Disabling Society*. Maidenhead: Open University Press.

CHAPTER 7

Mobility

Bhanu Ramaswamy and Diana Jones

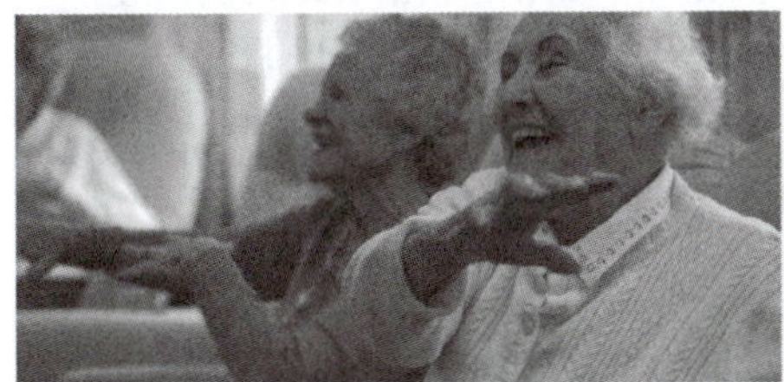
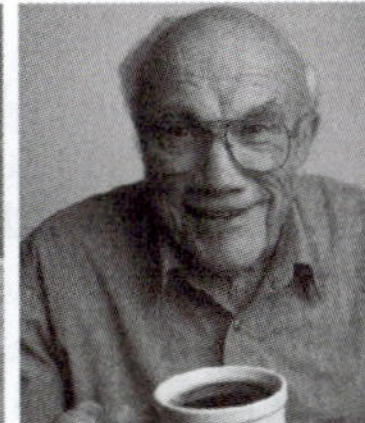
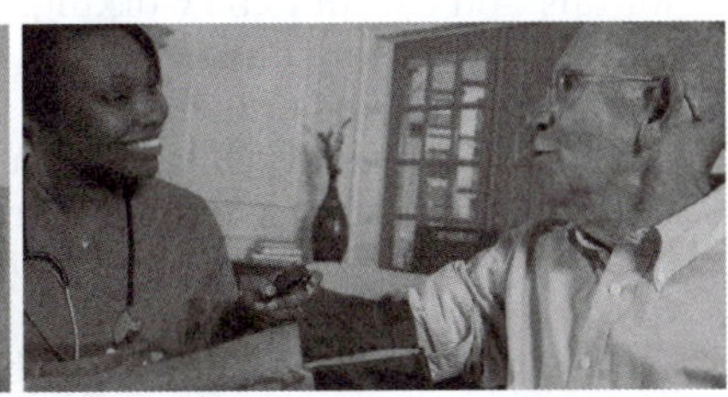

Learning objectives

At the end of this chapter, the reader will be able to:

- describe the individual and specific nature of the meaning of mobility in relation to the lives of in older people
- identify the domains of the World Health Organization (WHO) *International Classification of Functioning, Disability and Health* (ICF) (2001) and how they can be used to guide assessment, goal-setting and treatment planning in relation to mobility
- know of the range of assessment areas linked both directly and indirectly with mobility
- describe therapeutic interventions to meet mobility needs
- identify available resources or colleagues from other disciplines that might contribute to the assessment and management of mobility in older people

'We both feel that mobility relates to being able to get about by walking, although my wife includes a wheelchair and other forms of transport in her definition. We live in a terraced house in a city. I'm 76 years old and have had Parkinson's disease (PD) for 28 years. I've also got chest problems – COPD (chronic obstructive pulmonary disease) they call it. My wife is in her mid-70s too and has been increasingly troubled by arthritis over the last about 10 years – she can't carry things and pains in her back means she struggles to walk. She is having difficulty getting out of bed and low chairs, and she seizes up if she sits for a long time.

It's funny but walking about outside the house causes me less problems than moving about indoors. When I approach a door I often feel as if my feet are stuck to the floor. They call that 'freezing' and it comes with having PD. I know I shouldn't but I hold on to furniture for balance, and I even use a stick indoors on bad days. I always use one at night and outside – and so does my wife. We both use the stair lift, and the

(*continued*)

wife sends the laundry upstairs on it. She takes a trolley to the shops even if she's only getting a few things. Often when walking back from the local supermarket my wife has to alter her pace to match mine. I can walk one way OK but struggle on the return. Family and friends put her wheelchair in the car when we go on outings with them that may involve a long walk.

I'm worried because my wife has started to have dizzy spells and the pills she takes for this don't seem to be working. She becomes anxious in crowds and likes to hold on to someone for support. We've found that loud music, lots of noise, and people all talking at the same time make her walking worse. My wife recently fell on an escalator and damaged her shoulder; she has to travel 5 miles on the bus to go to physiotherapy. I do a weekly exercise class with other people with PD and my walking is better after the class. I don't think the local Trust can continue to provide professional input and the group may fold, which would be a shame. I also enjoy outdoor bowls and fishing.

We would both like to use the bus when out together but I feel unable to do so since one of my PD drugs was removed from the market. I haven't managed to maintain my level of mobility without it. I don't like to travel in taxis. I know my city and I think some taxi drivers take long routes to places. My wife thinks I'm just self-conscious about my mobility problems. The family keep telling us we should use taxis more often. They get frustrated with us.'

Introduction

The term 'mobility' is encompassed within a broad concept, and therefore nursing activity in relation to mobility needs to be multifaceted. Physical mobility is the action of moving from place to place, and often means different things to different people. Examples that underpin our ability to move around our environment and that form part of the wider picture of mobility include the skill of walking in different settings; of negotiating curbs, steps, stairs and escalators. If someone is housebound or frail, mobility may simply relate to the ability of getting into and out of chairs or the bed or to get to another room. Meanwhile, in relation to active older people this might also include the ability to get into a car as well as other modes of transport to travel.

Health clinicians are increasingly using the World Health Organization (WHO) *International Classification of Functioning, Disability and Health* (ICF) (2001) domains for assessments of people in their care. This framework can be a useful tool in raising awareness of the meaning of mobility in relation to the lives of older people and, most importantly, to discover how they use mobility to enable their social needs. If used to compliment subjective and observational elements of a nursing assessment, the ICF can be used to guide goal-setting and treatment planning in relation to mobility.

In the following sections of this chapter, the concept of mobility and aspects of nursing activity in relation to mobility and older people will be explored though a series of scenarios. The individuals described have mobility challenges arising from very different causes – secondary to a hernia, as a result of a stroke, and following a childhood illness. Each person has contributed their insight into why mobility is important to them, and in particular relates this to a period where they recently received health care (including nursing) intervention. At the end of the chapter, the main issues relating to mobility of these older subjects have been used to illustrate how they might sit within the ICF domains to develop a more complete assessment of their needs.

Common health conditions and associated impairments affecting mobility in older people: some facts and figures

With age, mobility-related problems increase. Forty-three per cent of people in England over 50 years of age already self-report limitation in physical function, 13 per cent of which relates to difficulty with mobility, with 13 per cent reporting difficulty with a basic activity of daily life (ADL) (self-care). In the English Longitudinal Study of Ageing (ELSA) (Banks et al., 2010), of the respondents in their 80s and older, 81 per cent recorded some physical difficulty with one basic ADL, with 50 per cent requiring help for this. Such limitations correlate to increasing expressions of depressive symptoms, decreased life satisfaction, quality of life and loneliness. Walking speed slowed dramatically with age (ELSA, 2002; Health Surveys for England (HSE) 2004), and on observation of the participants in the ELSA study, one in forty people aged between 60 and 64 walked more slowly than 0.4 metres/second, increasing to one in five at age 80 and over. These decreases were more notable in women than in men.

The HSE (2004) survey of people aged 65 and over also highlighted that 37 per cent of men and 40 per cent of women had at least one functional limitation; for example, vision, hearing, communication, walking, or using stairs, and both the number and degree of limitation increased with age. The most frequently reported limitation was difficulty in walking up a flight of 12 stairs without resting.

Older people were among the few who reported difficulty accessing local amenities, such as a post office or supermarket (Banks et al., 2010). It was noted that occupational class affected function in older life, with people who had manual occupations reporting up to twice as many difficulties with physical function as those with managerial or professional occupations (Banks et al., 2010).

Seventy-one per cent of both men and women aged 65 and over reported longstanding illness that limited their activities in some way. The prevalence of long-standing illness and limiting long-standing illness increased with age in both sexes; the most common types reported among those aged 65 and over were musculoskeletal problems, heart and circulatory diseases (including stroke), diabetes, arthritis and emotional/anxiety-related problems (Banks et al., 2010; HSE, 2004, 2005). These trends are not isolated to the UK (see Resources section).

Understanding mobility in the context of nursing activity with older people

Mobility in the context of nursing older people is based on an understanding of the individual's ability to undertake the tasks they *want* and *need* to perform; for example, doing a personal care task, preparing a meal, walking to the shops or socializing (Squires and Hastings, 2002). Pain or another condition, whether psychological or physical, might also affect their experience of mobility. Whether community dwelling or in a care setting, the maintenance of mobility essentially underpins a person's ability to remain independent, with freedom to make choices about their activities (Bourret et al., 2002).

Key point

Mobility in the context of nursing older people is based on an understanding of the individual's ability to undertake the tasks they *want* and *need* to perform.

Scenario 7.1 describes a mobility issue which was disregarded by the health professionals during this individual's period of hospitalization.

Scenario 7.1

David is a 63-year-old university lecturer living in a city in the north of England. His mobility was compromised due to an inguinal hernia that was repaired two years ago. Increasing groin pain caused limitations in David's otherwise active lifestyle. He therefore underwent several investigations, initially through his GP, then a surgical consultant, and was finally provided with a date for elective admission to his local hospital for the surgery. Following a successful operation David was discharged with one follow-up out-patient appointment. There is no past medical or medication history of note.

Socially, David lives in a house with his partner. He is an avid runner and since the operation has returned to running and over the past year has built up his distance so that he is able to run 7 miles. David also cycles to and from work. He is a political activist and keen photographer – both activities take him out and about nationally and internationally.

The aspect of mobility most affected – David was disappointed and annoyed that all staff underestimated his need to carry on with running as a hobby and for fitness, plus a return to cycling as a means to get to work. Staff were only interested that he had regained sufficient mobility to walk and thus return home, and were unable to provide advice on when or whether he should resume running and cycling. Although not overtly ageist, no consideration was given to his prior physical ability and activity levels. He sees it as an achievement that he has returned to full ability despite lack of support and advice from health care staff.

- *What steps could you take to ensure that you know what level of activity an older person wishes to have?*
- *How could David have been better supported to achieve his goals?*

In a concept analysis of the term 'mobility', Rush and Ouellet (1993) identified four common attributes. These are:

- freedom and independence of movement within all aspects of life;
- the purposefulness (or goal-directedness) of movement;
- awareness of the competence to move about in relation to the environment;
- adaptability in familiar and new environments.

These attributes emphasize the dynamic nature of mobility, and the likelihood of a change in relation to ageing, a person's health status and changes in the context of an individual's life. On reading Scenario 7.1, it is clear where the staff have underestimated important mobility-related attributes, so David's needs to regain peak fitness and regain his pre-surgery lifestyle go unrecognized and ignored. Further issues pertaining to David's mobility are considered in the following section.

Conceptualizing mobility challenges in the context of ageing

The ICF (WHO, 2001) offers a conceptual framework that enables health care professionals and older people to consider the effect of multiple impairments on mobility (Figure 7.1). The impairments often impact on activities of daily living and how the person can participate in societal roles in later life (Izaks and Westendorp, 2003). The ICF framework also considers issues in context; for example, environmental (physical and attitudinal) and personal (medication, support) factors. These can act either as barriers or facilitators in the analysis and the subsequent planning of appropriate nursing interventions and support. As a point of interest, many hospitals now use the related International Classification of Diseases and Related Health Problems (ICD-10) to code patients' problems on admission.

Using the ICF to explore the causes and effects of the mobility problems experienced by David we can see that the area requiring greatest assessment would be David's fitness level (Impairments). His motivation to return to peak fitness is a potential facilitator of mobility and would be recorded in the 'Personal factors' section.

It is important to remember that few professions work in isolation within the health and social care setting. If the issue of David's future fitness needs had been picked up by the ward staff, although they may not have been the appropriate people to answer David's questions or if it was deemed too soon for him to start exercise at a higher level, the staff

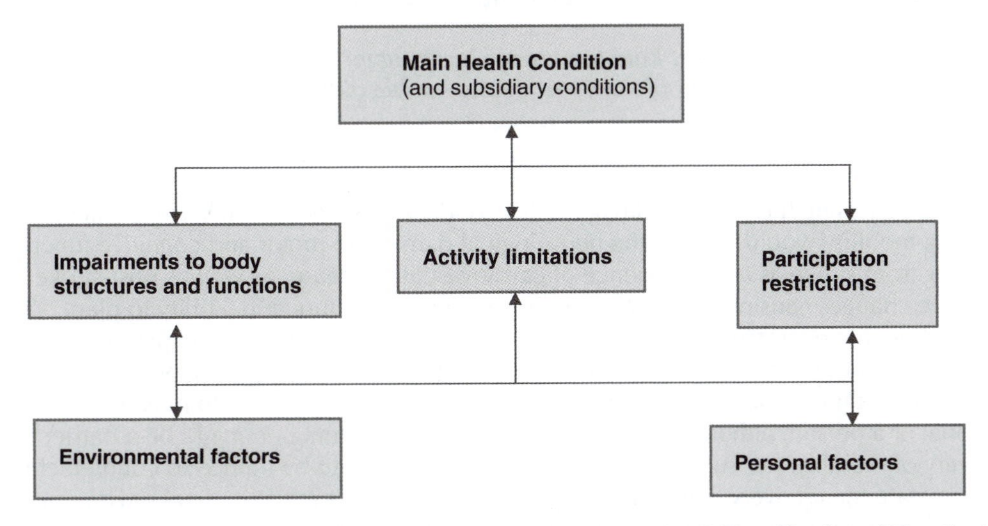

Figure 7.1: Interactions between the components of the International Classification of Functioning

Source: Reproduced with permission from WHO. Short version booklet of the *International Classification of Functioning, Independence and Health* (WHO, 2001: 26). Available online at www.who.int/classifications/icf/en/; ISBN/WHO Reference Number 92 4 154544 5

could have referred David to the therapy services. This may have been to the community or the out-patient physiotherapy department to ensure David's physical progress was managed and monitored to his satisfaction as his operation scar healed.

Scenario 7.2 describes mobility-related concerns about encountering unknown, challenging factors in the physical environment.

Scenario 7.2

Kate is a 75-year-old housewife living in a city in the English Midlands. Her mobility was affected by a stroke one year ago; she has since almost regained the speech and language skills she lost, has recovered 95 per cent of the motor skills on her right side that were lost for at least three months post-stroke, but still has mild sensory impairment. When tired however all Kate's symptoms are worse. Her past medical history includes hypothyroidism, Vitamin B12 deficiency and high blood pressure and her medication regime attempts to maintain a stable condition.

Socially, Kate lives in a house with her husband and oldest daughter (a retired nurse); she has been able to return to most aspects of her life; for example, shopping, cooking, gardening, but has now stopped driving, and has agreed to employ a weekly cleaner for major housework.

The aspect of mobility most affected – although mobility has returned it is compromised by major fatigue. Kate has some apathy and difficulty in motivating herself to remain as physically active as she was before the stroke. She lacks confidence in her physical ability. This affects travel and use of transport both at home and internationally, as she still makes an annual trip to India. She is proud of the fact she still travels but is now acknowledging she has become less adventurous and independent and finds the multiple logistical issues daunting (e.g. environmental issues in relation to hotel layout and location). While confident to go to the familiar GP surgery, any unaccompanied hospital visits cause panic.

- *How would you support Kate to manage her fatigue?*
- *What services are available in your area to enable older people get around in the community?*

In terms of using the ICF model (Figure 7.1) to identify issues for Kate, 'impairments' affecting mobility would include the neurological damage to motor and cognitive function resulting from stroke as a consequence of cardiovascular disease, as well as post-stroke cognitive changes causing apathy and diminished executive function (ability to plan). We can see how her expressed concerns about encountering challenges in the physical environment would fit into the section on 'Environmental factors'. Having noted earlier that professionals should use networks in the health and social care setting to maximize the potential of a person, although Kate's apathy and executive function might be a barrier to recovery of mobility, her supportive and engaged family could be trained to counteract this and facilitate the recovery. Kate's family outlook forms part of the attitudinal environment around her and is recorded as a positive 'Environmental factor'.

Kate is not alone in her concerns about negotiating the outdoor environment. A study of older people living in the community (Shumway-Cook et al., 2003) found that mobility disability is characterized by reduced willingness to encounter environmental challenges, with implications for physical fitness and social interaction. By including questions about environmental factors in nursing assessment, options could be identified for therapeutic strategies in care plans to help maintain participation in the world outside the home post-discharge. This is particularly important in the light of research on life-space mobility after hospitalization of older people (Brown et al., 2009). Life-space is a helpful measure of physical function in terms of participation, measuring where someone goes, how frequently and how independently. Patients requiring surgery will experience greater immediate decline but more rapid recovery (as with David in Scenario 7.1) compared with non-surgical patients, whose decline might be viewed as modest (as with Kate in Scenario 7.2) but who might show slow recovery over extended follow-up.

Nurses respond to the mobility issues of older people in a full range of settings – in hospital out-patient clinics, accident and emergency departments or wards; in community in health centres and the home; and in care homes. Older people not only visit health care facilities to address their own needs but to support their partners and families, often at facilities distant to their homes. They can be concerned about the availability of parking to attend an appointment, about finding their way in unfamiliar surroundings; accessing a wheelchair and help to push it; the efficacy of medication wearing off and affecting mobility; and the need to use stairs or lifts. Mobility concerns also exist in the community in relation to accessing GP surgeries, podiatry services or obtaining prescriptions. Nurses with a sound knowledge of the mobility needs of older people, together with older people themselves and the groups representing them, can feed in to service improvement initiatives and planning of new facilities to ensure their specific needs are met (Department of Health (DoH), 2008).

Key point

Older people visit health care facilities not only to address their own needs but to support their partners and families.

Assessing mobility

To better illustrate the multifactorial nature of mobility assessment, various forms used by nurses across one Primary Care Trust were identified and the key areas of nursing assessment in relation to older people's mobility were isolated. Mobility issues may be central to domains of certain assessment; for example, when determining level of dependence, or when completing a moving and handling or a falls risk form. Other areas of assessment may have implications for mobility; for example, toileting and skin integrity. It is important that information gathered during assessments of issues directly related to mobility is linked to assessments in areas with an indirect link to mobility to ensure that an overall understanding of the individual's mobility status is gained (Weaver, 2005). Appropriate nursing and multidisciplinary strategies can then be put in place to support and promote mobility.

Assessment domains that focus on mobility directly

Moving and handling

Specific moving and handling risk assessments are undertaken to highlight physical safety from the point of view of older people and staff. Personal handling assessment will note details of the level of independence of the individual.

If the person is dependent on some assistance, the following should be recorded:

- the number of carers;
- the handling method;
- any aids and equipment needed.

Personal handling forms are often completed in collaboration with other professions; for example, physiotherapists. Risk assessment will include consideration of a wide range of factors that contribute to safe moving and handling, and would include:

- communication issues;
- cognition;
- comprehension;
- sight/hearing;
- attitudes and appropriate behaviour;
- history of falls/seizures;
- medication;
- posture;
- transfers and balance (including involuntary movements);
- strength;
- range of movement or flexibility;
- pain;
- skin condition.

Older people may ask for help to move or the provision of bedrails. It is important for nurses to consider their need at a particular point in time, and also their progression towards increasing independence and discharge. If the older person being nursed has a main carer at home who would also need to help in aspects of their mobility, it is important to review any moving and handling issues in the context of this partnership. This is particularly the case if the carer will need to facilitate an individual to get out of bed to access the toilet at night. The interruption of the sleep pattern of the carer is likely to directly affect their energy levels, general health and psychological well-being.

Risk assessment is a dynamic process subject to ongoing updating and review. Review can highlight that progression is limited by poor cognition or insight which puts the person at risk of falls or injury. Sensitive communication is needed to ensure individuals understand the balance between the physical improvement observed by the nurses, which would indicate a move to greater independence, and the perceived role of the nurse to help and offer care. This can be particularly challenging in a rehabilitation setting where the promotion of independence is likely to be a central goal.

Falls

Falls are a major cause of disability and death in people aged over 75 years in the UK, while falls prevention was a standard within the National Service Framework for Older People (DoH, 2001). The National Institute for Health and Clinical Excellence (NICE) falls guideline (NICE, 2004) highlighted risk identification and multifactorial falls risk assessment linked to multifactorial interventions as key priorities. These have been prominent features of subsequent guidance, such as the Falls and Fractures Prevention guidance for commissioners of health and social care for older people (DoH, 2009).

Specific falls risk assessments often overlap with manual handling assessments. Many risk tools place the person into one of three risk categories – low, medium and high, with recommendations for staff to follow according to the category. A basic assessment should take the following into account:

- history of falls;
- number and frequency;
- causes;
- intervention to date;
- number and type of medication, including alcohol intake and whether they suffer form postural hypertension;
- nutrition and particularly bone health;
- problems affecting vision or hearing;
- the condition of feet and footwear;
- problems with balance, transfers and walking (including walking aids used);
- the environment (institutional and home);
- confidence to move;
- if they have coping strategies – e.g. getting up off the floor;
- memory/comprehension.

Family carers may be able to provide important contextual information about falls in the home, especially if the person is unable to provide accurate details. Multidisciplinary team colleagues may already be involved with the older person and updating them on the current episode of care may be important. Referral to other multidisciplinary colleagues, for example, dietician, audiologist or local emergency alarm specialist, may be appropriate. Decision-making around falls prevention involves balancing risks, rights and responsibilities (as discussed in Chapter 13). Clarke (2003) suggests that service users and carers, the public and professionals should adopt a more realistic view of risk acceptance to counteract extreme risk-management solutions that threaten civil liberties. A diagnosis of dementia may result in a gradual loss of safe mobility and performance of unaided everyday tasks (Oddy, 2003). Falling often becomes common when the person becomes unable to perceive a risk, such as poor balance on standing, and at this point consideration of a chair alarm may be necessary. This might act as a cue to remind the individual that they should not get up by themselves, or alert a nearby staff member that the person is trying to move. An occupational therapist or physiotherapist can give advice about equipment and adaptations to aid mobility and make the person's surroundings safer. If the person with dementia becomes confined to a bed or chair, carers will need advice on how to help individuals to move without injuring themselves. Scenario 7.3 describes a person with long-standing mobility issues that require staff to consider utilizing manual handling methods, and whose physical condition and cognitive decline place her in the higher category of falls risk.

Scenario 7.3

Shona is a 74-year-old female from a rural area in the north of England. Since the age of eight she has had musculoskeletal problems in her lower limbs following childhood measles. Difficulties caused by arthritis have necessitated numerous

(continued)

operations (including replacements of both knees and both hips). She has been transferred from the acute hospital where her most recent surgery and recovery took place to a community hospital bed for rehabilitation.

In addition to her orthopaedic problems, Shona is currently on medication to treat depression, a gastric ulcer (in the previous year) and hypertension. Socially, Shona lives alone in a bungalow and although she admits to being a little forgetful was previously able to go out to visit friends weekly, to walk about and to go shopping with her daughter.

The aspect of mobility most affected – Shona has been what she classifies as 'disabled' all her life, recognizing the unusual/unconventional way she tackles mobility-related activities. She has fought to retain independence over the years, and finds it very difficult to understand concerns about her current abilities and future mobility as she sticks rigidly to a daily routine. Her declining mobility is of key importance to her daughter. She raises most concerns as she is the person who neighbours ring if they fear Shona will fall and injure herself when they see her out shopping. The Single Assessment Process completed on initial acute hospital admission did not highlight Shona's lack of insight into her declining mobility status. Mobility issues related to a safe discharge home were therefore not identified until specialist assessment by therapy staff when Shona was transferred for further rehabilitation.

- *How could staff work together and with Shona to manage her discharge home from hospital?*
- *How could you build on Shona's lifelong experience of living with limited mobility?*

Using the ICF model, the impairments affecting Shona's mobility include her long-term musculoskeletal deficits that have necessitated orthopaedic surgery and that compromise manual handling techniques. Recovery from surgery is complicated by Shona's mental health diagnosis and identification of her lack of realism about the current reduced ability to foresee falls risks. Her daughter's concerns and stress could be placed in the 'Environmental factors' section (attitudinal environment). If falls safety issues are not addressed holistically and Shona's daughter is not included throughout the planning and decision-making process, her concerns may prove a barrier to recovery of her mother's mobility.

Taking these issues into consideration, and when reviewing both the manual handling and the falls assessment lists, Shona would fall into a category of high falls risk. A compromise is needed to ensure a safe discharge that permits Shona her right to return home as she has the capacity to make that decision. A social care package will be necessary to minimize personal risks through her poor mobility with referral to community rehabilitation to ensure graded improvement is facilitated on her return home.

Assessment domains with an indirect link to mobility

Assessment and interventions that reduce the risk of major decline in mobility are likely to require attention to psychosocial as well as health issues (Ayis et al., 2006). Table 7.1 identifies and explores assessment domains that are often overlooked in terms of their indirect, yet important link to mobility.

Breathing	Deconditioning can cause breathlessness when a person walks; if they are fearful of being breathless (e.g. after an asthma attack) the person may become more self-limiting. Assessment is cyclical and should determine whether an approach of reassurance and slower movement, but firmness in making the person do an activity, permits them to complete a task they would otherwise have left to the staff to do for them with your assistance. This approach also becomes the first step in showing the person how to achieve completion of a task themselves. If a person has heart failure, they may appear to be out of breath while doing very little on observation, yet actually do not perceive themselves to be breathless as this is their norm.
Eating and drinking	Monitoring weight and dietary intake is important to ensure the availability of energy and state of hydration. The sense of smell of older people is often decreased and affects their appetite. As well as affecting kidney function necessary in the elimination of many metabolized medications, weight loss and dehydration have implications on both physical and mental health.
Elimination	Bowel function needs to be measured against its normal pattern and confusion and pain can occur with constipation. As falls risk is known to increase if urinary incontinence is a problem, assess for night time polyuria as this can also adversely affect sleep patterns and a person may be more prone to falling if sleepy or tired.
Hygiene and dressing	Consider the impact of the person's balance mechanism and flexibility as these may hinder someone getting to their feet. Consider whether for safety they should sit to put shoes and socks on. Do they have the ability to bend down all the way to cut toenails or should they lift one leg up to rest on the other thigh if bending makes them dizzy or breathless?
Controlling body temperature	Cold extremities indicate poor circulation and can result in decreased sensitivity to touch, make muscles stiffer and joints less flexible, thus affecting mobility. Someone too hot may be at risk of fainting.
Skin integrity	If the person has swollen ankles, leg ulcers or other skin conditions, assess if there are impediments to movement around the ankle, especially if pain is an issue or if they have to have an ulcer dressed.
Expressing sexuality	This is an area that is poorly assessed due to potential embarrassment of either the assessor or person being interviewed. Remembering that intimacy is not solely an issue of the young, and a professionally approached discussion may at least trigger a referral to a specialist such as a urologist, gynaecologist, or sexual health specialist.
Sleeping	The pattern of sleep alters with age, and any additional interruptions such as getting up at night to use the toilet, or an inability to turn due to joint pain or stiffness, will further affect this. A referral to a physiotherapist or occupational therapist may be indicated if equipment is deemed of benefit to assist in movement at night.
Medication	It is important to understand if the person is taking their medication as prescribed as many people are admitted to hospital on the basis of uncontrolled symptoms. With progressive conditions such as arthritis, heart disease, Parkinson's Disease and so on, has the medication been increased over time to counteract the deterioration? Also assess if the person is taking sedatives that are no longer effective yet may result in falling at night.
Pain	Assess whether pain is causing inhibition of movement. Referral may be needed to increase analgesia temporarily while mobility is being improved, especially after an acute injury. Referral to a physiotherapist for assessment of a (more) suitable mobility aid may be relevant.
Mental state – mood memory	Assess the person with wandering tendencies and the risks they may place themselves in, in their home environment. Those with low mood may be too apathetic to be active and thus become weaker through lack of exercise and poor appetite/diet; those with a poor memory may not remember to eat or take medications, risking malnourishment and undermedication.

Table 7.1 Assessment domains with an indirect link to mobility

Managing mobility

Planning nursing interventions in relation to mobility

A range of terms are used in relation to planning interventions; for example, developing nursing diagnoses, care planning and goal-setting (Kneafsey, 2007). Comprehensive assessment is a necessary precursor in formulating patient-centred nursing goals; ensuring involvement of the older person in goal-setting promotes choice and participation in the process. This should minimize frustrations expressed by older people in relation to the lack of opportunity to be part of the planning of the (rehabilitation) process (Wallin et al., 2007).

As the pension age rises and people are expected to work later in life, mobility will need to be assessed and addressed efficiently to ensure return to work in a timely period. Assessment of personal interests and leisure activities can have important implications for mobility interventions (e.g. David's use of cycling to support his participation in both work and political activities). Likewise socio-cultural needs may have a mobility component (e.g. Kate's annual trip to visit relatives in India, and Shona's weekly trip shopping with her daughter). These areas of assessment and nursing strategies should be linked to the appropriate impairment, activity and participation domains on the ICF. Table 7.2 illustrates how this may be done using the three mobility case scenarios.

The importance of thinking more widely during the assessment process

Proformas designed for the collection of standardized data, perhaps by a range of individuals in relation to a single assessment process, may have restricted space and in turn can be limiting in terms of helping to make important links between domains of assessment. Making such links is an important step between collecting information and problem-solving at the level of the individual in relation to their mobility needs. There is also a danger of a restriction in thinking in relation to setting. For example, a nurse in an acute setting might not visualize the mobility needs of an older person on discharge. Alternatively, assumptions may be made that mobility and professionals in a different setting will deal with other issues without explicit referrals being made to ensure that matters are passed on. This was the case with David; while nursing intervention ensured optimal post-hernia recovery of mobility and self-care to permit a return home, it was assumed the ward physiotherapists would take into account David's love of running. As nothing specific was mentioned to the physiotherapists, however, this was not considered and David was discharged without information regarding his chosen interest.

Promoting health benefits for mobility

Kneafsey (2007) and Weaver (2005) stipulate that the nursing goals aimed at promoting maximum health benefit in relation to mobility should include the promotion of:

- as normal a movement pattern and posture as can be regained;
- sufficient balance to minimize falls risks;
- independence and maximal mobility potential;
- sufficient sleep and rest;

- activity tolerance balanced against conservation of energy thus minimizing fatigue;
- interaction with others;
- minimizing pain and risks such as cardiovascular problems and pressure sores.

It is always important when discussing and agreeing goals with the older person, or when considering how to meet the goals, not to attempt to work in isolation but to link with other professionals who might already be involved in the care of the older person; for example, a dietician, an occupational therapist or social services personnel. There is strong evidence of

Scenario 7.1–David	*Scenario 7.2–Kate*	*Scenario 7.3–Shona*
Main assessment and intervention focus: multifactorial – post-operative pain, medications, immobility, fear/uncertainty about movement permitted post-operatively	Main assessment and intervention focus: post-stroke mobility and falls risk	Main assessment and intervention focus: post-operative hip precautions
Impairment: Pain control via opioids, with nurses monitoring for constipation as well as for post-operative thromboembolism risk	**Impairment**: Falls risk recorded at least weekly on a chart to review progress and to gauge whether the risk posed a threat when planning for discharge	**Impairment**: Operation scar and weakened muscle joint integrity might mean that Shona was at risk of dislocation. Nurses had to monitor for post-operative wound management and for thromoembolism
Activity limitations from restricted mobility improved with reassurance from nursing staff as analgesia reduced. Initial fear of soreness on walking and of possible injury to the new scar also abated	**Activity limitations** recorded using manual handling charts completed as recovery of mobility was noted and Kate became physically stronger and capable of transferring herself	**Activity limitations** already being experienced due to previous history of orthopaedic surgery. Nursing staff were more vigilant when transferring – especially in and out of bed; ensured a higher chair and toilet seat and monitored for fatigue levels when walking
Participation: David soon regained confidence to walk on the ward by himself with no concerns related to discharge. He required initial assistance to put on anti-embolic compression stockings as he was unable to bend sufficiently	**Participation**: Overcoming fear of falling was the main issue – on the part of the staff, Kate herself as she regained balance senses and her family who had fears about whether obstacles around her home might make the environment less safe when considering her readiness for discharge	**Participation**: No issues with regard to participation except to monitor memory when adhering to post-operative precautions

Table 7.2 Nursing assessments and interventions related to mobility linked to ICF

the effectiveness of interdisciplinary team management in the rehabilitation of older people (Wells et al., 2003), and nurses and other professionals need to be clear about their input in relation to the goals of the team, the older person themselves and their carer.

Nursing strategies and interventions in relation to mobility

Just as assessment and goal-setting have a multidisciplinary component, strategies and interventions in relation to mobility benefit from drawing on a range of expertise and knowledge bases (Hubbard et al., 2004). There is a need for research to identify the most effective way of supporting older people's mobility, particularly in the context of the different perspectives on mobility held by the different members of the rehabilitation team (Kneafsey, 2007). Best practice will only be gained through collaboration, with each profession sharing their perspective in the context of the management of individual older people.

Brown Wilson (2002) reviewed the aspect of safer handling of nursing staff in the private sector following specific manual handling training. It was noted that in the people whose mobility improved, the trained nurses reported they assessed the client's ability to move each time while also involving the client in the decision on how to move. This form of problem-solving is essential in helping the older person make decisions that will affect both their autonomy and independence.

Nursing interventions to promote mobility

Nursing interventions to promote mobility identified in a systematic review of the literature (Kneafsey, 2007) include:

- the development of relationships with patients;
- the use of motivational and teaching skills;
- therapeutic positioning and transferring of patients;
- range of movement exercises to maintain and improve joint flexibility, strengthening exercises and general exercise programmes;
- the use of splints to treat and minimize spasticity and contractures.

Engaging people with dementia

When engaging people with dementia in mobility-related activities, Oddy (2004) states that consideration should be given to:

- providing frequent reminders about what to do;
- speaking clearly and ensuring requests are short and clear;
- using familiar words or cues;
- knowing a person's likes and dislikes;
- offering reassurance;
- checking issues such as postural hypotension and medication, in case drugs cause drowsiness and affect balance;
- checking that footwear is sensible.

From our scenarios it is clear that it is part of health care teams' interventions for mobility to provide older people with the support and encouragement they need to return to agreed levels of physical activity. This may actually result in an increase in activity, but should permit participation in activities they need, and wish to pursue. Improvements in functional status and quality of life are seen in older adults as a result of regular physical activity, even if this is taken up later in life. Physical activity and obesity are among the modifiable behavioural factors that are associated with the maintenance of health in older age (Burke et al., 2001). Activities recommended by health care professionals should always take into account health factors that could affect capability for safe performance; for example, aerobic fitness, and gender and cultural preferences. Older people take part in the full range of physical activities including walking, swimming, dancing and gardening as well as formal exercise sessions. The recommendation is that older adults should, if appropriate, engage in at least 30 minutes of moderate-intensity physical activity five days per week (DoH, 2004).

Evaluation of nursing goals

It is important to review the manual handling risk form and broader nursing goals on a regular basis. Nursing shift patterns can make it difficult for the member of staff who originally set a goal to review it. Colleagues of any profession should share this responsibility, especially as various team members address goals related to mobility. Ideally, the older person and perhaps their carer will have participated in goal-setting and they also need to be encouraged to monitor progression of goals, resetting them if necessary. The handover period between shifts is a key time to share patient goals. If an individual is being transferred to another care setting it is important to inform staff of the goals that have been set previously so they can review them in a new context.

An example of this is seen in the case of Shona. Her daughter expressed concerns to the nurses during her evening visit, causing them to question the reality of Shona's expectations to return to weekly shopping trips as soon as she was discharged. The information was communicated with the therapy staff the following morning and Shona's goals were revisited with her. As a consequence community rehabilitation was organized to provide discharge support and Shona was more realistic about her need to increase mobility once home before she could resume her previous trips out with her daughter.

Aids, equipment and adaptations to support mobility

Nurses have an opportunity to ensure that the health care settings within which they work with older people provide an environment that facilitates safe mobility. An uncluttered environment will be helpful to people with sight impairment; appropriate chairs will facilitate transfers; support rails will assist independence in toilet facilities. Early liaison with multidisciplinary colleagues will allow assessment for aids, equipment and adaptations necessary for timely discharge planning from a hospital setting.

Equipment used in the context of an acute hospital setting may not fit the confines of a home; for example, bariatric hoist and bed levers. It is imperative that both family and formal carers are trained in key manual handling techniques and equipment use prior to discharge. Shona has had adaptations to her bungalow to support her mobility, including a larger than normal wheelchair ordered specifically to accommodate her post-surgical condition. Her daughter, however, only had a small hatchback car and a low back condition that affected her ability to lift. She was therefore unable to transport her mother's new

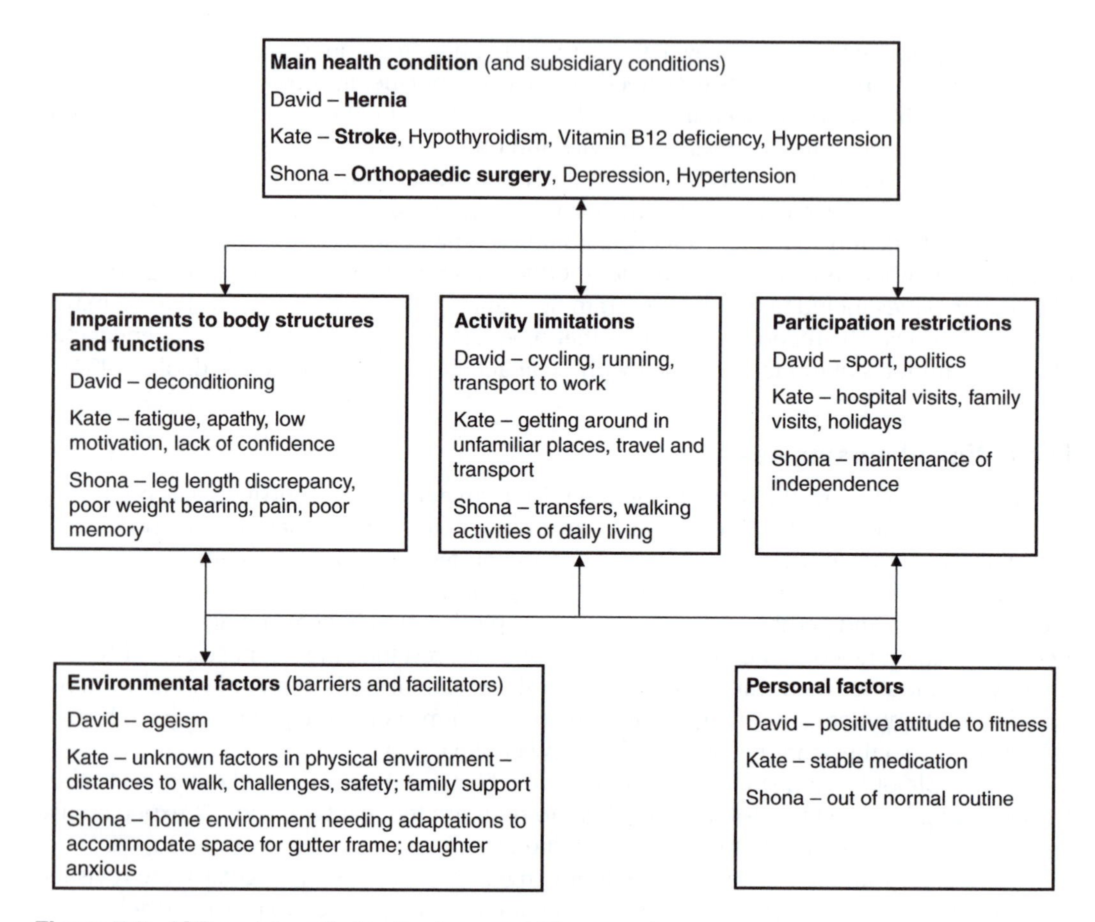

Figure 7.2: ICF model applied to the three mobility scenarios

wheelchair when they went out, and had to organize the availability of a hire chair prior to any trips to destinations other than the supermarket; she found this stressful.

Older people report that they are aware that their mobility is becoming compromised but they find it hard to make decisions about adapting the garden or house or changing their home altogether. It is often a crisis that precipitates the decision. Nurses and other members of the team need to be proactive in talking about mobility issues with older people in an attempt to avoid managing a crisis if preventative steps are not taken.

Figure 7.2 provides an overview of the ICF framework for the three case scenarios. It illustrates how such a model might be used to compliment the generic proformas used when recording assessment, ensuring a holistic management of the older person.

Travel and transport

The ability to travel is important to older people and serves a range of functions, including entertainment (getting out of the house); participation (in organizations and classes);

independence (not having to rely on others); and social interaction (the opportunity to meet people) (Department for Transport (DfT), 2001). Mobility in the labour force means that families are no longer likely to live nearby, necessitating travel to maintain contact. Fewer local shops and other facilities necessitate travel to main centres for shopping, recreation and education. Changing road layouts and rules of the road may mean older drivers feel less confident. For people with compromised mobility, walking around in large centres with few seats and toilets can be anxiety provoking. Younger generations may be perceived as not helpful or mistrusted if they do offer assistance. Health care professionals assessing mobility for older people need to have an understanding of the issues they face moving about in the wider world and the support available for getting about. This requires consideration if an older person has to travel to visit a relative in hospital, or for attendance at out-patient appointments for example.

A special mention is appropriate to be made of the challenges faced by people with memory loss and dementia, for whom even the simple act of walking can be regarded as 'wandering' and 'aimless'. Obviously, it is important to challenge any such assumptions and establish in the first instance what purpose the activity services – it may be that they are wanting to reach a shop, or ease a painful back. None the less, people with dementia and their supporters do worry about 'getting lost' and being unable to find the way back again if they go out. For some, a global positioning system (GPS) may be appropriate so that they can be found easily, or simply carrying a mobile phone so that they know they can seek support if necessary. Feeling disoriented can be very frightening and so people with dementia may avoid unfamiliar places, or, if uncertain of where they are, may be anxious and distressed. It is important that they are reassured and supported to feel safe again.

The transport needs of older people

A study into the transport needs and requirements of older people (DfT, 2001) investigated older people's experiences of, and aspirations for, transport systems. Declining driving ability, due to physical and cognitive problems and financial pressures, can result in individuals giving up their cars. A high proportion of older people become dependent on bus and rail services, yet many experience difficulty using these modes of transport. Older people highlighted the information about safe driving that they wanted access to as they got older: the need to address failing eyesight, strategies for driving at night and coping with congestion, and awareness of special car features; for example, automatic transmission and power steering. They saw a more formal role for doctors and opticians in deciding whether drivers were safe to continue to drive. Regular public transport users were concerned about customer care (including driving practices which increased risk of accident, such as moving off before people were seated; lack of handrails; overcrowding). Prompt repair of pavements was highlighted to reduce risk of falls. Personalized transport schemes such as Shopmobility, Dial-A-Ride and door-to-door transport schemes were valued.

Taxis are a key component of the travel and transport pathway. However, older people can experience anxiety about cost, the assistance they can expect from the driver, and concern about whether taxi design will accommodate their disability; for example, degrees of hip flexion after hip replacement or obesity. There is a clear need for a range of central and local government departments and transport operators,

(*continued*)

including community and voluntary providers and taxi firms, to work with older people's organizations and individuals to address broad mobility, travel and transport issues and offer a range of joined-up provision over the older age span.

Age UK update information on travel and transport, including parking, for older people on a regular basis and collate a fact sheet which is downloadable from their website (see Resources section).

Conclusion

This chapter has provided some context to the many meanings older people ascribe to mobility. An understanding of the domains in which mobility may be encountered in nursing practice will help guide assessment, goal-setting and treatment planning processes. By ensuring these are explored in relation to the needs of the individual, it will permit the person to retain some ability to complete self-chosen tasks and give them the freedom to live a preferred lifestyle.

In summary, mobility relates to our ability to move around our environment. Nurses encounter the mobility needs of older people in the full range of practice settings. The International Classification of Functioning (ICF) provides a clear framework with which to explore multiple factors that contribute to the experience of mobility and aspects of assessment may be directly (e.g. moving and handling) or indirectly (e.g. skin integrity) related to mobility. Teamwork, and in partnership with older people, is important when assessing, goal-setting and executing strategies to promote mobility in older people.

Acknowledgements

The authors wish to thank the older people who contributed their mobility narratives to this chapter. Recognition is also due to staff and students at Derbyshire County NHS Primary Care Trust for their insights and critical reading.

References

Ayis, S., Gooberman-Hill, R., Bowling, A. and Ebrahim, S. (2006) Predicting catastrophic decline in mobility among older people, *Age and Ageing*, 35: 382–7.

Banks, J., Lessof, C., Nazroo, J., Rogers, N., Stafford, M. and Steptoe, A. (2010) *Financial Circumstances, Health and Well-being of the Older Population in England*. The 2008 English Longitudinal Study Of Ageing (Wave 4). London: The Institute for Fiscal Studies.

Bourret, E., Bernick, L., Cott, C.A. and Kontos, P.C. (2002) The meaning of mobility for residents and staff in long-term care facilities, *Journal of Advanced Nursing*, 37(4): 338–45.

Brown, C., Roth, D., Allman, R.M., Sawyer, P., Ritchie, C.S. and Roseman, J.M. (2009) Trajectories of life-space mobility after hospitalization, *Annals of Internal Medicine*, 150(6): 372–80.

Brown Wilson, C. (2002) Safer handling practice: influence of staff education on older people, *British Journal of Nursing*, 11(20): 1332–9.

Burke, G., Arnold, A., Bild, D.E., Cushman, M., Fried, L.P., Newman, A. ,Nunn, C. and Robbins, J. (2001) Factors associated with healthy aging: the cardiovascular health study, *Journal of The American Geriatrics Society*, 49: 254–62.

Clarke, J. (2003) The concept of risk and older people: implications for practice, *Gerontological Nursing Practice*, 15(7): 14–18.

Department for Transport (DfT) (2001) *Older People: Their Transport Needs and Requirements – Main Report*. Available online at www.sortclearinghouse.info/research/228/; accessed 12 January 2011.

Department of Health (DoH) (2001) *National Service Framework for Older People*. London: Her Majesty's Stationery Office (HMSO).

Department of Health (DoH) (2004) *At Least 5 a Week: Evidence on the Impact of Physical Activity and its Relationship to Health. A Report from the Chief Medical Officer*. London: HMSO.

Department of Health (DoH) (2008) *Real Involvement: Working with People to Improve Health Services*. London: HMSO.

Department of Health (DoH) 2009) *Prevention Package for Older People Resources*. London: HMSO.

English Longitudinal Study of Ageing (ELSA) (2002) Available online at www.ifs.org.uk/elsa/; accessed 30 May 2009.

Health Survey for England (HSE) Available online at www.dh.gov.uk/en/Publicationsandstatistics/PublishedSurvey/HealthSurveyForEngland/index.htm; accessed 12 January 2011, utilizing data mainly from the Reports of 2004 and 2005.

Hubbard, R., O'Mahony, S., Cross, E., Morgan, A., Hortop, H., Morse, R. and Topham, L. (2004) The ageing of the population: implications for multidisciplinary care in hospital, *Age and Ageing*, 33: 479–82.

Izaks, G. and Westendorp, R. (2003) Ill or just old? Towards a conceptual framework of the relation between ageing and disease, *BMC Geriatrics*, 3: 7.

Kneafsey, R. (2007) A systematic review of nursing contributions to mobility rehabilitation: examining the quality and content of the evidence, *Journal of Nursing and Healthcare of Chronic Illness in association with Journal of Clinical Nursing*, 16(11c): 325–40.

National Institute for Clinical Excellence (NICE) (2004) *Clinical Practice Guideline for the Assessment and Prevention of Falls in the Elderly*. London: Royal College of Nursing. Available online at www.nice.org.uk/nicemedia/pdf/CG021fullguideline.pdf; accessed 12 January 2011.

Oddy, R. (2003) *Promoting Mobility for People with Dementia: A Problem Solving Approach*. London: Age Concern England.

Oddy, R. (2004) Promoting success in mobility for residents with dementia, *Nursing & Residential Care*, 6(3): 124–7.

Rush, K. and Ouellet, L. (1993) Mobility: a concept analysis, *Journal of Advanced Nursing*, 18: 486–92.

Shumway-Cook, A., Patla, A., Stewart, A., Ferrucci, L., Ciol, M.A. and Guralnik, J.M. (2003) Environmental components of mobility disability in community-living older persons, *Journal of The American Geriatrics Society*, 51: 393–8.

Squires, A. and Hastings, M. (2002) *Rehabilitation of the Older Person: A Handbook for the Interdisciplinary Team*. Cheltenham: Nelson Thornes.

Wallin, M., Talvitie, U., Cattan, M. and Karppi, S-L. (2007) The meanings older people give to their rehabilitation experience, *Age and Society*, 27: 147–64.

Weaver, D. (2005) Helping individuals to maintain mobility, *Nursing and Residential Care*, 7(8): 43–5.

Wells, J., Seabrook, J., Stolee, P., Borrie, M.J. and Knoefel, F. (2003) State of the art in geriatric rehabilitation. Part I: review of frailty and comprehensive geriatric assessment, *Archives of Physical Medicine and Rehabilitation*, 84: 890–7.

World Health Organization (WHO) (2001) *International Classification of Functioning, Disability and Health*. Geneva: WHO.

CHAPTER 8

Nutrition, including food preparation and planning

Angela Dickinson

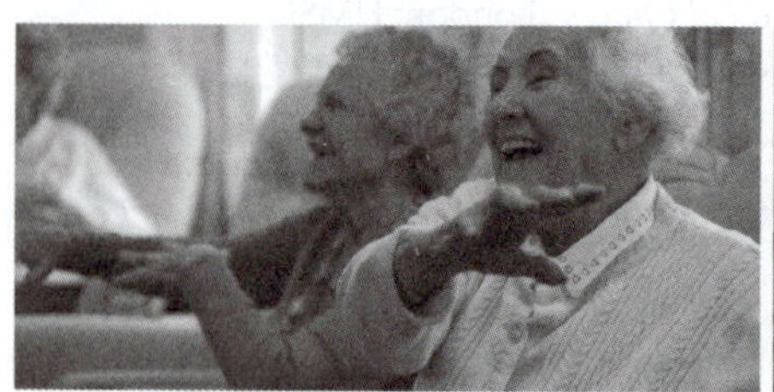
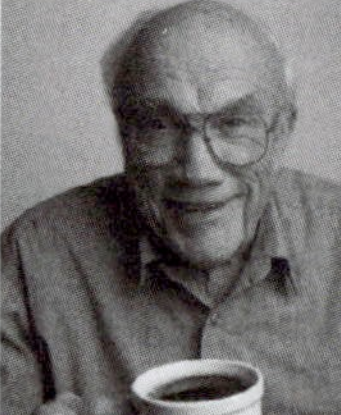
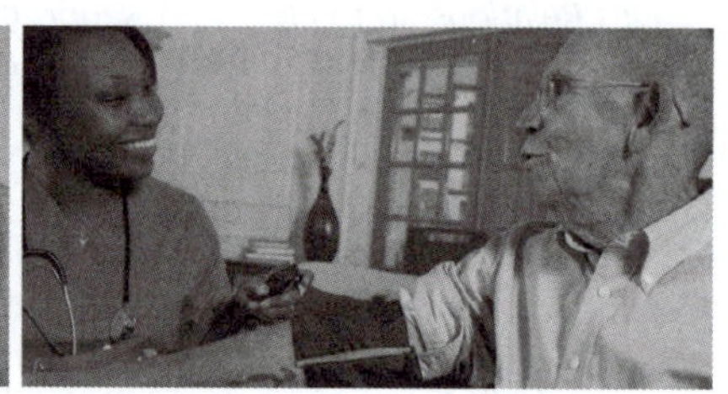

Learning objectives

At the end of this chapter, the reader will be able to:

- understand how the heterogeneous nature of the older population makes it impossible for a one size fits all approach to meeting the nutritional needs of older people
- describe why nutrition needs to be approached in a broad and interdisciplinary way
- identify how the cultural and social aspects of food and eating contributes to older people's well-being and makes a person-centred approach essential
- understand why nutrition and hydration are important aspects of older people's nursing and social care in all care settings
- be aware of the purpose and importance of screening for nutritional risk
- describe the nurse's role in the nutritional well-being of older patients

Daphne Westwood (Member of the Public Involvement in Research Group, Centre for Research in Primary and Community Care, University of Hertfordshire) comments as follows:

'Most older people are well aware of the benefits of eating nutritious food, and five different fruit and vegetables a day, but with two million pensioners living below the poverty line (recent statistics) and with additional difficulties such as poor health and solitary living, many are finding these benefits difficult to achieve. Most have spent their former years bringing up families, shopping and cooking as economically as possible, and it is difficult to change the habits of a lifetime.

Buying and cooking for just one or two is not easy. Meat, fish and eggs can be bought in smaller quantities, but pre-packed vegetables and fruit, greens and salad usually contain far more than older people can eat before the contents start to deteriorate, and to buy smaller amounts often makes shopping more expensive. Supermarkets' own brand basic foods do sometimes help but flavour and quality are often sacrificed. Ill health and lack of mobility are also major factors for many not being able to enjoy shopping for or cooking good food.

Many local authorities provide meals-on-wheels, or transport to centres that provide wholesome food, and these often have the advantage of having other social activities available. Yet these services are often dependent on government funding, or the work of voluntary bodies, and churches. They often provide good, economical, subsidised meals for older people, and some, who perhaps have the money, go regularly to more than one centre on different days each week (people older than some of the customers often staff these centres!).

Most people enjoy well-cooked and nutritious food, and for older people it is an important part of life. It is even more important when loneliness is a major factor. Some older people who I know look forward each week to going to a local church café. They plan, share taxis, or walk together to go there, socialise, and afterwards discuss the meals. It is a very anticipated outing. But what about breakfast and supper? And the other days of the week?'

Diane Munday (Member of the Public Involvement in Research Group, Centre for Research in Primary and Community Care, University of Hertfordshire) comments:

'Having been diagnosed with Type 2 diabetes thirty five years ago and, despite having progressed through diet only, tablets and now tablets and insulin, I have remained free of any of the complications that can arise from poor control. So, either I have been lucky or I am getting it right!

I like to think that it is the latter and, as I am a couch potato by nature and heartily dislike "exercise", it is keeping active in everyday living alongside understanding about food and watching what I eat that is really important to me.

Most people know that a healthy diet – one that is low in sugar, low in saturated fat and high in fibre as well as limited in overall quantity – is what we should all aim for. And it is no different for people with diabetes except that we should be even more careful about avoiding added sugar.

Fortunately there are many low sugar products on the market and a little knowledge about how to read food labels (such as knowing that manufacturers can be crafty and disguise sugar with all sorts of fancy names like glucose, dextrose, invert sugar) helps me to shop healthily. Even more importantly I have learned to always take a list and never to shop for food on an empty stomach when everything looks tempting.

I still really like eating and for many elderly people it is one of life's remaining pleasures. Unfortunately I still have a sweet tooth but, unlike when I was diagnosed in the 1970s, there are sugar substitutes that can be used for sweetening drinks and with a little experimenting for cooking favourite recipes.

(*continued*)

I firmly believe that everybody needs the odd treat and I have found that breaking the rules occasionally, particularly if I am "good" most of the time, does not affect my overall control but hugely improves my quality of life generally. So if I go out for a meal I really enjoy it and having eaten some "forbidden" foods am more careful than usual about what I eat the next day.'

Introduction

The above two examples both illustrate the importance of food and eating in the everyday lives of older people. Daphne explains how the experience of social isolation, particularly when this is compounded by other factors such as low income and poor mobility, affect the whole process which culminates in eating. She explains how both statutory and voluntary sector providers can have a positive experience in the lives of older people. Diane describes her experience of living with a long-term condition – diabetes – which has a direct influence on her experience of eating. She described the strategies she has developed over the years to manage her condition, and how despite dietary restrictions, food provides great pleasure and contributes greatly to her quality of life. All of these factors will be explored in further detail in this chapter.

Dietary intake, nutritional status and the social and cultural context of eating are fundamental to the physical health, quality of life and well-being of older people. The older population is an extremely heterogeneous group with diverse resources (e.g. income, skills, education, health, etc.) and needs (e.g. information, support, skills, etc.).

Key point

Dietary intake, nutritional status and the social and cultural context of eating are fundamental to the physical health, quality of life and well-being of older people.

Understanding the eating practices and habits of current generations of the older population is of great interest as during their lifetimes they have experienced what is historically one of the most rapidly changing periods in terms of food supply. Older people have lived through extreme changes in food availability during their lifetimes, from scarcity during and following the war years to the seeming overabundance of recent times. Rapid developments in food technology, agriculture and retailing have made these changes possible.

As the population of the world ages, older people increase in number and their importance as consumers, both of food and health care. The later stages of the life are also associated with major social changes; for example, retirement and, for some, loss of a partner, all of which might be expected to affect eating habits.

As nurses we need to understand and take account of the dietary intake and nutritional status of older people in order to provide the care they need, whether this is for health education information at one end of the spectrum to physical and/or emotional support with eating at the other end. This need is also supported by epidemiological data, such as that provided in a recent report that has estimated that at any point in time, more than three million people in the UK will be either malnourished or at risk of malnutrition. Most of the people affected (93 per cnt) live in the community (this includes about 2–3 per cent who are living in sheltered housing), about 5 per cent living in care homes and 2 per cent being cared for in hospital settings. The authors estimated the cost of disease-related malnutrition in the UK in 2007 at over £13 billion per annum, with about 80 per cent of this cost in England (BAPEN, 2009).

Approaches to understanding nutrition

The majority of research interest into nutrition and eating has been within nutritional science, sociology, anthropology and psychology. Each of these disciplines brings a distinct focus and makes a specific discipline-based contribution to our understanding of nutrition. All of the approaches add different facets to our understanding and subsequent practice, and will be examined only very briefly here.

The biomedical scientific perspective

The nutritional (biomedical) perspective has dominated research into food and eating and concentrates on the physiological and biochemical mechanisms of eating, such as the essential nutrients (how they work and which foods they are obtained from); and the delay and prevention of degenerative disease by dietary modification. Nutritional science has helped to uncover links between diet and health (Germov and Williams, 1996).

Within the nutritional science perspective, food choice is perceived in terms of achieving the optimal physiological state of the organism in order to maximize health and longevity. This approach often paints a rather negative view of nutrition in old age, tending to study nutrition in terms of a decline in physiological functioning; for example, focusing on areas such as anorexia, declining taste and smell, constipation, malnutrition, diseases and physical problems.

> “This mechanistic and disease-orientated view of health inevitably paints a bleak and negative view of the prospects for health in old age. Later life is portrayed as a time of declining strength and increased frailty as organs and tissues wear out or succumb to disease and degeneration.
>
> (Sidell, 1995: 4)”

Psychological approaches

Psychology describes itself as the science of behaviour, and attempts to explain why an organism does what it does (Logue, 1986).

Psychologists researching food choice work on various aspects, from the sensory aspects of food choice, examining the effect of food on mood, learning and experience, measuring attitudes and beliefs and predicting behaviour. Some psychologists have attempted to develop predictive models of food choice with varying degrees of success. Difficulties arise in the development of such models due to the large range of potential factors which affect food choice. The models assume that food choice is a 'reasoned action' but other evidence suggests that many influences play a part (such as access to and availability of food). What people choose to eat is not always rational and often depends on the context of eating (e.g.

people tend to eat more when they eat with others compared to when they eat alone), thus models tend to predict the choice of some but not all foods (Shepherd and Raats, 1996).

Psychology research again tends to concentrate upon the negative aspects of ageing, such as a decline in sensory taste, smell and vision, role loss, depression and loneliness therefore reflecting the negative perceptions of society. Booth (1994) described eating habits as being deeply ingrained and inflexible in later life.

Sociological and anthropological perspectives

The nutritionally based research perspective tends to separate food intake from the social aspects of eating and that for humans 'the physiological dimension of food is inextricably intertwined with the symbolic' (Lupton, 1996: 8). This means that though people are generally aware of the rules of healthy eating, they do not put them into practice and the social sciences try to explain why this is.

Despite food being such a central part of everyday life, or perhaps because of this fact, research into food use in older age has been relatively unexplored by sociologists. Food and eating generally take place within the privacy of the household with the associated work being viewed as women's work and consequently devalued by society (Van Esterik, 1997).

There appears to be a growing interest and recognition of the need to have a wider understanding of the role played by food in people's lives. Fieldhouse (1995) lists a wide range of influences on food selection, including physical availability, political, economic, cultural and religious factors, socio-psychological reasons and individual choice.

Each of these theoretical approaches adds a different, but complementary understanding and enables nurses to draw on knowledge from both biomedical science and social science to improve our understanding of the nutritional care we can provide to people as they age.

Nutritional requirements in older age

There is room here for only a brief summary of the nutritional requirements for older adults (for more detailed information see Stanner et al., 2009).

Fluid intakes

Fluid intake is an often disregarded, but important aspect of nutrition. Older people are particularly vulnerable to dehydration due to factors such as:

- reduced thirst mechanism (less likely to feel thirsty);
- increased fluid loss (poorer renal function);
- medication such as diuretics, laxatives, hypnotics;
- swallowing difficulties;
- incontinence;
- dementia or stroke (can result in insensitivity to thirst);
- poor mobility/dexterity;
- poor access to toilets (conscious restriction of fluids);
- living in an institution.

Factors such as vomiting, diarrhoea, fever and high environmental temperatures increase requirements for fluids. There is evidence that adequate hydration can help prevent pressure ulcers, urinary infections, heart disease, low blood pressure and diabetes, as well as reduce risks of developing some cancers (bowel, breast, prostate) and reduce the risk of developing kidney stones and coronary heart disease (Royal College of Nursing (RCN) and National Patient Safety Afency (NPSA), 2007). Dehydration is one of the risk factors for falls in older people, due to its effects on mental state, as well as increasing risks of dizziness or fainting. Water in hard water areas also provides significant levels of dietary calcium (essential for bone mineral density). Dehydration also affects mental performance and leads to chronic constipation.

Alcohol

Moderate intakes of alcohol can have a positive health effect throughout the adult lifespan including into old age. Metabolism of alcohol is affected by age, sex (women metabolize alcohol more slowly) and health status. However, excessive intake affects numerous organs and can interact with medication (see de Morais et al., 2009 for a useful review).

No specific recommendations are set for older people in the UK, but there is some agreement that this should be lower than for younger adults. Other countries have set lower levels, including the USA which recommends older people limit their intake to one alcoholic drink per day (de Morais et al., 2009).

Energy intakes

The body requires energy in order to fulfil functions such as maintaining physiological equilibrium, digesting and absorbing food, regulating body temperature as well as fuelling physical activity. Total energy expenditure tends to decrease as we age. Body composition changes with age, so that for a given weight, the body will have less muscle and more body fat, which reduces the basal metabolic rate (BMR). As people age there is a tendency for them to become less physically active which reduces energy expenditure. However, we should be careful not to generalize and stereotype older people. For example, a study in the USA found that on retirement, people increased their activity levels and participation in sport (Evenson et al., 2002). Current recommendations for energy intakes in the UK for older people are lower than those of younger adults, based on the above assumptions (Department of Health (DoH), 1991).

Actual requirements for energy will be influenced by activity levels, as well as any concurrent disease, especially if there is metabolic stress, fever or muscular spasms, all of which will increase energy requirements.

Maintaining body weight

Although the NHS costs associated with under- rather than over-nutrition are greater for this age group, recommendations to maintain healthy body weights are just as relevant to older people as other groups of the population. Undernutrition increases the risk of disease, affects the immune system, delays recovery from illness and has an adverse effect on clinical outcomes. Being obese increases the risk of developing a number of chronic diseases such as type two diabetes.

Macronutrients

For fat, carbohydrate and dietary fibre the dietary recommendations for older people in the UK are the same as for the younger adult population (DoH, 1991).

Protein intake

Increased levels of protein are required in older people in the presence of illness, infection and wounds, including pressure ulcers, surgery or trauma. If older people consume too little protein, over a period of time this will result in loss of muscle mass, poor wound healing and impaired immune function.

In the absence of the above, protein requirements are recommended to be at the same level as younger adults (0.75g protein/kg/day).

Micronutrients

Recommendations for levels of micronutrients (vitamins and minerals) in older age remain unchanged from the adult population, apart from the requirements for vitamin D (See Table 8.1). This change in recommendation assumes that older people will be exposed to lower levels of sunlight and are less efficient at manufacturing vitamin D from sunlight than adults aged under 65.

Older adults living in care homes or who are unable to move outside without assistance will be particularly prone to vitamin D deficiency and may need dietary supplementation. Vitamin D is essential to bone health as it is promotes absorption of calcium from the gut and is involved in the process of bone formation and maturation. Vitamin D supplementation has been shown to reduce the risk of falling, both for older people living in institutions and those who live in their own homes, through reducing muscle weakness, thus improving balance and mobility (Bischoff-Ferrari et al., 2004).

Nutritional screening and assessment

Malnutrition is present in the older adult population particularly in those who are likely to come into contact with health services, therefore nutritional assessment and screening tools can be useful to identify those in need of nutritional care. Rapid and early detection of undernutrition is important to prevent downward spirals in health. Malnutrition has a number of causes, some of which will be visited later in this chapter. The term 'anorexia of ageing' is frequently used and refers to the reduced appetite and energy intakes sometimes seen in older people which leads to being underweight, malnutrition and increased risk of disease (Morley, 1997).

The causes of 'anorexia of ageing' are well documented and a useful mnemonic 'MEALS ON WHEELS' to help remember these has been developed by Morley (1997) (see Table 8.2). It could be useful for nurses to bear these risk factors in mind when screening and assessing patients.

Clinically, there are a number of ways that undernutrition can be assessed and determined. These range from the low-tech methods of weight and height measurement, through to more complex, high-tech methods of computerized tomography (CT scans), and so on, which are expensive and unsuitable for use in everyday practice. Biochemical indicators are used in clinical settings but their use is limited as many also indicate non-nutritional pathological processes.

Nutrient	*RNI Men*	*RNI Women*
Vitamins		
Thiamine	0.9 (mg/d)	0.8 (mg/d)
Riboflavin	1.3 (mg/d)	1.1 (mg/d)
Niacin	16 (mg/d)	12 (mg/d)
Vitamin B6	1.4 (mg/d)	1.2 (mg/d)
Vitamin B12	1.5 (μg/d)	1.5 (μg/d)
Folate	200 (μg/d)	200 (μg/d)
Vitamin C	40 (mg/d)	40 (mg/d)
Vitamin A	700 (μg/d)	600 (μg/d)
Vitamin D	10 (μg/d) (after 65 years)	10 (μg/d) (after 65 years)
Minerals		
Calcium	700 (mg/d)	700 (mg/d)
Phosphorus	550 (mg/d)	550 (mg/d)
Magnesium	300 (mg/d)	270 (mg/d)
Sodium	1600 (mg/d)	1600 (mg/d)
Potassium	3500 (mg/d)	3500 (mg/d)
Chloride	2500 (mg/d)	2500 (mg/d)
Iron	8.7 (mg/d)	8.7 (mg/d)
Zinc	9.5 (mg/d)	7.0 (mg/d)
Copper	1.2 (mg/d)	1.2 (mg/d)
Selenium	75 (μg/d)	60 (μg/d)
Iodine	140 (μg/d)	140 (μg/d)

Source: Department of Health (1991)

Table 8.1 Reference nutrient intakes (RNI) for adults aged over 50, vitamins and minerals

Anthropometry

Loss of body weight is the most important way to determine undernutrition. Weight losses of 10 per cent over six months, 7.5 per cent in three months or 5 per cent in one month are related to significant mortality and morbidity (Morley and van Staveren, 2009).

Body mass index (BMI) is a useful measure of desirable weight, and is calculated by measuring weight in kilograms and dividing it by the square of height (kg/m^2). For example, a 70 kg man who is 1.8 metres in height, would have a BMI of $80 \div (1.8 \times 1.8) =$ **21.6**. In practice these calculations are made easier by the use of readily calculated BMI grids.

Other factors can affect interpretation of weight loss such as dehydration, oedema and ascites, so should be checked for in older people.

Identification of under- and overnutrition is through measurement of the BMI, which is calculated from an individual's height and weight. For the general population underweight is defined as having a BMI of less than 18.5 kg/m^2, while overweight is a BMI 25–29.9 kg.m^2 and obese, above 30 kg/m^2. BMI is used in a number of screening tools to calculate risk of malnutrition, including the UK Malnutrition Universal Screening Tool (MUST) (BAPEN,

M	Medications (digoxin, theophyline, fluoxetine)
E	Emotional causes (depression)
A	Alcoholism
L	Late-life paranoia
S	Swallowing problems
O	Oral problems
N	No money
W	Wandering and other dementia-related problems
H	Hyperthyroidism
E	Enteral problems
E	Eating problems
L	Low salt (in general therapeutic diets)
S	Shopping and cooking

Table 8.2 **'MEALS ON WHEELS'** mnemonic to assist recall of the causes of anorexia of ageing

2003), which we look at later. Body mass index is thought to be a less reliable tool in older people due to loss in height and changes in body composition. However, in the absence of other easily obtained measures, BMI is still used, though using different cut off points to define underweight (less than 24 kg/m^2) and the range of healthy weights being 24–29 kg/m^2 have been proposed (Beck and Ovesen, 1998). It is sometimes difficult to measure height accurately if someone is unable to stand, so other proxy measures of height can be used. These include demi-span, ulnar length and knee height (all of which can be used to determine a MUST score for an older person).

Nutritional screening and nutritional assessment are often used interchangeably but actually mean different things. Definitions from the *Essence of Care* are useful to consider to distinguish between nutritional screening and assessment (DoH, 2003, 'Benchmarks for Food and Nutrition': 2):

> “ Screening: A process of identifying patients who are already malnourished or who are at risk of becoming so. Those at high level of risk require referral for a further comprehensive nutritional assessment. (Unqualified staff, students, carers can screen patients if they have received the necessary education and training and have been assessed as competent to undertake the assessment, but accountability remains with the registered practitioner). ”

> “ Assessment: is a more detailed process in which a range of specific methods can be used to identify and quantify impairment of nutritional status (assessment is undertaken by registered practitioners who have received the necessary education and training and have been assessed as competent to undertake the level of assessment required e.g. registered nurse, dietitian). ”

Assessment should take into account the patient's physical, religious, cultural, age related and special needs, requirements and requests.

	Factor	*Benchmark of best practice*
1	Screening and assessment	Nutritional screening progresses further to identify patients' assessment for all patients identified as nutritional needs 'at risk'
2	Planning, implementation	Plans of care based on ongoing nutritional assessment and evaluation of care assessments are devised, implemented and for those patients evaluated who require a nutritional assessment
3	A conducive environment (acceptable sights, smells and sounds)	The environment is conducive to enabling the individual patients to eat
4	Assistance to eat and drink	Patients receive the care and assistance they require with eating and drinking
5	Obtaining food	Patients and/or carers, whatever their communication needs, have sufficient information to enable them to obtain their food
6	Food provided	Food that is provided by the service meets the needs of individual patients
7	Food availability	Patients have set meal times, are offered a replacement meal if a meal is missed and can access snacks at any time
8	Food presentation	Food is presented to patients in a way that takes into account what appeals to them as individuals
9	Monitoring	The amount of food patients actually eat is monitored, recorded and leads to action when there is cause for concern
10	Eating to promote health	All opportunities are used to encourage patients to eat to promote their own health

Source: Essence of Care, (DoH, 2003)

Table 8.3 The essence of care benchmark for food and nutrition

Screening

There are a number of screening and assessment tools which claim to be useful in the older population. Seventy one of these were reviewed by Green and Watson (2006) who concluded that many tools failed to report validity and/or reliability testing but were used clinically. Screening tools available include the Mini Nutritional Assessment, the Subjective Global Assessment, and many others. However the MUST (BAPEN 2003) is one of the tools which is becoming the mostly widely adopted in clinical settings and is well validated across a range of care settings (available online at www.bapen.org.uk/pdfs/must/must_full.pdf).

Essence of care

A benchmarking tool has been developed for use in primary, secondary and tertiary settings and with all patient and/or carer groups, including mental health settings in the UK to support quality improvements and one of the benchmarks focuses on food and nutrition (DoH, 2003; see Table 8.3).

Assessment

Dietary intake can be assessed using a number of tools. These include using food records – where everything that is eaten and drunk is recorded, although unfortunately these are frequently poorly maintained, even in clinical settings. Diet histories can be taken, and are often carried out by dietitians, but are time-consuming. Food frequency questionnaires explore how often foods are eaten, and 24-hour recall methods collect information over a short period. However, both of these methods rely on memory and the accuracy of reporting.

Summary

Despite a range of tools to assist practitioners in screening and assessing patients for nutritional risk, in a recent study more qualitative approaches to assist in understanding of, for example, what kind of food people liked and for those with cognitive problems, exploring with them, their family and carers how best to assist them with eating were felt by nurses to be just as important (Dickinson et al., 2008). Nurses then need to draw on a range of techniques, both formal and informal, in order to find out as much as possible about people as individuals in order to provide the best care possible.

Key point

Nurses need to draw on a range of techniques to find out as much as possible about people as individuals in order to provide the best care possible.

Nutrition: older people in community settings

We begin this section with a scenario.

Scenario 8.1

Mrs Lyle lives on her own since her husband died five months ago. She has come to the surgery to have an influenza vaccination. You notice that she looks very depressed, and she tells you that she is missing her husband and finding it hard to cope. Her clothes appear very loose, indicating recent weight loss. On weighing her you find that she has lost 7 kg (she is 1.64 metres in height, and now weighs 50 kg).

- *What other information would you collect?*
- *What further action would you take?*
- *How would you evaluate the effectiveness of your actions?*

Background

The most recent large-scale survey of the diets and nutritional status of older people in the UK (Finch et al., 1998) found that the majority of the older people sampled were adequately nourished, deriving adequate amounts of the majority of vitamins and minerals from their diets. The diets of some subgroups, however, gave cause for concern; for example, those from low socio-economic groups, older age groups and those who live in institutions.

Energy intake of older people had decreased by 15 per cent since the previous Government survey (Department of Health and Social Security (DHSS), 1979). Despite the low energy intake, many older people were found to be overweight or obese (63 per cent of women and 67 per cent of men, defined by a BMI greater than 25) which indicates that energy intake was sufficient to meet their requirements. A small proportion were underweight (6 per cent of women and 3 per cent of men, having a BMI of less than 20). If older people have low energy intakes, their diets could also be deficient in other nutrients.

For older people the main concerns from a nutritional perspective were the relatively high saturated fat content of the diet (14.6 per cent of food energy for men and 15.3 per cent for women; these levels exceeding COMA recommended levels of 11 per cent; DoH, 1991), low vitamin D intake and high levels of anaemia. High levels of salt intake were also a concern. Eleven per cent of women and 9 per cent of men were anaemic, and these rose to 37 per cent of women and 16 per cent of men aged 85 and over.

A new report from GNASH (Group on Nutrition and Sheltered Housing 2009) led by BAPEN has established that 14 per cent (about 1 in 8) of people living in sheltered housing in England are at risk of malnutrition, with 9 per cent at high risk.

Risks factors for poor nutrition

Reduced consumption of fruit and vegetables in low income groups results in lower intakes of antioxidants and other vitamins and minerals (Donkin et al., 1998; Finch et al., 1998). The evidence base means that the association between low income and a poor diet is indisputable (e.g. Lilley and Hunt, 1998). Other risk factors for poor nutrition are indicated in Table 8.4, along with possible solutions that could be considered or provided by nurses.

Food safety

Food-borne illnesses affect large numbers of older people each year. These are estimated to affect 3.5 million British, 76 million US and 130 million European older people (Gettings,

Risk to adequate diet	*Possible solutions*
Poverty	Refer for benefits check
Bereavement and loss	Social support, bereavement counselling
Poor access to low-cost and nutritious food	Supporting community food schemes
Transport problems	Schemes such as 'Dial a Ride'
Inability to shop for themselves	Referral to voluntary sector for support/assistance
Social isolation	Information about community lunch groups/other opportunities to socialize in the community
Poor motivation to cook for themselves	Information about community lunch groups Encouragement to cook for friends/family
Unable to cook for themselves	Information about 'Meals on Wheels' and other food delivery schemes
Poor cooking skills	Community education classes
Poor nutritional knowledge	Culturally appropriate health education advice, including written information

Table 8.4 Some risk factors for poor nutrition in community dwelling older people

Food practice
Fridge not at 5°C or less
Eating soft cheeses, paté
Using unpasturized milk and milk products
Storing raw meats uncovered near cooked food
Contamination of cooked food with raw, through not thoroughly cleaning preparation surfaces, knives, and so on in hot soapy water
Eating raw/undercooked eggs

Table 8.5 Some risky food practices

2009). Risks of developing food-borne illnesses increase with age, and the consequences of contracting these infections are more severe than in younger adults. Recently, the UK Food Standards Agency has reported that one of these diseases – listeriosis bacteraemia – has increased three-fold from the 1990s to the present for those aged 60 or above in England and Wales (Food Standards Agency (FSA), 2008). Worryingly, some of these infections were contracted during stays in hospitals and care homes.

For listeriosis bacteraemia, consumption of contaminated food is thought to be the main route of infection. Ready-to-eat foods with an extended shelf life such as cooked meats, paté and sandwiches are thought to be the main contaminated foods. Other pathogens which are cause for concern in older people include: Campylobacter, Salmonella, E. Coli and Novovirus.

Food safety in the home is affected by both the knowledge and practice of food safety handling techniques. Research has found discrepancies between food safety knowledge and self-reported behaviour (Williamson et al., 1992) as individuals tend to feel safe when handling food in their own home. However, Worsfeld and Griffiths (1997) estimate that 60 per cent of all food poisoning occurs in the home.

Other factors increasing risk include:

- medications with immunosuppressant effects, (including statins) (Bitar and Patil, 2004);
- overuse of H2-receptor antagonist medication and antacids and prolonged use of antibiotics;
- changes in intestinal motility and production of antibodies in the gut (Buzby, 2002);
- changes in sensitivity to taste and smell as well as visual acuity (Nordin, 2009).

Diminished eyesight can contribute to reducing food safety, as food labelling on packaging is often illegible to the older person (Hudson and Hartwell, 2002). There is also poor understanding of food labelling which affects adherence to 'sell by' and 'use by' dates on food which is affected by their relatively recent introduction – within older people's lifetimes (Dickinson, 1999).

There is clearly a role to play for health professionals in providing information about the risks associated with food (see Table 8.5), and their prevention through proper food storage and food preparation.

Further information can be obtained from local Environmental Health Departments (UK), the Food Standards Agency (UK) (www.food.gov.uk/safereating), and the US Department of Agriculture's (USDA) food safety inspection service, www.fsis.usda.gov.

Healthy nutrition in primary care settings

We begin this section with a scenario.

Scenario 8.2

Jenny lives alone in her house in the countryside. Because the shops are quite far away and she has no transport, she shops infrequently, and buys little food when she does.

Her current weight is 49 kg and her height is 1.4 metres.

- *What is her current BMI?*
- *What is her MUST score?*
- *What immediate action would you take?*
- *What would be your longer-term action plan?*
- *How would you evaluate the effectiveness of your plan?*

There is a clear case for opportunistic nutritional screening of older people when they come into contact with primary care services so that appropriate interventions and health promotion activities can be focused on those who need them.

Standard eight of the UK *National Service Framework for Older People* (NSFOP) (DoH, 2001) highlights the importance of health promotion activities with older people, activities which are further emphasized in the UK government white paper, *Our Health, Our Care, Our Say* (DoH, 2006). Nutrition is also one of the domains included in the UK single assessment process (DoH, 2001).

Practice nurses may be ideally placed to develop their health promotion skills within primary health care, and may be perceived by patients to be more approachable than GPs. Health visitors are trained to undertake health education and health promotion activities within the community. However, much of their work is with families with children under the age of five years (Pursey and Luker, 1993). There is currently no requirement to offer routine health screening to older people within the UK through the Quality Outcome Framework (DoH, 2003), a national pay for performance scheme that rewards GP practices on the basis of the quality of the care they provide to their patients as measured through achievement on a series of clinical indicators. This incentivizes GP practices through financial reward for achieving targets which include health promotion activities such as smoking cessation. However, lack of a specific target does not preclude health promoting activities.

Influences on uptake of nutrition education programmes

A review of what components influence the successful uptake of nutrition education programmes has identified the following factors (Sahyoun and Anderson, 2009):

- Objectives/messages should be:
  - tailored to individual needs;
  - clear;
  - simple;

(*continued*)

  - practical;
  - limited in number.
- frequent access to well-trained health professionals;
- participant involvement in goal-setting;
- behaviour modification based on theoretical models;
- material incentives;
- creation of support groups;
- recruitment of significant others;
- enlistment of local grocery stores.

Healthy nutrition in hospital settings

Scenario 8.3

Mr Miller was admitted to the ward with a chest infection. He has COPD and has lost 10 kg over the last three months. He is currently being treated with antibiotics which make him feel nauseous.

His current weight is 59 kg and his height is 1.8 metres.

- *What is his current BMI?*
- *What is his MUST score?*
- *What immediate action would you take?*
- *What would be your longer term action plan?*
- *How would you evaluate the effectiveness of your plan?*

Poor nutrition has been recognized as a problem in the hospital setting for decades (e.g. see Hill et al., 1977; Coates, 1985; Lennard-Jones, 1992; McWhirter and Pennington, 1994). Many years before this Florence Nightingale was concerned about patient nutrition and highlighted the important role nurses had to play in improving matters in her book *Notes on Nursing* (Nightingale, 1860).

Older patients are especially susceptible to undernutrition (Lehmann et al., 1991; Tierney, 1996). In addition to the consequences of poor nutrition discussed previously in this chapter, undernutrition increases both the length of hospital stay and the chance of readmission (Department of Health, 2001). Figures from 2008 estimate the prevalence of poor nutrition on admission to acute, mental health and care home settings at 28 per cent in the UK. This varied depending on where patients were admitted from, with levels as high as 52 per cent for patients admitted to hospital from a care home, and 32 per cent of those aged over 65 were malnourished (BAPEN, 2009). However, although knowledge of the prevalence of undernutrition in institutional settings is widely available, the problem remains.

Over the years a number of reasons have been proposed for undernutrition in hospitals. These include the notion that nurses have become less actively involved with mealtimes in recent years, often due to changes in meal delivery systems divorcing nurses from both the process of mealtimes and the associated patient care (Carr and Mitchell, 1991) and the demise of the hospital matron (Department of Health, 2003). Others argue that poor hospital food and inflexible catering (Association of Community Health Councils, 1997), and inadequate nutritional education of both nursing (Palmer, 1998) and medical staff (Royal College of Physicians, 2002) contribute. Currently, responsibilities around food, mealtimes and nutrition are complex and ill defined (Manthorpe and Watson, 2003) with different tasks falling across and between both professional disciplines and departments (Leat, 1998). Helping patients with eating is frequently delegated to less qualified staff, which can further reinforce the idea that mealtime care is an unskilled and unimportant activity.

Others have commentated on the impact that the historical origins of older people's care continues to have on current practice, with the needs of older people taking second place to those of the organization (e.g. McCormack, 2004).

Eating 'space'

Another important, and neglected aspect of mealtimes, is the space in which eating takes place. Institutions 'are symbolically associated with the loss of autonomy and independence' (Wiles, 2005: 105). Recently, there have been calls for work to explore and understand the importance of place to the experiences of older people as well as the nurses caring for them (Wiles, 2005; Andrews et al., 2005). Many hospital wards have 'lost' dayrooms and dining rooms – spaces where patients could eat together away from the hospital bed. Recently, evidence has shown that people eat significantly more when they eat together (e.g. Nijs et al., 2006; Wright et al., 2006).

Solutions to the problem have focused on developing and using tools to identify those patients at risk of undernutrition (Lehmann, 1989; Lennard-Jones, 1992; Closs, 1993), using specific interventions, such as refeeding regimens (Lehmann, 1989) and supplemental feeds (Bastow et al., 1983; Delmi et al., 1990; Woo et al., 1994), and improving hospital food, introduced in the NHS Plan outlined by the Department of Health (2000). More recently, the UK DoH (2003) have developed an initiative that aims to improve standards of fundamental aspects of care through the use of a benchmarking tool; benchmark three focuses on food and nutrition and was discussed earlier. In the UK, the issue of patient nutrition now falls under the direction of the National Patient Safety Agency (NPSA). Other initiatives supported by organizations such as Age UK through campaigns including 'Hungry to be heard' include the use of protected mealtimes and serving meals on 'red trays' to alert staff to a patient's need for help.

Hickson et al. (2004) introduced health care assistants who were supernumerary and had been trained to assist with feeding into the hospital setting. However, this intervention failed to have any impact on nutritional status or length of hospital stay for patients. They concluded that improving nutritional care is 'not as simple as employing more staff' (p. 77). Approaches of this type are also unlikely to be feasible in the current economic climate and are unlikely to re-engage nurses with the complexities of mealtime care.

Applying evidence to practice

The application of nutritional evidence to practice can be difficult; for example, Gosney (2003) found that supplemental feeds are wasted more often than they are drunk, and introducing nutritional assessment on its own does little to improve practice at mealtimes or nutritional status (Jordan et al., 2003). Although the idea of protected mealtimes is presented as a new idea, Florence Nightingale could be seen as the originator of this idea. As early as 1859, she wrote: 'Nothing shall be done on a ward whilst patients are having their meal'.

Thus, although there is some evidence on which to base changes in practice, and the policies and initiatives offer structures and processes, the problem at the frontline of practice remains. Food still fails to reach the stomachs of patients, indicating that the complexity of mealtime care in institutional settings has not been sufficiently addressed. However, eating is a complex activity with associated social, psychological and biological aspects, and hospital mealtimes take place within the complex arena of, and thus are influenced by, clinical practice that has been described as a 'swampy lowland' (Schön, 1983).

If the patients' experience of mealtimes is to be improved, it is important that nurses become re-engaged in the process. The importance of food and mealtimes has to be recognized and prioritized by all members of the multidisciplinary team as well as the individual departments which impact on nutritional care. Cultural changes may also be necessary. This may feel like an impossible task. However, it is possible to make changes to improve patient's mealtime experience (e.g. Dickinson et al., 2008).

Key point

The importance of food and mealtimes has to be recognized and prioritized by all members of the multidisciplinary team.

Nursing interventions

Campaigns such as that being led by the UK Royal College of Nursing highlight a number of interventions that nurses can be involved in.

Activities which could be considered by nurses wishing to improve patient care at mealtimes include:

- nutritional screening;
- 'red tray' system;
- protected mealtimes;
- ensuring nursing staff are available to assist patients who need help;
- training and education;
- improving the mealtime environment;
- administration of prescribed supplements;
- provision of adapted equipment if required;
- provision of handwashing facilities before meals;
- use of volunteers to support mealtime care;
- essence of care benchmarking.

In summary, nurses working in hospital settings *can* make a difference to patients' experience of mealtimes, eating, and thus nutritional status, and are ideally placed to screen patients to identify those at nutritional risk.

Care home settings

We begin this section with a scenario.

Scenario 8.4

Mrs Jones, aged 79, has been admitted to the care home directly from the hospital setting and is very tearful and distressed when you meet her on arrival. She was admitted to the acute hospital following a stroke, which has left her without function in the limbs on the right side of her body. She is right-handed and embarrassed by what she perceives to be the messiness of her eating – she frequently spills food onto her clothes while attempting to feed herself. During her hospital stay of four weeks she has lost 8 kg and now weighs 44 kg. She is unable to stand, so her height has been estimated at 1.58 m using a proxy measure of her knee height.

Her family are very concerned at her weight loss and her low mood, which they think is contributing to her poor appetite. Before the stroke she was very active, and helped to care for her neighbours for whom she would do shopping and provide other help.

- *What screening/assessments would you undertake?*
- *What would be your immediate plan of care?*
- *How would you evaluate the effectiveness of the care you provide?*

Background

Older people who live in care homes can enjoy a good quality of life; however, they have high levels of health care need, due mainly to chronic, progressive disease and multiple disabilities, which often includes cognitive as well as physical difficulties (Help the Aged, 2007).

The most recent UK BAPEN survey (BAPEN, 2009) found that 42 per cent of people on admission to care homes were 'malnourished'. In a study in Finland (Suominen et al., 2005) one-third (29 per cent) of the studied residents suffered from malnutrition, and 60 per cent were at risk. Staff working in care home settings should be aware that almost half of their residents will be malnourished as they arrive into the setting. This requires immediate assessment, followed by a plan of action, evaluation and monitoring (Kumlien and Axelsson, 2002).

Often poor nutrition is a result of disease processes, but frequently is caused by difficulties with eating and the nutritional care received. For example, a study in Sweden (Kumlien and Axelsson, 2002) found that more than 80 per cent of residents with strokes in nursing homes were assessed as having dependence in eating. Residents had between one and seven different eating disabilities. Dysphagia was reported in almost a quarter of the residents with stroke and almost a third had poor food intake or poor appetite. Despite these difficulties, few weights were documented in the nursing records and there were no nutritional records.

However, despite the often bleak picture painted of nutrition in care homes, there are examples of good practice and care; for example, providing fresh, wholesome food and paying attention to the needs of residents as a central aspect of care (Jones, 2006).

There is a great deal that nurses can do to improve the nutritional status of older people in care homes.

Assistance with eating

Some studies have shown that many residents need help with eating, but this is frequently not given (Kayser-Jones and Schell, 1997). The time taken to help someone to eat can average less than 10 minutes per resident. Help is frequently physical, with neglect of verbal prompting or social stimulation which can increase both independence and quality of life during mealtimes (Simmons and Rahman, 2009).

A number of interventions have resulted in improved food intake. Residents with all types of eating difficulties have been found to require 35–40 minutes of staff time per meal (Simmons et al., 2007). Grouping residents who need help together increases efficiency of feeding assistance. Training non-nursing staff who work in care homes to assist at mealtimes to work as 'feeding assistants' was one development used successfully in the USA. The quality of care provided compared favourably with the level of care given by care assistants (Simmons et al., 2007). Residents eat more if encouraged to eat together in the dining room, and are more likely to receive help from staff and have their food intake documented accurately (Simmons and Levy-Storms, 2006). Other activities which can improve care include:

- giving liquid dietary supplements between meals rather than with meals;
- providing opportunities for the daily outdoor exposure necessary for sun exposure – (vitamin D) (Cederholm, 2009);
- observing residents' reaction to provided foods (they often do not like to complain if they do not like the food they are served);
- improving the ambience of food consumption (improves nutritional status and stabilizes the health of nursing home residents) (Mathey et al., 2001).

In summary, interventions to improve food intake need to focus on improving quality of life as well as quality of mealtime care.

Overview of nutritional care

Interventions by nurses need to be tailored to both the population group they are working with, and individuals within these broad demographic groups. A diagrammatic summary of both the needs of older people and health professional response at each of the levels are summarized in Figure 8.1. The pyramidal approach demonstrates that most older people will be living in their own homes, and the focus of health professionals working in these settings should aim to promote independence and health. At the top of the pyramid are older people in long-term care settings who will have very different needs, and are often dependent on the physical support provided by caregivers.

Older people with cognitive problems including dementia

Difficulties with eating develop in the later stages of dementia and frequently result in a great deal of distress to families and carers. A report by the Alzheimer's Society (2000) shows that around 80 per cent of persons with dementia have eating difficulties that place them at risk from malnutrition. Because of this risk, the usual focus of care is on increasing calorie intake, but carers often struggle with this task and mealtimes and eating become a source of stress and tension in the caregiving relationship. Common eating problems associated with dementia that can lead to poor nutrition include forgetting to eat, forgetting that they have just eaten, failing to recognize food items and eating things that are not food. Difficulties with tasks such as removing food packaging, knowing what utensils are for and

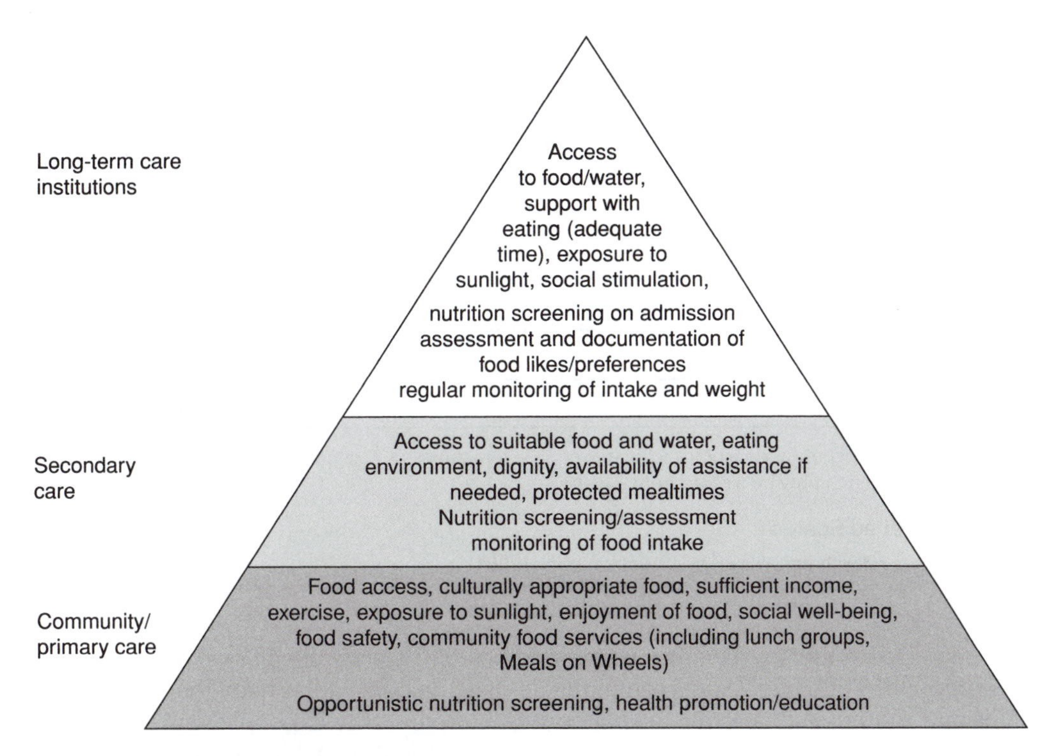

Figure 8.1: A pyramidal approach to nutritional care

using them, moving food or fluid to their mouth, chewing and swallowing problems may also be present. There may be difficulty initiating the eating process, or they may start eating, get distracted, and fail to finish (Trinkle et al., 1992).

Other factors which affect nutritional intake in the general population also affect those with dementia, but their cognitive and communication difficulties may make it harder for them to cope with them. Patients with dementia may not be able tell anyone they are hungry or that they need help with eating or more time to chew and swallow. When people try to help with eating, some patients with dementia will resist, by pushing the food away, refusing to open their mouths, or spitting food out (Watson et al., 2001).

If older people move to an unfamiliar environment, existing eating difficulties are likely to worsen in the new setting (this includes settings such as a hospital or care home) due to unfamiliar place, and different mealtime routines and foods. However, social skills can be preserved, even in the later stages of dementia. Continuing to observe the rituals associated with mealtimes, such as setting the table and eating with others, can provide essential cues to eating for people with cognitive impairment.

Assessment of eating difficulties of people with dementia

The Edinburgh Feeding Scale (The EdFed Scale #2) (Watson et al., 2001; see Figure 8.2) is a tool which enables practitioners to determine the level of impairment with eating as well as evaluate the need for possible psychosocial and clinical interventions, such as

Item	*Never* (Score 1)	*Sometimes* (Score 2)	*Often* (Score 3)
Leaving mouth open			
Refusing to swallow			
Spitting			
Turning head away			
Refusing to open mouth			
Refusing to eat			
Total			

Scoring: Items are scored on a 3-point scale (never = 1; sometimes = 2; often = 3) and the individual item scores are summed to provide a score from 3 to 18.

Figure 8.2: EdFed Scale #2

Source: Reproduced with permission from Watson et al. (2001)

referrals for speech therapy, environmental modification, dietary alterations, environmental modification, diet alterations, and communication techniques. It has been found to be a reliable and valid tool to describe the pattern of eating difficulty in people with dementia (Watson et al., 2001). Repeating the assessment over time also enables reassessment and documentation of level of function and planning of suitable care.

The use of the tool ensures that observation of the patient is as unobtrusive as possible. It is recommended that the person completing the assessment does not actually assist with the meal being observed or interact with the patient/carer during the observation. The meal being observed should also take place where the person usually eats. The observer should note how often (or if) the specific behaviours described in the tool occur during the meal. After the observation, the observer should talk to the patient's caregiver to check how often and under what circumstances the observed behaviours occur in order to complete the baseline assessment.

For institutional settings, undertaking Dementia Care Mapping (Brooker, 2005) will provide additional contextual information about both the environment and a measure of how person centred care at mealtimes is.

Specific nursing interventions for dementia

Green and Watson (2006) undertook a systematic review of interventions which could enable nurses to help older people with dementia to eat. A number of interventions were found to have been studied, including changing meal service systems, staff assignment, introducing nutritional assessment and subsequent food provision, changing food texture, occupational and behavioural interventions, using music and making environmental changes to dining rooms. They concluded that the current evidence for the effectiveness of interventions is poor and argued for further studies, both qualitative and quantitative.

Some of the studies identified showed some promise, such as those suggesting that dinner music, particularly soothing music, can reduce irritability, fear or panic and depressed mood and can stimulate patients with dementia in a nursing-home ward to eating more (Ragneskog et al., 1999). Music also affected the behaviour of staff, increasing the time they spent with older people and possibly increasing the amount of food they served (Ragneskog et al., 1996). Changing meal patterns could be of benefit if the changes increased communication between older people with dementia and between them and nurses.

There is also evidence that nurses' interpretations of the aversive behaviour of patients with dementia relating to eating differ (Pasman et al., 2003). The authors recommended that the behaviour of particular patients should be discussed by nurses with each other, physicians, other disciplines and the patient's family to obtain more insight into all its potential causes and to determine together the most likely interpretation and appropriate way in which to deal with the aversive behaviour. This could give nurses more confidence and improve the quality and continuity of care provided.

More recently, providing training to nursing assistants improved their knowledge, attitudes and behaviour and increased the eating time for patients with dementia (Chang and Lin, 2005). Young et al. (2005) found that increasing the carbohydrate content of dinner increases food intake for people with dementia. Interestingly, Dunne et al. (2004) found that food and liquid intake increased by a mean 25 per cent for food and 84 per cent for liquid, through using a simple and inexpensive intervention of introducing high contrast tableware (red and blue) for patients with advanced Alzheimer's disease.

Use of finger food is recommended for people with dementia who have difficulty using utensils or who are reluctant to sit down to eat so they can eat as they walk. Food and snacks should be readily available (Voices, 1998).

End of life, eating and dementia

Food and eating often present ethical dilemmas, particularly towards the end of life (Aveyard, 2000; Barratt, 2000). Wasson et al., 2001 advise involving all members of the multidiscliplinary team, including speech and language therapists and dieticians, and make the following specific recommendations for providing food to people in end-stage dementia:

- Think about whether the cessation of eating is linked to an overall deterioration.
- Exclude the possibility of infections that could affect cognitive ability, willingness to eat and that may require treatment.
- If the patient appears to be dying, although not immediately, continue to offer small amounts of food and fluids without giving up too easily or using undue force.

In summary, although there are no definitive answers of which interventions have most to contribute to the improved nutritional care of older people with cognitive problems and dementia, and which are supported by a strong evidence base, there are clearly activities which can make a difference to the individual experiences of this patient group. Interventions to support the diverse and changing needs of this group of people are likely to be multifactorial and there is unlikely ever to be a one-size-fits-all intervention. More research is clearly needed but, in the meantime, there is scope for imaginative and creative nursing practice which supports the dignity and needs of older people and their family carers.

Conclusion

Eating is a complex activity with social, psychological and biological aspects. Therefore any attempt to improve the health of older people through better nutritional care has to draw on a broad evidence base and take a wide focus in order to address this complexity. Acknowledgement of this complexity, as well as the recognition that changing practice is far from a straightforward and linear process, needs to underpin any changes to clinical practice which I hope reading this chapter has inspired you to consider.

This chapter has touched lightly on the complex subject of nutrition in older people. The chapter has not considered the specific dietary needs of people with long-term conditions, such as diabetes, who require specific nutritional advice and care. There is much research still to be done, but even that which we do know is too broad and vast to be covered in one chapter.

Florence Nightingale should perhaps have the final words of this chapter, which highlights the fact that nutritional care has been an issue of concern throughout the history of modern nursing practice.

> “If the nurse is an intelligent being, and not a mere carrier of diets to and from the patient, let her exercise her intelligence in these things.
>
> (Nightingale, 1860)”

References

Alzheimer's Society (2000) *Food for Thought*. London: Alzheimer's Society.

Andrews, G., McCormack, B. and Reed, J. (2005) Editorial: the importance of place in older people's care: three papers developing the geographies of nursing work, *International Journal of Older People Nursing*, 14(8b): 98–99.

Association of Community Health Councils (1997) *Hungry in Hospital?* London: Association of Community Health Councils for England and Wales.

Aveyard, H. (2001) Is there a concept of autonomy that can usefully inform nursing practice? *Journal of Advanced Nursing*, 32(2): 352–58.

BAPEN (2003) *Malnutrition Universal Screening Tool* (MUST). Available online at www.bapen.org.uk/pdfs/must_full.pdf.

BAPEN (2009) *Combating Malnutrition: Recommendations For Action. Report From The Advisory Group On Malnutrition*. Redditch: BAPEN.

Barratt, J. (2000) A patient with Alzheimer's disease, fed via percutaneous endoscopic gastrostomy with personal reflections on some of the ethical issues arising from this case, *Journal of Human Nutrition and Dietetics*, 13(1): 51–54.

Bastow, M.D., Rawlings, J. and Allison, S.P. (1983) Benefits of supplementary feeding after fractured neck of femur: a randomised controlled trial, *British Medical Journal*, 287: 1589–92.

Beck, A. and Ovesen, L. (1998) At which body mass index and degree of weight loss should hospitalised elderly patients be considered at nutritional risk? *Clinical Nutrition*, 17: 195–98.

Bischoff-Ferrari, H.A., Dawson-Hughes, B. and Willett, W.C. et al. (2004) Effect of vitamin D on falls: a meta-analysis, *Journal of the American Medical Association*, 291: 1999–2006.

Bitar, K.N. and Patil, S.B. (2004) Ageing and gastrointestinal smooth muscle, *Mechanisms of Ageing and Development*, 125(12): 907–10.

Booth, D.A. (1994) *Psychology of Nutrition*. London: Taylor & Francis.

Brooker, D. (2005) Dementia care mapping: a review of the research literature, *The Gerontologist*, 45(special issue 1): 11–18.

Buzby, J.C. (2002) Older adults at risk of complications from microbial foodborne illness, *Food Review*, 25(2): 30–35.

Carr, E.K. and Mitchell, J.R.A. (1991) A comparison of the mealtime care given to patients by nurses using two different meal delivery systems, *International Journal of Nursing Studies*, 28(1): 19–25.

Cederholm, T. (2009) Nutrition and bone health in the elderly, in M. Raats, L. de Groot and W. van Staveren (eds) *Food for the Ageing Population*. Woodhead Publishing, Cambridge: 252–70.

Chang, C-C. and Lin, L-C. (2005) Effects of a feeding skills training programme on nursing assistants and dementia patients, *Journal of Clinical Nursing*, 14(10): 1185–92.

Closs, S.J. (1993) Malnutrition: the key to pressure sores? *Nursing Standard*, 8(4): 32–36.

Coates, V. (1985) *Are they Being Served?* London: Royal College of Nursing.

de Morais, C., Afonso, C. and de Almeida, V. (2009) Older people's consumtion of alcoholic beverages: the social significance and health implications, in M. Raats, L. de Groot and W. van Staveren (eds) *Food for the Ageing Population* (pp. 128–52). Cambridge: Woodhead Publishing.

Delmi, M., Rapin, C.H., Bengoa, P.D. et al. (1990) Dietary supplementation in elderly patients with fractured neck of femur, *Lancet,* i: 1013–16.

Department of Health (DoH) (1991) *Dietary Reference Values for Food Energy and Nutrients for the United Kingdom. Report on Health and Social Subjects, No 41* London: Her Majesty's Stationery Office (HMSO).

Department of Health (DoH) (2000) *NHS Plan*. London: DoH.

Department of Health (DoH) (2001) *National Service Framework for Older People*. London: DoH.

Department of Health (2003) *Essence of Care*. London: DoH.

Department of Health (DoH) (2006) *Our Health, Our Care, Our Say: A New Direction for Community Services*. London: Her Majesty's Stationery Office (HMSO).

Department of Health and Social Security (DHSS) (1979) *Nutrition and Health in Old Age. Report on Health and Social Subjects, No. 16)* London: HMSO.

Dickinson, A. (1999) The food choices and eating habits of older people: a grounded theory. Unpublished PhD Thesis, Buckinghamshire Chilterns University College.

Dickinson, A., Welch, C. and Ager, L. (2008) No longer hungry in hospital: improving the hospital mealtime experience for older people through Action Research, *Journal of Clinical Nursing*, 17(11): 1492–502.

Donkin, A.J.M., Johnson, A.E., Lilley, J.M., Morgan, K., Neale, R.J., Page, R., and Silburn, R.L. (1998) Gender and living alone as determinants of fruit and vegetable consumption among elderly people living alone in urban Nottingham, *Appetite*, 30: 39–51.

Dunne, T.E., Neargarder, S.A., Cipollonid, P.B., Cronin-Golombc, A. (2004) Visual contrast enhances food and liquid intake in advanced Alzheimer's disease, *Clinical Nutrition*, 23: 533–38.

Evenson, K., Rosamund, W., Cai, J. et al. (2002) Influence of retirement on leisure-time physical activity: The Atherosclerosis Risk in Communities Study, *American Journal of Epidemiology*, 155: 692–99.

Fieldhouse, P. (1995) *Food and Nutrition: Customs and Culture*, 2nd edn. London: Chapman & Hall.

Finch, S., Doyle, W., Lowe, C., Bates, C.J., Prentice, A., Smithers, G. and Clarke, P.C. (1998) *National Diet and Nutrition Survey: People Aged 65 Years and Over*. London: The Stationery Office.

Food Standards Agency Advisory Committee on the Microbiological Safety of Food (2008) Report on the Increased Incidence of Listeriosis in the UK. FSA.

Germov, J. and Williams, L. (1996) The epidemic of dieting women: the need for a sociological approach to food and nutrition, *Appetite*, 27: 97–108.

Gettings, M.A. (2009) Food safety and older people, in M. Raats, L. de Groot and W. van Staveren (eds) *Food for the Ageing Population* (pp. 501–24). Cambridge: Woodhead Publishing.

Gosney, M. (2003) Are we wasting our money on food supplements in elder care wards?, *Journal of Advanced Nursing*, 43(3): 275–80.

Green, S.M. and Watson, R. (2006) Nutritional screening and assessment tools for use by nurses: literature review, *Journal of Advanced Nursing*, 54(4): 477–90.

Group on Nutrition and Sheltered Housing (GNASH) (2009) *Screening for Malnutrition in Sheltered Housing*. Redditch: BAPEN.

Help the Aged (2007) *Quality of Life in Care Homes: A Review of the Literature* (prepared for Help the Aged by The National Care Homes Research and Development Forum). London: Help the Aged.

Hickson, M., Bulpitt, C., Nunes, M., Peters, R., Cooke, J., Nicholl, C. and Frost, G. (2004) Does additional feeding support provided by health care assistants improve nutritional status and outcome in acutely ill older in-patients? – A randomised controlled trial, *Clinical Nutrition*, 23: 69–77.

Hill, G.L., Pickford, I. and Young, G.A. (1977) Malnutrition in surgical patients: an unrecognised problem, *Lancet*, i: 689–92.

Hudson, P.K. and Hartwell, H.J. (2002) Food safety awareness of older people at home: a pilot study, *Journal of the Royal Society for the Promotion of Health*, 122(3): 165–69.

Jones, V. (2006) Fresh inspiration, *The Guardian*, Wednesday, 17 May. Available online at www.guardian.co.uk/society/2006/may/17/longtermcare.guardiansocietysupplement; accessed December 2010.

Jordan, S., Snow, D., Hayes, C. et al. (2003) Introducing a nutrition screening tool: an explanatory study in a district general hospital, *Journal of Advanced Nursing*, 44(1): 12–23.

Kayser-Jones, J. and Schell, E. (1997) The effect of staffing on the quality of care at mealtime, *Nursing Outlook*, 45: 64–72.

Kumlien, S. and Axelsson, K. (2002) Stroke patients in nursing homes: eating, feeding, nutrition and related care, *Journal of Clinical Nursing*, 11(4): 498–509.

Leat, D. (1998) Food choice and the British system of formal and informal welfare provision: questions for research, in A. Murcott (ed.) *The Nation's Diet* (pp. 289–301). London: Longmans.

Lehmann, A.B. (1989) Review: undernutrition in elderly people, *Age and Ageing*, 18: 339–53.

Lehmann, A.B., Bassey, E.J., Morgan, K. and Dallosso, H.M. (1991) Normal values for weight, skeletal size and body mass indices in 890 men and women aged over 65 years, *Clinical Nutrition*, 10: 18–22.

Lennard-Jones, J.E. (1992) A positive approach to nutrition as a treatment. Report of a working party on the role of enteral and parenteral feeding in hospital and at home, London: King's Fund.

Lilley, J. and Hunt, P. (1998) *Opportunities for and Barriers to Change in Dietary Behaviour in Elderly People*. London: HEA.

Logue, A.W. (1986) *Psychology of Eating and Drinking*. New York: W.H. Freeman.

Lupton, D. (1996) *Food, the Body and the Self*. London: Sage Publications.

Manthorpe, J. and Watson, R. (2003) Poorly served? Eating and dementia, *Journal of Advanced Nursing*, 41(2): 162–69.

Mathey, M-F., Vanneste, V.G., de Graaf, C., de Groot, L., and van Staveren, W.A. (2001) Health effect of improved meal ambiance in a Dutch nursing home: a 1-year intervention study, *Preventive Medicine*, 32(5): 416–23.

McCormack, B. (2004) Person-centredness in gerontological nursing: an overview of the literature, *International Journal of Older People Nursing*, 13(3a): 31–38.

McWhirter, J.P. and Pennington, C.R. (1994) Incidence and recognition of malnutrition in hospital, *British Medical Journal*, 308: 945–48.

Morley, J.E. (1997) Anorexia of aging: physiologic and pathologic, *American Journal of Clinical Nutrition*, 66: 760–73.

Morley, J.E. and van Staveren, W.A. (2009) Undernutrition: diagnosis, causes, consequences and treatment, in M. Raats, L. de Groot and W. van Staveren (eds) *Food for the Ageing Population* (pp. 153–68). Cambridge: Woodhead Publishing.

Nightingale, F. (1860) *Notes on Nursing. What It Is, and What It Is Not*. New York: Appleton & Co. Available online at www.digital.library.upenn.edu/women/nightingale/nursing/nursing.html; accessed December 2010.

Nijs, K.A.N.D., de Graaf, C., Kok, F.J., and van Staveren, W.A. (2006) Effect of family style mealtimes on quality of life, physical performance, and body weight of nursing home residents: cluster randomised controlled trial, *British Medical Journals*, 332: 1180–184.

Nordin, S. (2009) Sensory perception of food and ageing, in M. Raats, L. de Groot and W. van Staveren (eds) *Food for the Ageing Population* (pp. 73–94). Great Abingdon: Woodhead Publishing.

Palmer, D. (1998) The persisting problem of malnutrition in healthcare, *Journal of Advanced Nursing*, 28(5): 931–32.

Pasman, H. R. W., The, A. M., On wuteaka-Philipsen, B.D., van der Wal, G. and Ribbe, M.W. (2003) Feeding nursing home patients with severe dementia: a qualitative study, *Journal of Advanced Nursing*, 42(3): 304–11.

Pursey, A.C. and Luker, K.A. (1993) Assessment of older people at home: a missed opportunity? in J. Wilson-Barnet and J. Macleod Clark (eds) *Research in Health Promotion and Nursing* (pp. 132–39). London: Macmillan Press.

Ragneskog, H., Bråne, G., Karlsson, I. and Kihlgren, M. (1996) Influence of dinner music on food intake and symptoms common in dementia, *Scandinavian Journal of Caring Sciences*, 10(1): 11–17.

Ragneskog, H., Kilgrhen, M., Karlosson, I. and Norberg, A. (1999) Dinner music for demented patients, *Clinical Nursing Research*, 5: 262–82.

Royal College of Nursing (RCN) and National Patient Safety Agency (NPSA) (2007) *Water for Health: Hydration Best Practice Toolkit for Hospitals and Healthcare*. London: Royal College of Nursing.

Royal College of Physicians (2002) *Nutrition and Patients: a Doctor's Responsibility*. London: Royal College of Physicians.

Sahyoun, N.R. and Anderson, A.L. (2009) Developing nutrition education for older people, in M. Raats, L. de Groot and W. van Staveren (eds) *Food for the Ageing Population* (pp. 525–38). Cambridge: Woodhead Publishing.

Schön, D.A. (1983) *The Reflective Practitioner*. London: Temple Smith.

Shepherd, R. and Raats, M.M. (1996) Attitudes and beliefs in food habits, in H.L. Meiselman and H.J.H. MacFie (eds) *Food Choice, Acceptance and Consumption* (pp. 346–64). London: Blackie Academic and Professional.

Sidell, M. (1995) *Health in Old Age: Myth, Mystery and Management*. Maidenhead: Open University Press.

Simmons, S.F. and Levy-Storms, L. (2006) The effect of dining location on nutritional care quality in care homes, *Journal of Nutrition, Health and Aging*, 9(6): 434–39.

Simmons, S.F. and Rahman, A. (2009) Quality of feeding assistance care in nursing homes, in M. Raats, L. de Groot and W. van Staveren (eds) *Food for the Ageing Population* (pp. 539–59). Cambridge: Woodhead Publishing.

Simmons, S.F., Bertrand, R., Shier, V., Sweetland, R., Moore, T., Hurd, D. and Schnelle, J.F. (2007) A preliminary evaluation of the Paid Feeding Assistant regulation: impact on feeding assistance care process quality in nursing homes, *The Gerontologist*, 47(2): 184–92.

Stanner, S., Thompson, R. and Buttriss, J.L. (eds) (2009) *Healthy Ageing: The Role of Nutrition and Lifestyle*. Chichester: Wiley.

Suominen, M., Muurinen, S., Routasalo, F., Soini, H., Suur-Uski, I., Peiponen, A., Finne-Soveri, H. and Pitkala, K.H. (2005) Malnutrition and associated factors among aged residents in all nursing homes in Helsinki, *European Journal of Clinical Nutrition*, 59: 578–83.

Tierney, A.J. (1996) Undernutrition and elderly hospital patients: a review, *Journal of Advanced Nursing*, 23: 228–36.

Trinkle, D.B., Burns, A., Levy, H. (1992) Brief report: abnormal eating behaviour in dementia – a descriptive study, *International Journal of Geriatric Psychiatry*, 7: 799–803.

Van Esterik, P. (1997) Women and nurture in industrialised societies, *Proceedings of the Nutrition Society*, 56: 335–43.

Voices (1998) Eating well for older people with dementia: a good practice guide for residential and nursing homes and others involved in caring for older people with dementia. *London: Voices and Gardner Merchant Healthcare Services*.

Wasson, K., Tate, H. and Hayes, C. (2001) Food refusal and dysphagia in older people with dementia: ethical and practical issues, *International Journal of Palliative Nursing*, 7(10): 465–71.

Watson, R., Green, S.M. and Legg, L. (2001) The Edinburgh Feeding Evaluation in Dementia Scale #2 (EdFED #2): inter- and intra-rater reliability, *Clinical Effectiveness in Nursing*, 5(4): 84–96.

Wiles, J. (2005) Conceptualizing place in the care of older people: the contributions of geographical gerontology, *International Journal of Older People Nursing*, 14(8b): 100–8.

Williamson, D.M., Gravani, R.B. and Lawless, H.T. (1992) Correlating food safety knowledge with home food preparation practices, *Food Technology*, 46(5): 94–100.

Woo, J., Ho, S.C., Mak, Y.T. et al. (1994) Nutritional status of elderly patients during recovery from chest infection and the role of nutritional supplementation assessed by a prospective randomised single-blind trial, *Age and Ageing*, 23: 40–48.

Worsfeld, D. and Griffiths, C.J. (1997) Food safety behaviour in the home, *British Food Journal*, 99(3): 97–104.

Wright L., Hickson, M. and Forest, G. (2006) Eating together is important: using a dining room in an acute elderly medical ward increases energy intake, *Journal of Human Nutrition and Dietics*, 19(1): 23–96.

Young, K.W.H., Greenwood, C.E., van Reekum, R. and Binns, M.A. (2005) A randomized, crossover trial of high-carbohydrate foods in nursing home residents with Alzheimer's disease: associations among intervention response, body mass index, and behavioral and cognitive function, *The Journals of Gerontology Series A: Biological Sciences and Medical Sciences*, 60: 1039–45.

CHAPTER 9

Continence management

Jo Booth

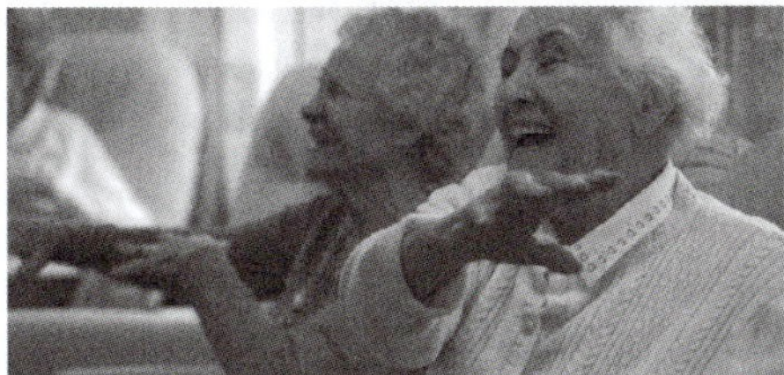 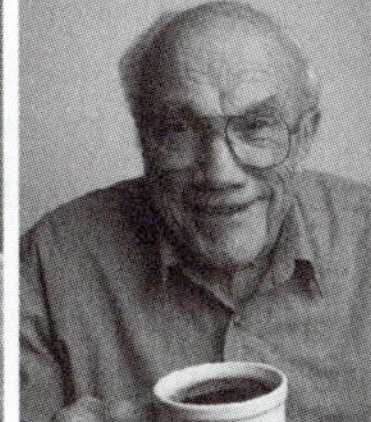 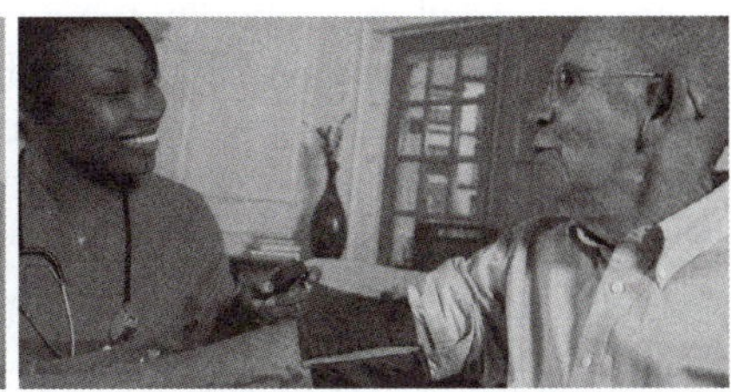

Learning objectives

At the end of this chapter, the reader will be able to:

- understand the extent and impact of continence difficulties in older people
- recognize the role of assessment in identifying the specific type of continence problem and the appropriate approach to intervention
- appreciate how active continence promotion may be empowering and the many and varied approaches by which older people can be helped to achieve continence

Mr Durrani, a 75-year-old gentleman attending a local continence promotion clinic, comments as follows:

'I need help nurse . . . this urine thing is really getting me down. I keep needing to pee. I play golf but I just can't even think about going out on a golf course as I keep needing the toilet. . . . Golf is my life. I really don't want to give it up but I just don't know what else to do. My wife made me come here in case there was some pills I could take or even some pads to wear. . . . I'll do anything. . . . It is so embarrassing. Sometimes I wet myself if I can't find a toilet quick enough. Once it starts, I can't seem to stop it. I've stopped going out for a pint with my mates cos that just makes me worse. Once I start going to the toilet, I'm there every 5 minutes. They joked and laughed about it but I was just dead embarrassed. What if I start to smell? My missus says I am dead grumpy in the morning. I think it is cos I keep waking up to pee. I am so tired and I can't always get back to sleep . . . and so is she cos I keep disturbing her.'

Introduction

This commentary illustrates the impact that continence difficulties can have on many aspects of an older person's life including their physical, social and emotional functioning and their family relationships. It also highlights the stigma of continence dysfunction and the disempowerment that is experienced by those with such conditions.

Continence involves elimination, which is the term used to describe the discarding of waste materials from the body in the form of urine and faeces. Successful elimination is fundamental to our overall health, well-being and quality of life and is achieved by controlled and appropriate bladder and bowel functioning, which we call continence. Not being in control of our bodily functioning, especially elimination is disempowering. One of our earliest human developments, which usually occurs in our pre-memory period, is to develop independent control of our bladder and bowel functioning. To lose this has connotations of infancy and dependency and is associated with feelings of shame and stigma (Shaw, 2001; Norton, 2006).

Elimination involves 'hidden' activities that are rarely discussed, even in close relationships. They are also 'hidden' geographically, as they usually take place in private, behind a closed and usually locked door. Equally such activities are hidden socially in the sense that anything to do with toilet-related activities is rarely discussed, especially if it includes bowel functioning. Where there is discussion, it usually takes the form of a joke or humorous interaction. Open discussion of bladder and bowel function is taboo in most societies with the consequence that reporting of problems, opportunities for in-depth assessment and the availability of person-focused evidence to inform nurses' practice is limited. There is very little written about toilet-related activities despite the fact that they are an essential aspect of human functioning undertaken by each of us every day.

Management of bladder and bowel elimination is primarily a nursing responsibility in all care contexts (Cheater et al., 2008; Heckenberg, 2008; Booth et al., 2009) and forms a major part of nurses' work with older people. Morris et al. (2004) showed that 13 per cent of staff time in a subacute care setting was spent on continence care tasks.

Given the level of responsibility and proportion of time nurses are engaged with continence-related practice it might reasonably be expected that they demonstrate competence and expertise in managing elimination problems experienced by older people. However, evidence suggests that nurses often demonstrate:

1. **Ageist attitudes** – an acceptance of inevitability and decline, especially among older people who have dementia or mental health conditions (Dingwall and McLafferty, 2006; Brittain and Shaw, 2007).
2. **A predominant use of containment products** rather than active bladder and bowel rehabilitation techniques aimed at promoting continence (Wagg et al., 2008; Booth et al., 2009).
3. **Overuse of indwelling urethral catheters** especially in acute areas.
4. **Disinterest in helping older people recover bladder and bowel function** as such activities are seen as low priority (Dingwall and McLafferty, 2006; Booth et al., 2009).

Such behaviour is surprising because conservative interventions designed to promote continence in older people are successful in the majority of cases. An estimated 70 per cent of older people will recover continence or significantly improve their symptoms using simple lifestyle advice and behavioural approaches that are delivered by nurses (Borrie et al., 2002; Williams et al., 2002; Byles et al., 2005). This chapter is written from the position that activities to promote urinary and faecal continence empower older people and should be prominent in nurses' repertoire of knowledge and skills.

Bladder and bowel problems experienced by older people

As we age we may experience a range of difficulties with elimination. Nurses may only associate urinary incontinence, regardless of type, with older people. However, it is important to highlight that urinary incontinence is *not* an inevitable consequence of ageing. Urinary incontinence is just one of a number of lower urinary tract symptoms (LUTS), and other bladder and bowel problems which older people experience across all health and care contexts (Box 9.1).

Box 9.1 Lower urinary tract symptoms (LUTS)

Storage symptoms

Urinary incontinence – the involuntary leakage of any urine.

Frequency – the person considers that he/she voids too often by day.

Urgency – a sudden compelling desire to pass urine which is difficult to defer.

Nocturia – waking at night one or more times to void.

Voiding symptoms

Hesitancy – difficulty in initiating micturition resulting in a delay in the onset of voiding after the individual is ready to pass urine.

Intermittency – urine flow which stops and starts, on one or more occasions, during micturition.

Straining – the muscular effort used to either initiate, maintain or improve the urinary stream.

Slow stream – a perception of reduced urine flow, usually compared to previous performance or in comparison to others.

Post-micturition symptoms

Incomplete emptying – a feeling experienced by the individual after passing urine.

Post-micturition dribble – involuntary loss of urine immediately after finishing passing urine, usually after leaving the toilet in men, or after rising from the toilet in women.

International Continence Society (2005)

Lower urinary tract symptoms (LUTSs) are more common and more bothersome to older people than urinary incontinence alone (Figure 9.1), but it is rare that such symptoms are reported and treated before actual leakage is experienced. This is because older people commonly underreport urinary and bowel symptoms (Horrocks et al., 2004; Rodriguez et al., 2007) and most do not seek support until they consider that the symptoms are severe enough to warrant taking up what they regard as 'valuable professional time' (Hagglund and Ahlstrom, 2007; Booth et al., 2010).

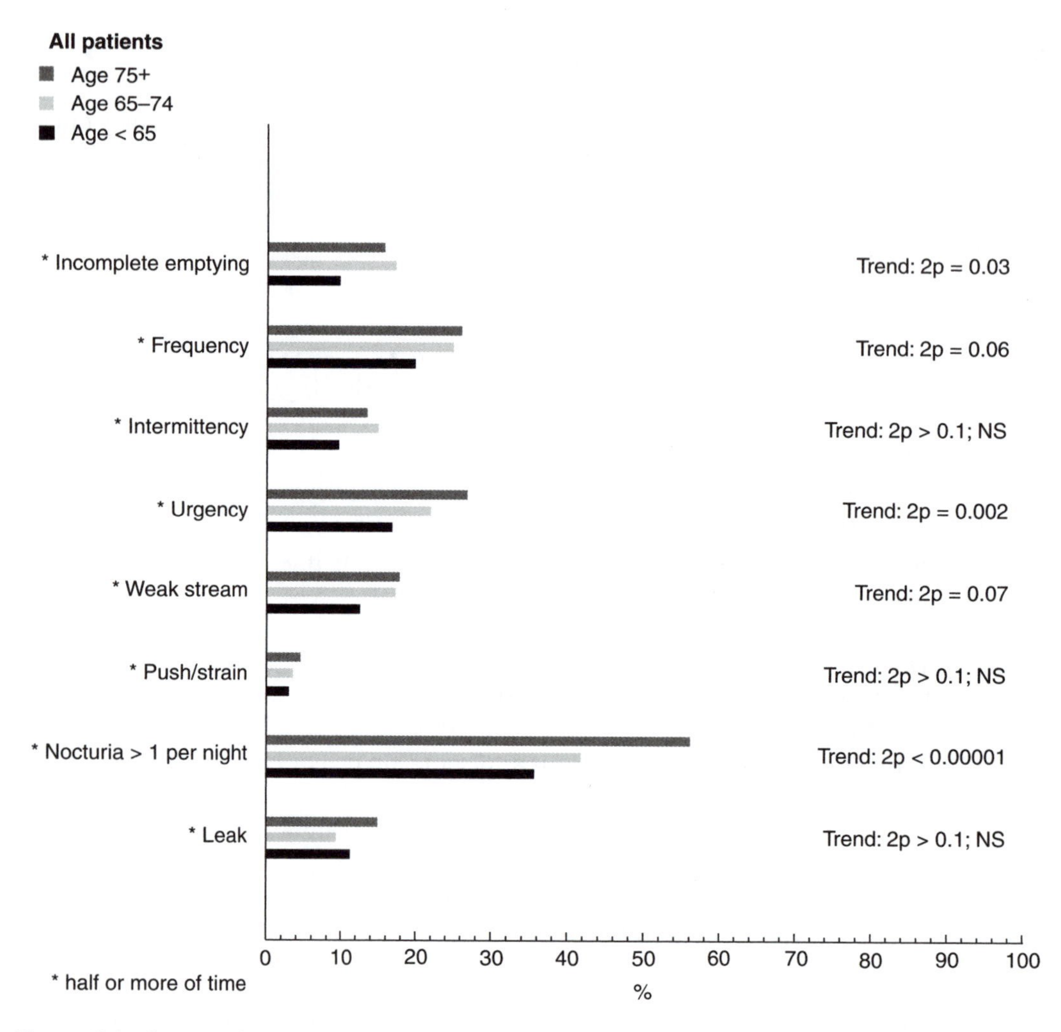

Figure 9.1: Lower urinary tract symptoms experienced by community living older people

Despite the focus of many nurses on incontinence, the two conditions experienced most frequently by older people are overactive bladder syndrome (OAB) and benign prostatic hyperplasia (BPH). Overactive bladder is defined as urgency, with or without urge incontinence, usually with frequency and nocturia in the absence of local pathological or hormonal factors (Kavia and Mumtaz, 2005) and is experienced by both men and women alike. It is the result of detrusor muscle instability of unknown cause or secondary to neurological conditions such as Parkinson's Disease, stroke or multiple sclerosis. BPH is an enlargement of the prostate gland, which typically affects men as they get older. Around the age of 40 the prostate begins to grow. From 45 onwards the growth of the prostate may accelerate and start to compress the urethra. This can lead to urinary problems, including both storage and voiding symptoms and possible bladder and kidney damage if left untreated. However, when diagnosed and treated early, there is a low risk of developing complications. Like most urinary dysfunction, BPH is not a life-threatening condition but it can negatively impact on quality of life. In addition, it should be noted that 70 per cent of men with bladder outflow obstruction (voiding symptoms) will have some symptoms of an overactive bladder (storage symptoms) (Dmochowski and Staskin, 2002).

Nevertheless, despite their prevalence these two conditions of overactive bladder and benign prostatic hypertension remain poorly recognized, with a lack of research detailing the impact on older people, their experiences and priorities for intervention. In a study of the effects of nocturia it was found to impact on many aspects of the older person's daily living and profoundly affect their relationships, participation and quality of life (Booth and McMillan, 2009).

Prevalence of bladder and bowel dysfunction in older people

Older people are at greater risk of developing difficulties with elimination for a variety of reasons relating to their physical, cognitive, motivational and functional status as well as any presence of co-morbid medical conditions and associated medications (DuBeau, 2007; Wagg et al., 2008). However, the epidemiology of bladder and bowel dysfunction in different care contexts is not fully understood as studies use a variety of different definitions, are often cross-sectional and reliant on self-report by older people. We know this results in under-reporting and an under-representation of hard to reach groups, such as older people with dementia or those who are frail and housebound. Despite these limitations it is accepted that the highest prevalence of elimination difficulties is found in care homes, where prevalence of urinary incontinence ranges between 43–77 per cent (Offermans et al., 2009) and constipation is present in 50 per cent residents (Bosshard et al., 2004).

For older people living in the community, the EPIC study, which included five countries across Europe, showed urinary incontinence in 19 per cent of women and 10 per cent men (Irwin et al., 2006). Prevalence figures for older people in secondary care are few as there is no mechanism to routinely record this data; however, the UK Royal College of Physicians continence audit (Wagg et al., 2008) highlighted the significant levels of cognitive (53 per cent) and functional impairments (72 per cent) associated with the high rates of incontinence found.

While it is important to be aware of the extent of elimination problems in different care contexts, for practitioners it is the *types* of problem that need to be understood if interventions are to be appropriately targeted and thus likely to be of most benefit.

Types of urinary incontinence (UI)

Before the type of urinary incontinence can be identified, a decision must be reached on whether the condition is *transient* or *established*. Transient urinary incontinence is reversible, usually with simple treatments and attention to the underlying acute medical condition. The most common causes may be remembered using the mnemonic 'DRIP' and are listed in Box 9.2.

Box 9.2 Causes of transient urinary incontinence

D – Delirium, Depression, Disorientation
R – Reduced mobility, acute Retention
I – Infection, Impaction of stool
P – Pharmaceuticals, Polyuria

Adapted from Sander (1998)

Where the urinary incontinence is established, it is not considered directly reversible and may be classified as one of the following types:

- **Urge urinary incontinence (UUI)** – involuntary leakage accompanied by, or immediately preceded by, a sudden compelling desire to pass urine which is difficult to defer (urgency). This is the single most common type of urinary incontinence experienced by older people, particularly older women.
- **Stress urinary incontinence (SUI)** – involuntary leakage on effort or exertion, or on sneezing or coughing. This type of UI is associated with younger women following childbirth and those who are overweight. Pure stress UI is less common in older people than urge and mixed UI.
- **Mixed urinary incontinence** – involuntary leakage associated with urgency and also with exertion, effort, sneezing or coughing. This type of UI is commonly found in older populations, particularly older women.
- **Functional urinary incontinence** – involuntary leakage associated with the inability to reach or use toilet facilities. It is the result of physical, cognitive or communicative impairment and is commonly found among older people often following an acute illness or event, or in those who are frail.
- **Overflow urinary incontinence** – involuntary leakage associated with an inability of the bladder to empty completely, overdistension of the bladder and overflow leakage of urine. The most common cause of this is bladder outlet obstruction (BOO) in men with BPH.

Much of the literature focuses on UI as a single entity, largely ignoring other LUTS and showing little consideration for the interactions and potentially cumulative effects of urinary and bowel symptoms with other syndromes commonly experienced by older people such as cognitive impairment, delirium and falls (Coll-Planas et al., 2008).

Bowel problems

Constipation – is a symptom not a disease and increases in prevalence with age. There is no universal definition of constipation in older people and most will complain of straining, a sense of incomplete emptying and hard stools rather than infrequency.

Faecal incontinence (FI) – in older people this is most commonly the result of faecal impaction and overflow of liquid stools, although massive faecal loading and impaction with soft stool can also occur. Other causes of FI in older people are severe diarrhoea, anorectal muscle weakness, neurological conditions such as stroke, dementia and Parkinson's Disease.

Impact of elimination difficulties

A difficulty with bladder and bowel control carries stigma and is ultimately a disempowering experience (Norton, 2006). The effects of incontinence on self-image, emotional well-being and quality of life should not be underestimated. Despite being 'hidden', incontinence is known to negatively impact on self-esteem, mental health, personal relationships, sexual and social activities and lead to loneliness and isolation (Fultz and Herzog, 2001). This has been shown for older people with cognitive impairment as well as those without (DuBeau et al., 2006). People with incontinence are more depressed, more anxious, feel more stigmatized and have poorer life satisfaction than those who are continent (Shaw et al., 2001). Physically, elimination difficulties in older people are associated with impaired mobility (Fonda et al., 2005), falls and fractures (Brown et al., 2000), poor skin integrity, and functional and cognitive decline (Huang et al., 2007). Incontinence is often the key factor in the decision to institutionalize an older person and can prevent discharge from hospital to home (Thom et al., 1997). Urge and mixed urinary incontinence and their associated LUTS of frequency, nocturia and urgency, are more distressing and linked to poorer physical health and quality of life than stress incontinence (Monz et al., 2005).

Key point

The effects of incontinence on self-image, emotional well-being and quality of life should not be underestimated.

Sanctions may be applied to those who are unable to conform to expected societal norms around elimination. Many older people fear they may be subject to such sanctions and excluded from participating in their chosen activities if they are unable to control their bladder and bowels.

Examples of sanctions experienced by older people:

- A woman was asked to leave her lunch club as the other members complained about the smell of urine
- A man with urgency to void was stopped by the police for urinating behind a tree, as it was near a school.

Nurses' (and other health care professionals') attitudes towards elimination are profoundly influential on whether older people access appropriate health care or feel isolated and excluded.

Approach to continence promotion

The ability of the lower urinary tract and bowel to store and empty their contents appropriately is sufficient to maintain continence in younger people; however, a much more diverse range of conditions is essential to achieve the same status in older people, particularly those who are frail. Best practice in managing elimination difficulties in older people is a skilled and varied endeavour demanding a high level of knowledge, sensitivity and skill.

The conceptual model that underpins nurses' approach to managing elimination difficulties is key to understanding the older person's experiences of empowerment and disempowerment.

In a traditional medical model difficulties with elimination are considered an illness, and nurses' and others' interventions are aimed towards cure – the older person is the passive recipient of treatments, which are usually drug-based or surgical in nature. In a purely social model problems with elimination are contained using palliative approaches such as providing adaptive equipment; for example, absorbent pads to enable the person to continue to participate in their usual activities. There are no attempts to alter the person's bladder and bowel symptoms as the focus is on maintaining the person's social status. Neither of these models sits comfortably with the requirements of all older people experiencing elimination problems and a rehabilitation model is considered more appropriate for many. This approach views elimination difficulties as potentially disabling and considers a combination of education and other forms of support to facilitate the older person to change their behaviour, together with environmental adaptation and provision of appropriate equipment, to be empowering. The older person is supported to find effective strategies to regain control of their bladder and bowels. These three approaches are reflected in the Continence Paradigm (Fonda et al., 2005) – Figure 9.2 – which is a useful basis for goal-setting and care planning between the older person, the nurse and other family members where agreed and considered helpful to the process.

Assessment

Assessment is key to both the quality and outcomes of care provided, as it is essential to understand the older person's needs in their personal living, health and family context. The specific type and nature of the elimination problems experienced can only be accurately identified on the basis of a comprehensive assessment. All too often a continence assessment is seen as 'deciding which size pad to supply'. This negates the needs of the older person and undermines the knowledge and skills of the nurse. While the use of appropriate aids and equipment are essential elements in the process of continence promotion, such an approach is neither the only nor the best approach in every situation and should only be considered as part of a systematic and considered review of the older person in context.

The components of a comprehensive assessment are shown in Box 9.3.

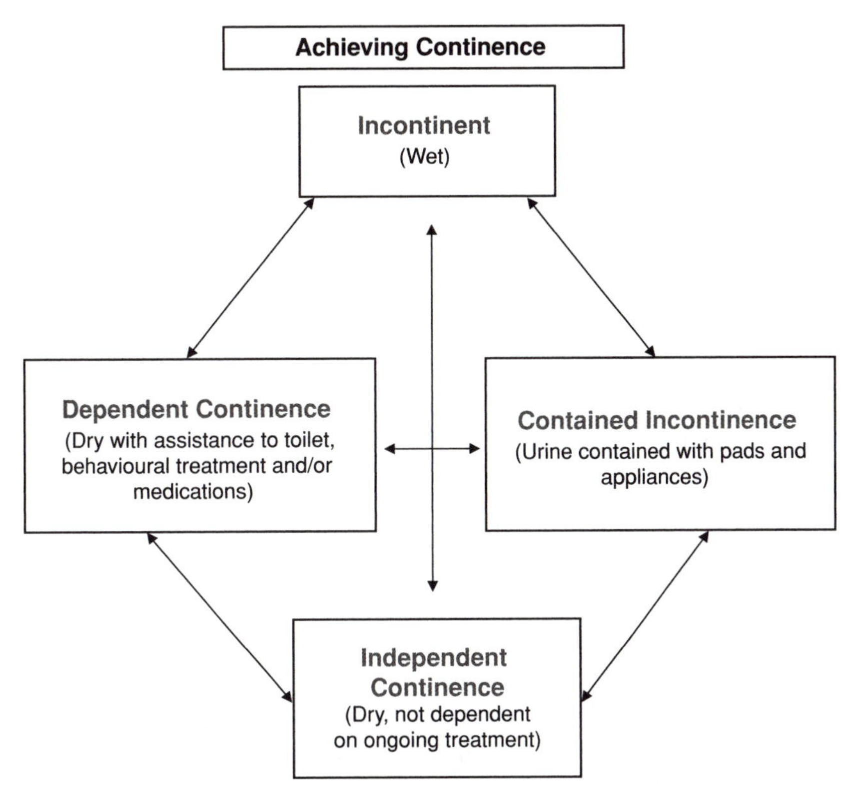

Figure 9.2: The continence paradigm and associated models of health care

Source: Adapted from *Incontinence* (2005), 1163–239 Plymouth, UK Health Publication Ltd.

Box 9.3 Components of an elimination assessment

History – from older person or if appropriate, carer.

- *Current bladder and bowel symptoms*

  Onset and duration?

  Frequency?

  Timing? (day/night)

  Associated with?/Precipitated by?

  Leakage? Amount? Type?

  Other symptoms (e.g. pain? bleeding?)

- *Previous continence status*
- *Elimination patterns*

  Usual bladder habits – daytime voids, nocturia

  Usual bowel habits – frequency, timing defeacation, constipation

(*continued*)

- *Functional status*

  Mobility, transfers, dexterity, balance, vision – day and night
- *Cognitive status*

  Comprehension, planning and sequencing, expressive ability, memory, orientation, mood
- *Medical history and current status*

  Chronic conditions (e.g. diabetes, neurological disease, musculoskeletal illness, cardiovascular disease, bowel conditions)

  Mental illness (e.g. depression)

  Acute medical illness

  Current medication
- *Surgical history*

  Previous genitourinary/abdominal/renal surgery
- *Obstetric history (women)*

  Number of births

  Trauma?
- *Environmental situation*

  Access and suitability of toilet, bed and seating arrangements, available support
- *Perceived cause*
- *Impact on quality of life* – perceived bother, social and psychological impact
- *Desire for treatment* – including motivation, willingness to follow proposed plans
- *Expectations of treatment effect*

Clinical assessment:

Urinalysis

Bladder diary or frequency/volume

Post-void residual urine

Physical examination

History taking

Recording an accurate and detailed history of the elimination problems being experienced by the older person is essential to enable you to begin to form your ideas on the likely nature of the problem(s) and therefore the range of interventions that you will recommend. Ideally, this will be undertaken during dialogue between you and the older person, but may involve asking relatives or carers, especially where the older person has cognitive impairment.

The most important aspect of the history relates to the current bladder and bowel symptoms, which need to be described in some detail to aid the correct identification of the problem. This is where knowledge and understanding of LUTS (Box 9.1) is invaluable. Specific symptom clusters, their duration, timing and frequency of occurrence can tell you a great deal. For example, descriptions of urgently needing to use the toilet 10 times daily and twice overnight, with no actual urinary leakage would alert you to the possibility of an overactive bladder. Similarly, an older man who complains of difficulty starting to pass urine and a slow stream, with lots of dribbling afterwards which continues for up to half an hour each time, would indicate the likelihood of prostate enlargement and the need to refer on for specialist assessment, particularly to exclude prostate cancer.

The current bladder and bowel symptom assessment provides you with a useful snapshot and initial thoughts on causation. However, it is important that the person's previous continence status, including their usual bladder and bowel habits and patterns of functioning, are also elicited as this adds a further layer to the overall picture that can be both revealing and guide the direction of intervention. An example would be a history of chronic constipation and its association with voiding difficulties due to the pressure on the urethra.

In older people the functional status can sometimes explain the cause of the elimination difficulties, especially when associated with a disabling condition such as stroke or dementia. It can also provide a good indication of often simple adaptive measures that can be taken to promote independent continence. A functional assessment should include cognitive, communicative and sensory functioning in addition to physical functioning as factors such as poor night time vision or inability to summon help quickly can dictate whether an older person is able to be continent or not. An intact lower urinary tract and bowel are insufficient to guarantee continence in older people who also require a certain level of functional ability within their particular environment in order to maintain or attain continence. It is thus important that functional assessment is undertaken in the older person's usual living environment. Assessing a person's ability to function within a hospital bathroom situation is unlikely to be reflected in their home situation and should be borne in mind in relation to care planning and discharge arrangements.

Similarly, cognitive status is a key determinant of intervention and the probability of effect. A diagnosis of dementia for instance does not preclude plans for active promotion of continence. However, it does suggest different approaches to those used with older people who have no cognitive impairment. For example, if using a scheduled voiding technique you would choose prompted voiding over bladder retraining. The mood of the older person is an important indicator of likely motivation to participate in active bladder or bowel rehabilitation approaches and indeed requires careful consideration, as perceived 'failure' may be more debilitating in terms of psychological recovery than more dependent approaches to managing incontinence that might be utilized.

You need to clearly document the person's previous medical, surgical and obstetric history. For example, you will be alert to medical conditions that potentially impair urinary tract function such as diabetes mellitus or previous renal disease. Cardiac conditions such as heart failure may cause fluid retention and an overnight diuresis, rheumatoid arthritis can cause severe mobility difficulties and pain, which mitigate against fast access to toilet facilities, and respiratory disease may need to be considered when climbing many stairs. Any bowel disorder including the commonly reported diverticular disease may lead to bowel symptoms such as constipation and diarrhoea. Previous abdominal surgery may cause adhesions that impact on bladder and bowel function. Pregnancy and vaginal delivery increase the risk of damage to the pelvic floor such that bladder and bowel functioning may be affected both immediately and after many years. Multiple pregnancies, large babies, traumatic deliveries and post-natal continence problems should all alert you to possible pelvic floor damage.

Obtaining a full history may be done over several interviews with the older person. In addition to the history, a comprehensive assessment also includes a clinical assessment and physical examination.

Clinical assessment

Urinalysis is a simple but essential part of the clinical assessment. It identifies the presence of a urinary tract infection (leucocytes, nitrite, protein) which is the most common and easily treatable cause of transient urinary incontinence. In addition it can indicate dehydration or a low fluid intake (specific gravity) or the potential presence of serious underlying medical conditions such as diabetes mellitus (glucose, ketones), liver disease (bilirubin, urobilinogen) and renal tract disorder (blood, protein, glucose).

Voiding diaries, sometimes known as frequency/voiding charts, are also an essential component of a comprehensive assessment. Over an agreed period (usually three days) the amounts and timing of bladder output and any incontinence episodes are recorded, together with the volumes and timing of fluid intake. The information provided by such charts is invaluable for diagnosing the type of bladder problem the person is experiencing. They also enable voiding programmes to be tailored to the individual's habits and needs.

The third component of the clinical assessment is to obtain an estimate of any post-void residual urine in the bladder. This can be achieved using an in-out urethral catheter or a portable ultrasound bladder scan (the preferred option since it is non-invasive). The definitive volume of post-void residual urine that would initiate further action to drain it has not yet been agreed. Figures of 100 ml, 150 ml and over 200 ml are found in different literature and guidelines. The important consideration is the person's symptom description; for instance, do they suffer from repeated urinary tract infections or do they complain of feelings of incomplete emptying?

Physical examination

A comprehensive assessment necessitates a physical examination. This includes a vaginal examination in women. This is carried out by a trained health care professional (a nurse, physiotherapist or doctor). The examination is used to check for uterine or vaginal prolapse, evidence of stress incontinence, to assess and monitor pelvic floor contraction, to check for signs of atrophic vaginitis and for a perineal and vulval skin assessment.

In men a digital examination of the rectum is performed, again by a trained health care professional. It is mainly used to assess for prostate enlargement, examine for rectal bleeding, assess for constipation, examine for any physiological changes related to altered bowel habit, to assess anal tone and strength and identify any infestation. Informed consent is always obtained prior to both of these examinations.

Goal-setting

One of the most important parts of the assessment and planning process is exploring with the older person their perceptions of their condition and their goals for any intervention offered. Arguably, the need for a partnership approach is greater for effective continence promotion than in almost any other aspect of nursing with older people as the mainstay of interventions lies in lifestyle and behavioural approaches which demand that the older person both acknowledges and owns the efforts required.

Interventions

Transient elimination difficulties in older people should be treated first. Common reversible conditions include infections, acute urinary retention, stool impaction and the side-effects of drugs.

Lifestyle interventions

Self-monitoring

Enabling older people to understand how their bladder and bowel work is an important part of effective continence promotion. There is evidence that self-monitoring techniques are effective when taught to older people as first line treatment for urinary incontinence (Kincade et al., 2007). This includes individual counselling about reducing caffeine consumption, ensuring appropriate fluid intake and avoiding constipation. These activities are simple, safe and inexpensive and can easily be taught by nurses as part of self-care (Pryor, 2009) for bladder and bowel health promotion.

> **Key point**
>
> Enabling older people to understand how their bladder and bowel work is an important part of effective continence promotion.

Fluid advice

Not drinking an adequate amount of fluid each day can increase the risk of dehydration and developing a urinary tract infection (Gray and Krissovich, 2003). It concentrates the urine, which irritates the bladder and thus causes it to be overactive as the bladder is 'trained' to hold smaller quantities of urine before the urge to go to the toilet is felt. Low fluid intake is also linked to constipation, which puts extra stress on the pelvic floor muscles. Older people should aim for 1.5–2 litres of fluid intake daily and should not be concerned that increasing their fluid intake will induce incontinence. Despite fears of increased frequency or incontinence a study among older women showed that adjusting fluid volumes within these guidelines resulted in neither (Tomlinson et al., 1999). Advice on fluid intake should include reducing specific bladder irritants such as caffeine, carbonated drinks and alcohol.

Scenario 9.1

Mrs Kennedy is a 66-year-old woman who was widowed in the previous year. She has been diagnosed with depression with one of her major complaints being poor sleep quality with numerous disturbances and long periods of sleeplessness. She complains she is up for most of the night as she has severe nocturia as well as urgency and daytime frequency. Assessment and a three-day frequency volume chart shows she has a reduced bladder capacity (maximum 180 ml) and frequency of 14–16 voids/24 hours. She drinks up to eight cups of coffee per day including overnight when she is unable to sleep. An agreed treatment plan began with lifestyle interventions – she agreed to replace all but two cups of coffee with hot blackcurrant juice or Horlicks for bedtime. An explanation of why her bladder capacity was low and the need for her to control and regulate the number of voids during the day was provided. Follow-up frequency volume charting after four weeks showed Mrs Kennedy had quickly increased her bladder capacity and the number of daytime voids had reduced by 2–4 per day. She continued to void 3–4 times nightly but felt that this was a result of her sleeplessness rather than being awakened by the urge to pass urine. Strategies to improve her sleeping are Mrs Kennedy's next goal.

- *What strategies to improve sleeping could you suggest?*

Diet

A healthy, well-balanced diet including five portions of fresh fruit and vegetables and wholegrain cereals is recommended to avoid constipation. Constipation is an important contributor to urinary retention in older men and women. Straining to pass a stool puts extra pressure on the pelvic floor, which can make stress urinary incontinence worse. It is important to ensure the stool is soft, which involves working with the older person or their carers to identify their most effective natural stool softener. Spicy foods and those high in fibre are usually the most successful but others include grapes, prunes, beans, and Indian and Thai dishes.

Weight management

Being overweight can increase the chances of experiencing stress and mixed urinary incontinence due to the accumulation of extra pressure on the pelvic floor and has been linked to the failure of surgical intervention. Losing weight can reduce the severity of symptoms.

Exercise

Forms of physical activity and exercise are recommended, not only for general health but particularly to manage and prevent constipation where it is an effective non-pharmacological intervention. There is debate on the role of physical activity in the treatment of urinary incontinence, where there is limited evidence of effect (Peterson, 2008).

Behavioural interventions

These include a range of conservative approaches targeted at particular types of incontinence. They are non-invasive and have no known detrimental effects, thus together with the lifestyle interventions previously outlined they should be implemented by nurses as their first line treatment with older people experiencing bladder or bowel incontinence.

Bladder retraining

This is a personalized voiding programme aimed at achieving independent continence by helping the older person to improve their control over an overactive bladder. This is achieved by increasing the intervals between voids, learning to suppress urge and increasing the functional bladder volume. The aim is to enable the bladder to hold more urine for longer periods. Prior to commencing a bladder retraining programme, a voiding diary is completed. This gives a starting point for the older person to work from and is a useful motivational tool as it enables progress to be monitored. Once the voiding diary has been analysed, the person aims to increase the amount of time between voids. One such programme might begin with hourly voiding, then add 15 minutes to this time each week until the agreed target has been reached (usually 3–4 hourly). It takes time and motivation, but can be very successful.

Understanding voluntary bladder control is important as it enables the older person to modify their behaviour in ways that support their chosen voiding interval. Thus, advising the person not to go to the toilet 'just in case', and educating them about the need to hold off when they experience urge, will help them to increase the bladder capacity over a period of time. Urge suppression, which includes distraction techniques, is a key component in bladder retraining. There is no single method that is effective for everybody. However, some people find counting backwards or reciting poetry helpful. Equally, it is useful to advise pelvic floor muscle contraction when urgency is experienced as this is considered one of the most effective means of suppression.

Scenario 9.2

Mr Johnson is a 78-year-old man with Parkinson's Disease, poor mobility, falls and shaky hands. As is commonly found in Parkinson's Disease he had urgency to void but usually no leakage. He was concerned he would become unable to reach the toilet in time as his walking was slowing down, especially at night, when he seemed to produce more urine than during the day. He wondered if he could have some pads to wear 'just in case he had an accident'. Following assessment and a full explanation of what was causing his urgency Mr Johnson agreed that a bladder retraining programme would help him maintain his bladder capacity and bladder control and that a urinal with a non-spill adapter would be more suited to his needs than absorbent pads for use overnight. Mr Johnson's initial voiding pattern was 2–3 hourly with strong urgency in the morning. He was taught to suppress his urge during the day using pelvic floor muscle exercises and deep breathing exercises. He was able to delay voiding by 15 minutes after two weeks and felt this would give him sufficient time to reach the toilet comfortably. He intends to continue with his urge suppression techniques and monitor his voiding pattern closely. The urinal for use in bed enabled him to regain his confidence and remain continent however Mr Johnson was unable to

(*continued*)

empty the urinal and was concerned it would overflow into his bed. He was given a second urinal and his carers emptied it when they visited.

- *What steps could be put in place to maintain Mr Johnson's dignity during this period of assessment?*

Prompted voiding

This is an active approach whereby older people with or without cognitive impairment are taught to initiate their own toileting through requests for help and receive positive reinforcement from carers when they do this. Although it is a resource-intensive process there is limited evidence of short-term effectiveness (Eustice et al., 2002). This is the only bladder re-education approach that is suitable for older people with dementia so it warrants consideration when continence (independent or dependent) is the goal.

Habit training

This is a voiding programme that attempts to determine the older person's usual pattern of micturition using a three-day frequency volume chart and then ensure the person is assisted to use the toilet in line with their usual pattern. It differs from prompted voiding and bladder retraining as it does not require active participation by the older person, and is thus nurse-led and therefore not an approach which could be considered empowering.

Timed voiding

Timed voiding is a fixed time interval toileting assistance programme (sometimes known as two-hourly toileting) that is used to manage urinary incontinence in older people who cannot participate in independent toileting. Although not a technique to promote continence it can be an effective method of ensuring dependent continence, providing staffing levels are adequate to maintain the programme.

Pelvic floor muscle therapy (PFMT)

PFMT is an effective, inexpensive treatment approach and is usually the first line treatment for stress urinary incontinence and may be combined with bladder training for urge or mixed urinary incontinence in older people (Wyman et al., 1998). Pelvic floor muscle therapy (PFMT) is also used effectively with men who experience urinary incontinence following prostatectomy. A structured PFMT programme aims at strengthening the muscles of the pelvic floor by contracting them in a timely and co-ordinated fashion. It is a learned technique that increases urethral resistance by increasing the peri-urethral muscle tension through repetitive voluntary contractions of the pelvic floor muscles. These exercises are usually taught by a continence nurse specialist or specialist physiotherapist. Pelvic floor muscle therapy (PFMT) has no adverse effects, although an improvement in symptoms might not be apparent for 6–8 weeks. Exercise programmes may last approximately 12–14 weeks, but there is a need to maintain this exercise approach regularly if sustained benefit is to be achieved.

Intermittent self-catheterization (ISC)

Intermittent catheterization (IC) is used when incomplete emptying and urinary retention cause problems including recurrent infections and overflow incontinence. It is suitable for those with urinary outflow obstruction, neurological disorders such as multiple sclerosis or stroke, and following surgery and spinal injuries. The catheter is inserted at intervals throughout the day depending on the severity of the symptoms. To learn ISC, the person must have manual dexterity, cognitive ability and good eyesight, plus good hygiene which is essential to reduce the risk of infection. This type of catheterization is increasingly favoured over indwelling catheterization, where the person can manage it, as it is associated with lower infection risk.

Advanced behavioural techniques

Other behavioural techniques to promote urinary and bowel continence may be implemented by continence nurse specialists and specialist physiotherapists. These include using electrical stimulation, weighted vaginal cones, biofeedback and anal irrigation techniques.

Medication

Medication may be of benefit in promoting continence when combined with behavioural interventions. However, it should be used carefully in older people as the side-effects may be more severe and there may be interactions with other medication.

- *Antimuscarinics* are prescribed for an overactive detrusor muscle and thus can be used to treat urge urinary incontinence, often in conjunction with bladder retraining. They can also help reduce nocturia and frequency. They have a number of side-effects which can result in poor tolerance among older people and high levels of discontinuation.
- *Vaginal oestrogens* are used in post-menopausal women where atrophic vaginitis is exacerbating a mixed or urge urinary incontinence.
- *Duloxetine hydrochloride* is a serotonin and noradrenaline reuptake inhibitor (SNRI) that increases neural input to the urethral sphincter, thereby relieving the symptoms of stress urinary incontinence. It is used to treat moderate to severe stress incontinence and should be combined with pelvic floor muscle training. However, this medication must be used under medical supervision and there is a high incidence of side-effects.
- *Laxatives* are a component in any bowel regime implemented to manage faecal loading in older people. They include bulk forming, stimulant, osmotic and stool softeners. Assessing the cause and type of constipation will determine which should be used.

Surgery

Surgery should only be an option when conservative approaches have failed. Age is not a barrier. However, minimally invasive techniques are preferable, especially in frail older people. Surgical intervention is most often used to treat stress urinary incontinence (SUI) and only rarely considered for urge urinary incontinence (UUI). There are many types of surgery, depending on the diagnoses, needs and health status of the person. However, it is beyond the scope of this chapter to discuss them in detail.

Type of medication	*Uses*
Alpha-blockers	Used in BPH to help relax the muscles in the bladder and the prostate, which then helps to reduce the pressure on the urethra
5-alpha-reductase inhibitors	Used in BPH to block the conversion of testosterone to DHT, which appears to stimulate overgrowth of prostate tissue
Antimuscarinics and antispasmodics	Used in BPH to treat urinary frequency and urgency

Table 9.1 Medication for improving urinary symptoms

Treating benign prostatic hyperplasia (BPH)

Minor symptoms of BPH usually do not require treatment but they may cause distress so why not? For moderate to severe symptoms, treatment is recommended. Both medication and surgery have their pros and cons. With the recent development of minimally invasive therapies (MIT), older men now have additional treatment options to accommodate their individual lifestyles and health needs. The aim is to achieve significant bladder symptom improvement less invasively than with surgery.

Medications

Medications are usually taken daily for a period of time – a few months to a few years (Table 9.1). These are aimed at improving the urinary symptoms experienced and are successful for 70–80 per cent of those who take them. Side-effects are common and may include: impotence, dizziness, headaches and fatigue.

Minimally invasive therapies (MIT)

These are non-surgical treatments, performed in a single session. They aim to reduce the tissue blocking the urethra by using energy and heat inside the prostate (thermal ablation). This can be achieved using different sources of energy and methods including transurethral needle ablation, transurethral microwave therapy, interstitial laser coagulation and transurethral water-induced thermotherapy.

Surgery for BPH

Transurethral resection of the prostate (TURP) is the standard invasive surgical treatment and involves passing a thin tube up the urethra through the end of the penis. The tube has a tiny camera and an eyepiece, so that the surgeon can see to pare away the enlarged prostate. Sometimes the person is left with urinary incontinence and erectile dysfunction following this surgery.

Containment There are many containment products available to manage both urinary and faecal incontinence. These include:

- disposable pads;
- washable pads;
- urosheaths;
- indwelling catheters – urethral and suprapubic;
- retracted penis pouch;
- pubic pressure appliance;
- penile clamp;
- urinals and uribags;
- drainable faecal collector;
- anal plugs.

A goal of contained incontinence does not involve active continence promotion and should be explored only when more rehabilitative approaches have been tried. Prior to use of any containment products, an assessment of individual needs must be carried out to ensure the product's suitability for the person's condition and context. It is vital that before supplying an older person with a containment product, clear instructions about the correct use, fitting, storage and disposal of the product are given.

Scenario 9.3

Mrs Robinson has Alzheimer's dementia and a poor short-term memory. She has a long-term history of stress urinary incontienence, which she managed with disposable pads but now has occasional urgency and thus a mixed incontinence. She has flooded her sheltered housing complex on two occasions by flushing pads down the toilet and has noticeable odour when she forgets to insert another pad. As she lives alone prompted voiding is not an option. Mrs Robinson's condition is managed using 'pull-up' pants, which successfully contain her incontinence while maintaining her dignity and 'normal' use of the toilet.

- *Think of an older person who you are nursing at present – is their continence being managed in a way that best maintains their dignity and the 'normal' use of a toilet?*
- *What could be done to improve this?*

For many people, the use of containment products allows them to lead a full life. The products are not a treatment but can successfully be used to control leakage and maintain dignity.

Conclusion

The importance of elimination to an older person's health and quality of life should not be underestimated; likewise, the benefits that accrue when nurses offer simple health promoting lifestyle advice and support for behavioural approaches to managing elimination difficulties. Working together with the older person to agree goals and select interventions is of fundamental importance, as when the person understands their body's functioning and what is required of them to change it successful outcomes are more likely to result.

References

Booth, J. and McMillan, L. (2009) Impact of nocturia on older people – implications for nursing practice, *British Journal of Nursing*, 18: 592–96.

Booth, J., Kumlien, S., Zhang, Y., Gustafson, B. and Tolson, D. (2009) Rehabilitation nurses practices in relation to urinary incontinence following stroke, *Journal of Clinical Nursing*, 18: 1049–58.

Booth, J., Lawrence, M., O'Neill et al. (2010) Exploring older people's experiences of nocturia: a poorly recognised urinary condition that limits participation, *Disability and Rehabilitation*, 32(9): 765–841.

Borrie, M.J., Bawden, M., Speechley, M. and Kloseck, M. (2002) Interventions led by nurse continence advisers in the management of urinary incontinence: a randomised controlled trial, *Canadian Medical Association Journal*, 166(10): 1267–73.

Bosshard, W., Dreher, R., Schnegg, J.F. and Bula, C.J. (2004) The treatment of chronic constipation in elderly people: an update, *Drugs and Aging*, 21(14): 911–30.

Brittain, K. and Shaw, C. (2007) The social consequences of living with and dealing with incontinence – a carers perspective, *Social Science and Medicine*, 65: 1274–83.

Brown, J.S., Vittinghoff, E., Wyman, J. et al. (2000) Urinary unconvinence: does it increase risk for falls and fractures? *Journal of the American Geriatrics Society*, 48: 721–25.

Byles, J.E., Chiarelli, P., Hicker, A.H., Bruin, C., Cockburn, J. and Parkinson, L. (2005) An evaluation of three community based projects to improve care for incontinence, *International Urogynaecology*, 16: 29–33.

Cheater, F.M., Baker, R., Gillies, C., Wailoo, A., Speirs, N., Reddish, S., Robertson, N. and Cawood, C. (2008) The nature and impact of urinary incontinence experienced by patients receiving community nursing services: a cross-sectional cohort study, *International Journal of Nursing Studies*, 45: 339–51.

Coll-Planas, L., Denkinger, M.D. and Nikolaus, T. (2008) Relationship of urinary incontinence and late-life disability: implications for clinical work and research in geriatrics, *Z Gerontology Geriatrics*, 41: 283–90.

Dingwall, L. and McLafferty, E. (2006) Do nurses promote urinary continence in hospitalised older people? An exploratory study, *Journal of Clinical Nursing*, 15: 1276–86.

Dmochowski, R.R. and Staskin, D. (2002) Overactive bladder in men: special considerations for evaluation and management, *Urology*, 60(5 Suppl 1): 56–62.

DuBeau, C. (2007) Beyond the bladder: management of urinary incontinence in older women, *Clinical Obstetrics and Gynecology*, 50(3): 720–34.

DuBeau, C., Simon, S.E. and Morris, J.N. (2006) The effect of urinary incontinence on quality of life in older nursing home residents, *Journal of the American Geriatrics Society*, 54(9): 1325–33.

Eustice, S., Roe, B. and Paterson, J. (2002) Prompted voiding for the management of urinary incontinence in adults, *Cochrane Database of Systematic Reviews*, Issue 2, Art. No. CD002113. DOI: 10.1002/14651858.CD002113.

Fonda, D., DuBeau, C., Harari, D. et al. (2005) Incontinence in the frail elderly, in P. Abrams, L. Cardozo and S. Khoury (eds) *Incontinence*, 3rd edn. (pp. 1163–239). Plymouth: Health Publication Ltd.

Fultz, N. and Herzog, A.R. (2001) Self reported social and emotional impact of urinary incontinence, *Journal of the American Geriatrics Society*, 49: 892–99.

Gray, M. and Krissovich, M. (2003) Does fluid intake influence the risk for urinary incontinence, urinary tract infection and bladder cancer? *Journal of Wound, Ostomy and Continence Nursing*, 30(3): 126–31.

Hagglund, D. and Ahlstrom, G. (2007) The meaning of women's experience of living with long-term urinary incontinence is powerlessness, *Journal of Clinical Nursing*, 16: 1946–54.

Heckenberg, G. (2008) Improving and ensuring best practice continence management in residential aged care, *International Journal of Evidence Based Healthcare*, 6: 260–69.

Horrocks, S., Somerset, M., Stoddart, H. and Peters, T.J. (2004) What prevents older people from seeking treatment for urinary incontinence? A qualitative exploration of barriers to the use of community continence services, *Family Practice*, 21: 689–96.

Huang, A., Brown, J., Thom, D., Fink, H. and Yaffe, K. (2007) Urinary incontinence in older community-dwelling women, *Obstetrics and Gynecology*, 109(4): 909 –16.

International Continence Society (2005) *3rd International Consultation on Incontinence*, Monaco, 26–29 June. Health Publication Ltd, Plymouth.

Irwin, D.E., Milson, I., Hunskaar, S. et al. (2006) Population-based survey of urinary incontinence, overactive bladder, and other lower urinary tract symptoms in five countries: results of the *EPIC Study of European Urology*, 50: 1306–15.

Kavia, R. and Mumtaz, F. (2005) Overactive bladder, *The Journal of the Royal Society for the Promotion of Health*, 125(4): 176–79.

Kincade, J.E., Dougherty, M., Carlson, J.R., Hunter, G.S. and Busby-Whitehead, J. (2007) Randomized clinical trial of efficacy of self-monitoring techniques to treat urinary incontinence in women, *Neurourology and Urodynamics*, 26: 507–11.

Monz, B., Pons, M.E., Hampel, C. et al. (2005) Patient reported impact of urinary incontinence: results from treatment-seeking women in 14 European countries, *Maturitas*, 52(Suppl): 24–34.

Morris, AR., Ho, M.T., Lapsley, H., Walsh, J., Gonski, P. and Moore, K.H. (2004) Costs of managing urinary and faecal incontinence in a sub-acute facility: a bottom-up approach, *Neurourology and Urodynamics*, 24: 56–62.

Norton, C. (2006) *Healthcare Professionals, Continence, Stigma and Taboos*. Stigma Conference Papers 2006. Available online at www.labelmenot.org/index_files/Page476.htm; accessed 17 June 2009.

Offermans, M.P., DuMonlin, M.F., Hamers, J.P. et al. (2009) Prevalence of urinary incontinence and associated risk factors in nursing home residents: a systematic review, *Neurourology and Urodynamics*, 28(4): 288–94.

Peterson, J.A. (2008) Minimize urinary incontinence: maximize physical activity in women, *Urologic Nursing*, 28(5): 351–56.

Pryor, J. (2009) Coaching patients to self-care: a primary responsibility of nursing, *International Journal of Older People Nursing*, 4: 79–88.

Rodriguez, N.A., Sackley, C.M. and Badger, F.J. (2007) Exploring the facets of continence care: a continence survey of care homes for older people in Birmingham, *Journal of Clinical Nursing*, 16: 954–62.

Sander, R. (1998) Promoting urinary continence in residential care, *Elderly Care*, 10(3): 28–35.

Shaw, C. (2001) A review of the psychosocial predictors of help-seeking behaviour and impact on quality of life in people with urinary incontinence, *Journal of Clinical Nursing*, 10(1): 15–24.

Shaw, C., Tansey, R., Jackson, C. et al. (2001) Barriers to help seeking in people with urinary symptoms, *Family Practice*, 18: 48–52.

Thom, D., Haan, M. and Van Den Eeden, S. (1997) Medically recognised urinary incontinence and risks of hospitalisation, nursing home admission and mortality, *Age and Ageing*, 26: 367–74.

Tomlinson, B.U., Dougherty, M.C., Pendergast, J.F., Boyington, A.R., Coffman, M.A. and Pickens, S.M. (1999) Dietary caffeine, fluid intake and urinary incontinence in older rural women, *International Urogynecology Journal*, 10: 22–28.

Wagg, A., Potter, J., Peel, P., Irwin, P., Lowe, D. and Pearson, M. (2008) National audit of continence care for older people: management of urinary incontinence, *Age and Ageing*, 37: 39–44.

Williams, K., Assassa, R., Smith, N., Rippin, C., Shaw, C. and Mayne, C. (2002) Continence management: good practice in continence care: development of a nurse-led service, *British Journal of Nursing*, 11(8): 548, 550, 552–9.

Wyman, J.F., Fantl, J.A., McClish, D.K. and Bump, M.D. (1998) Comparative efficacy of behavioural interventions in the management of female urinary incontinence, *American Journal of Obstetrics and Gynecology*, 179: 999–1007.

CHAPTER 10

Communication

Debbie Tolson and Christine Brown Wilson

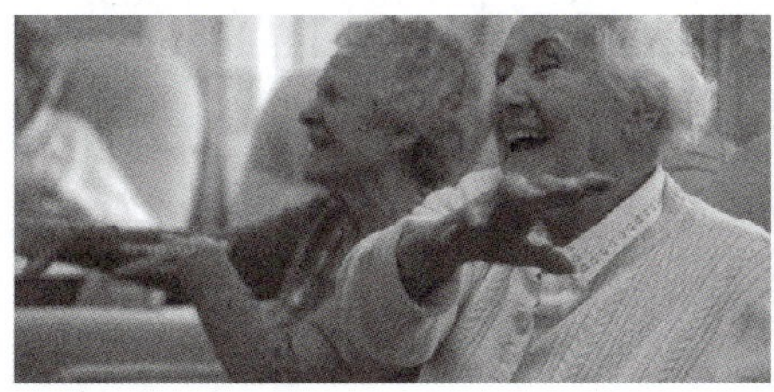
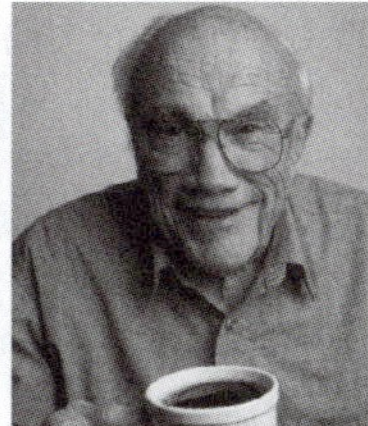
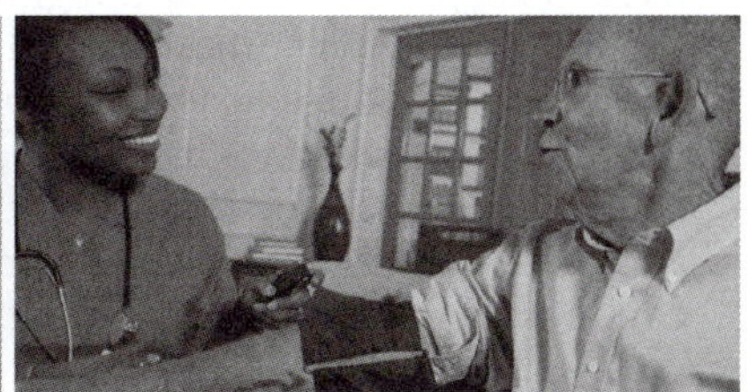

Learning objectives

At the end of this chapter, the reader will be able to:

- appreciate communication issues from an older person's perspective
- describe common challenges often reported by older people experiencing communication impairment due to age or long-term conditions
- reflect on strategies that may enable us to optimize the communication environment in a variety of nursing situations, including those which present particular complex challenges
- gain an insight into personal communicative style, strengths and areas for development

Mr R. Newman aged 79 years, London comments as follows:

'I'm no expert on communication but something happened to me about a year ago which I will never forget. I was in hospital, having my knee replaced. My wife can't manage on her own that's why I had to have my knees done and why I had put it off for so long. They only keep you in for a few days so I asked about getting help when I got home, meals and some help in the house you know just for the first few days. This young woman came to see me from social work and asked me a long list of questions. I wasn't feeling so bright you know, and she told me about all the assessments, the rules and what I could I get if I filled in all these forms. I couldn't follow it all, my mind just blurred. I couldn't take it in. It was my wife who has dementia not me but she said she was not eligible for help because she wasn't the patient, I wanted to scream that without me she soon would be . . . this young woman wouldn't stop talking at me about all the schemes including respite and what the GP should have done. That was not what we wanted and my daughter came down to stay. That girl, she just didn't get it, she, made me feel so stupid and ignorant as if I was begging for

(*continued*)

charity. I am glad she did not look at my face, I was filling up. All I wanted to know was if she could help me make some arrangements. She gave me a carrier bag full of leaflets, forms and books and told me everything I needed to know was in there and left. I was shaking... If that wasn't bad enough I tipped out the leaflets onto the bed and the one that struck me cold was about funeral plans. All I had wanted was to know if we could get meals delivered until I was back on my feet so that I wouldn't have to keep bothering my daughter. The staff nurse came over, she didn't say much, she just pulled the curtains round, put the bag of papers in the locker and held me. Bless her, that nurse just understood, she knew when words were not enough. I guess that's about it really for me, good communication is showing you care, really care and respecting people and their dignity. If you don't really care then there is a problem and that's when you make someone feel needlessly vulnerable, that's when communication goes badly wrong. You can have all the words but you need to care.'

Introduction

> "The problem with communication... is the illusion that it has been accomplished.
> George Bernard Shaw (1856–1950)"

To every situation we all bring different hopes and fears, abilities and ways of doing and being with others. As adults, many of us take for granted the ease at which we can converse, send messages and keep in touch with events at work, in the family, between friends and in the news more generally. The sophistication of our personal communication, spoken language, reading and writing abilities and our command of interpersonal communication skills in many ways defines the adults we become and the opportunities we have to participate in society. Throughout our lives the relationships we form with individuals, groups and agencies are to a large extent rooted in the effectiveness with which we communicate; sending and interpreting an array of intentional and unintentional messages to each other, some of which are forgotten in an instant and others, like those described above, to be endured and remembered for a long time. What we learn from Mr Newman's account is that we need to appreciate the what, the how, the how much, and the when of communication. In addition, we need to connect with people, display sensitivity and we need humility when we get it wrong. The nurse's response highlights the importance of different, non-verbal forms of communication, essential in those moments that are beyond words. There are no hard and fast rules about how to communicate but there are principles which can be applied, and evidence that we can draw upon to inform strategies to maximize communication opportunities for individuals experiencing communication challenges, particularly those associated with age or long-term conditions.

This chapter seeks to bring to the fore some of the communication issues that matter most to older people, expose some of the common age-related problems and offer discussion of nursing strategies for assessment, care planning and person-focused evaluation. We have chosen three scenarios to illuminate the complexity of negotiating communication-based care solutions in everyday nursing care scenarios. We are not offering a definitive text on communication, but insight into common communication challenges that exemplify those frequently encountered by nurses who work with older people. Each of these scenarios and suggested strategies for care have been developed in partnership with people experiencing these difficulties:

- **Lydia** has very little expressive speech due to aphasia following a stroke but is a skilled communicator and provides her 'ten top tips'.
- **Peter,** who lives with dementia, has provided a wealth of advice in some of the common pitfalls when communicating with people experiencing dementia.
- **Emily** is frustrated by others who see it as their right to tell her that she must get a hearing aid.

After a brief consideration of the nature of communication, and communication dynamics, we examine communication in a modern world. Information technology may not be at the fore of our thinking when we assess an older person's communication needs, but in relation to activities of daily living and as an adjunct to independent living, information communication technologies may, for some people, old or young, play a crucial role.

The nature of communication

Communication is about sending and receiving messages by means of our sensory and expressive systems. Effective communication between people involves the transmission of the intended message between the sender and recipient. It follows that ineffective communication involves errors that may occur either with the reception of incoming signals or due to problems with outgoing responses. Human communication is complex and optimal function requires sensori-perceptual, language, cognitive and motor skills to all work together (to be integrated) in addition to motivation (Le May, 2006: 166–67). There are many facets of communication, including speech, writing, reading, gesture and understanding the spoken word. The sophistication of our sensory systems and emotional responses to the communications we receive from the people and the environment we interact with influences our sense of worth, our personal identity and opportunities for fulfilment. Thus, the integrity of our communication systems is a major determinant of the quality of our lives.

Some time ago Gravell (1988) importantly noted that absence of the opportunity or desire to communicate can be as limiting for an older person as the common age-related changes that affect the auditory and visual systems (e.g. presbycusis and presbyopia) and condition specific difficulties that might arise following a stroke. In many ways, communication can be thought of as a continuous loop of transmitting, perceiving and receiving signals.

Figure 10.1 provides a simplified communication chain influenced by Gravell's original work. Breakdown at any point in this chain for intrapersonal reasons (within the person) or external reasons (behaviour of others, communication environment) potentially creates communication problems. When thinking how to support the communication needs of older people it is therefore important to identify the source or problem so that possible solutions can be explored. Remember that the solution does not always rest with the older person but sometimes the people with whom they regularly interact, including nurses, may need upskilling.

There is enormous potential for nurses to work with older people to find acceptable solutions to many communication problems while drawing on the wider expertise of the multidisciplinary health and social care teams. Sometimes the solution rests in individual

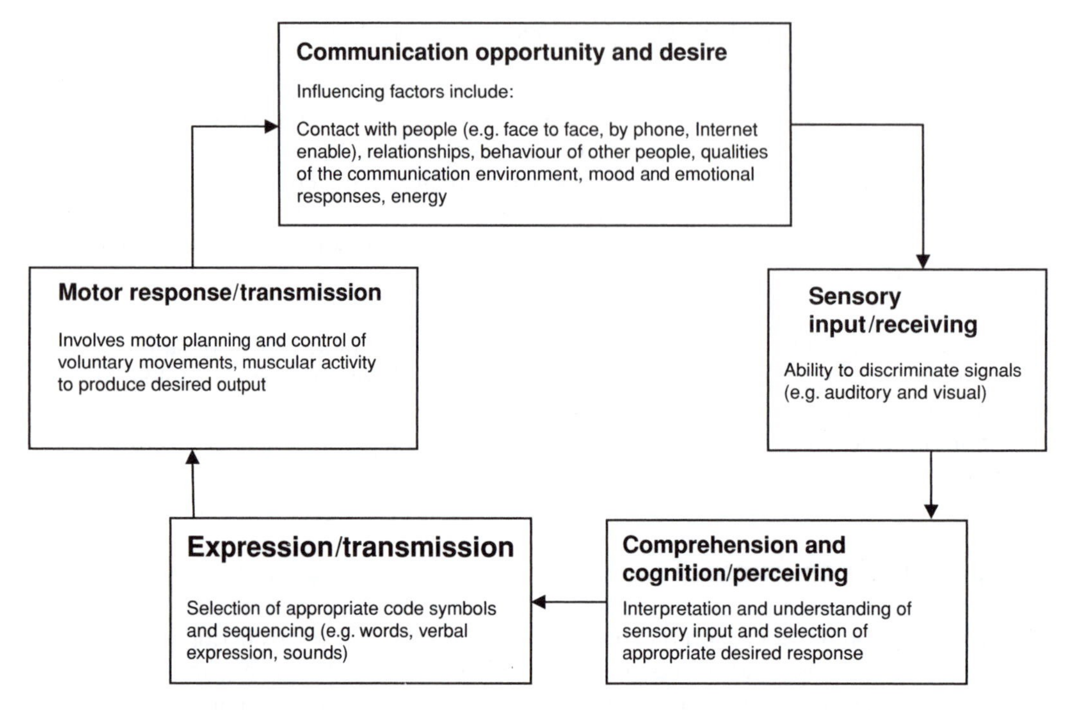

Figure 10.1: An overview of the communication chain

therapies, but often it involves others (communication partners) understanding the nature of the problem and adapting their own approaches to communication. Communication partners tend to primarily be family carers and friends who are considered central in supporting the person in everyday interactions. We would also suggest that nurses have a valuable role in enabling older people to interact more effectively in everyday situations, which could be enhanced by adopting the role of communication partner. Being aware of and making adjustments to the communication environment, such as reducing background noise, improving lighting and ensuring information is provided in accessible formats, also facilitates effective communication.

Key point

Nurses have a valuable role in enabling older people to interact more effectively in everyday situations, which could be enhanced by adopting the role of communication partner.

The ability to communicate is now recognized as an important component of healthy ageing and influences perceptions of the quality of an individual's life. Communication, for example, is required to participate in such things as activities of living, establishing and maintaining friendships, receiving quality care, maintaining social networks, facilitation of adaptation to change, discovery, involvement in decision-making, and relieving loneliness, depression, and anxiety (Worrall and Hickson, 2003).

When we invited older people to identify a key message to give nurses about communication: it was that it is central to feeling cared for and that communication is a continuous event.

Key point

The communication needs of older people are no different from younger people. Everyone needs social contact, explanation, advice, education, comfort and reassurance.

Adjusting the communication dynamic in later life

It is often age-related changes that are seen as the central challenges with communication in later life. We wish to explore the question of what creates the challenges in the communication process as we age. A common way of approaching this question is to focus on the conditions resulting in communication impairment. These conditions may be due to changes in physical function due to the ageing process (such as presbycusis) or long-term conditions (such as stroke or dementia). An alternative perspective of enhancing communication in later life might be to consider the context in which communication takes place and how the perception and (mis)interpretation of the changes to physical function alters the relationship between the older person and health and social care professionals.

For health care professionals, communication, whether spoken, written, or non-verbal, could be described as occurring in a 'moment'. However, as the model in the preceding section suggests, this moment of communication can be quite complex. For this reason we see communication as a dynamic process, where each person brings their own history and expertise to the 'moment' of communication in a health care context. Therefore, we suggest that communication in health and social care requires nurses, in particular, to see beyond the moment of communication, to understand the significance of what is being communicated in the context of the life of the older person and those who support them.

To this end, it may be helpful to consider communication in a biographical context, with the period of later life being seen as a time of development where older people hold aspirations, rather than a perception of this period as one of decline (Clarke and Warren, 2007). Indeed, it has been found that older people (and their families) actively use storytelling to engage with staff and communicate what is important in their lives (Brown Wilson et al., 2009). Furthermore, staff have been found to use this information to identify significant details in people's personal routines, creating opportunities for conversations (Brown Wilson and Davies, 2009).

It is important to recognize that communication performs a social role and subsequently supports a person's self-identity, while building and maintaining relationships (Garcia, 2008). This suggests the importance of conversation in communicating what is important in people's lives and subsequently how this information might be used by nurses to promote care that supports the older person's personal aspirations. We engage in different types of conversation depending on who we are speaking to and how well we know them, which suggests the value of developing trusting relationships between older people and professional carers (Brown Wilson and Davies, 2009). If nurses were to consider themselves as communication partners, as previously suggested, this would give both the nurse and older person an equal opportunity to contribute to the social process involved. Being a communication partner recognizes that there is joint responsibility for the success of the 'moment' of communication.

> **Key point**
>
> Communication performs a social role and subsequently supports a person's self-identity, while building and maintaining relationships.

Communicating in a modern world

An increasing number of everyday tasks are becoming technology-focused. Take a moment and think of all the aspects of daily life that are dominated by some form of technological device. This might include everyday appliances like microwaves, mobile phones, computers and ATMs (Automated Teller Machines). Imagine not being able to use any of these items and the impact this might have on your life. Slegers et al. (2009) undertook a controlled trial that assessed some of the common problems older people had in accessing these devices and found two areas of cognitive processing that caused older people difficulty: cognitive flexibility when having to switch between tasks, such as remembering your first choice when using a voice menu on the telephone; and cognitive speed – when processing information some devices automatically time out when delays occur. They suggested that to facilitate the use of technological devices that maintain an older person's autonomy, a logical series of comprehensive steps should be developed, reducing dependence on cognitive flexibility for the successful use of technology.

Older people may or may not have an interest in technology. However, it is becoming a crucial way in which in families and friends stay in touch, using email, text messaging and web-based social networking sites. It is also becoming more important to access lifestyle choices, such as online supermarket shopping and holidays. Older people who do not have access to such technologies or know how to use them may be at increased risk of social isolation. Support is being offered to older people in accessing web-based information through the emergence of websites such as Silver Surfers, which provides a portal for information suitable for the over 50s.

People with communication impairment may experience other problems when using everyday technological devices. For example:

- *people with aphasia* might not be able to process text or images and may have difficulty spelling accurately;
- *people with hearing impairment* are unable to access auditory clips without text captioning;
- *people with memory impairment* may struggle with retaining what they are doing while being asked to switch tasks.

Facilitating the use of web-based resources

Suggestions to facilitate the use of web-based resources for older people experiencing some of these issues include:

- having an option on websites for easier accessibility that breaks down the information from one page into a number of manageable sections for people who are unable to process large amounts of text;
- spelling accurately, so having a search engine to say 'did you mean' is particularly helpful;
- websites that enable the font and background colour to be changed to support engagement and facilitate use;
- breaking text up with relevant pictures or symbols to facilitate understanding;
- boxes showing lists is easier than drop-down menus;
- customized web browsers depending on disability – not one size fits all.

Health information is becoming increasingly web-based (e.g. see the websites of NHS Direct and Patient Choice). However, the potential benefits of engaging with technology may not be available to people with disabilities due to poor technology access or poor web design (Elman et al. 2003).

Promoting self-determination and health literacy

Maintaining effective communication to allow the older individual to receive and retain information about their health and care options is critical to working in partnership with people and understanding their preferences. In addition to appreciating how age-related changes and conditions may affect the flow of information and capacity for and speed of information processing, it is important for nurses to have insight into the psychological mechanisms that underlie people's choices and judgements.

There is accumulating evidence that age-related differences in deliberative and affective processes (cognitive and motivational) interplay in ways that are not fully understood or appreciated by the older individual, or indeed nurses, in terms of making decisions and judgements (Peters et al., 2007). Many of us can think of examples where an older person we know seems to make an unusual or unexpected choice; that is, when we weigh up the information and choices presented from our own vantage point. The review by Peters et al. highlights the possibility that older adults selectively use their deliberative capacities based on their level of motivation to make decisions, and research suggests there is a tendency among some older people to be swayed by the emotional content of information. Decision-making at any age involves the head and the heart, and it is easy to underestimate the impact on older people of emotive information and the powerful influences in the marketplace and within families. It is not unusual for practitioners and families to underestimate an older individual's capacity to make decisions and express preferences when communication impediments exist, and to question the appropriateness of decisions and judgements made by anyone who reaches a conclusion that does not coincide with their own.

Key point

It is easy to underestimate an older individual's capacity to make decisions and express preferences when communication impediments exist.

The Mental Capacity Act

The Mental Capacity Act (2005) provides some very clear guidance in the role of others to support the decisions of people. The five core principles are:

1. A person must be assumed to have capacity unless it is established that he lacks capacity.
2. A person is not to be treated as unable to make a decision unless all practicable steps to help him to do so have been taken without success.
3. A person is not to be treated as unable to make a decision merely because he makes an unwise decision.
4. An act done, or decision made, under this Act for or on behalf of a person who lacks capacity must be done, or made, in his best interests.
5. Before the act is done, or the decision is made, regard must be had to whether the purpose for which it is needed can be as effectively achieved in a way that is less restrictive of the person's rights and freedom of action.

Tuckett (2005) offers an insightful discussion about the importance afforded by nurses to honesty and information sharing, and brings to the fore a tendency among nurses working with dependent older people to use communication strategies that control the care encounter. He contends that nurses afford a lower priority to truth telling than the older people for whom they purport to care. A possible contributing factor to this may be a failure to appreciate the capacity a person has to process information or to express their point of view. Alternative explanations might include prevailing paternalistic cultures of care that do not foster meaningful and equal partnerships. In a recent study of influences on nurse communication with older people at the end of life, Clarke and Ross (2006) revealed that often relatives, but not the individual, were informed, which conflicts with current palliative care guidance which places the individual in receipt of care centrally, irrespective of age.

The link between an individual's ability to comprehend and use health information relates to opportunities for self-determination, notions of self-care and health literacy. In describing health literacy, Speros (2005) highlights the many factors that may influence how people relate to relevant health messages and their capacity to act upon accessible information. Accumulating evidence suggests that older people are particularly vulnerable to low health literacy and that nurses have yet to grasp the opportunity that they have to improve this situation (Tolson, 2008). Improving levels of health literacy among older people will in part depend on nurses acquiring age-appropriate communication strategies and deploying these effectively (whether seeking to communicate at an individual or at a population level).

Negotiating age-related hearing problems

Age-related hearing impairment (presbycusis) is one of the most common impediments to communication in later life and for most people it can be effectively managed. Empowering older people to adjust to presbycusis begins with appreciating and understanding the functional difference between hearing and listening. Hearing is essentially a passive activity as the volumes and frequencies that are audible to us cannot be consciously adjusted; listening on the other hand is active. Our listening behaviours and our capacity to listen can change and are affected by the listening environment in which we find ourselves (Tolson and Swan, 2006: 184). In situations where listening requires more effort it is likely that the desire to communicate will diminish (see Figure 9.1).

Difficulty with hearing is not an inevitable consequence of getting old, but epidemiological data demonstrates that prevalence escalates with advancing age; 37 per cent of people aged between 61–70 years increasing to 60 per cent in those aged 71–80 years (Davis, 1995). Estimates of prevalence among dependent older people receiving long-term nursing care suggests that those not suitable for a hearing aid may be as high as 90 per cent (Tolson, 1997; Tolson and Stephens, 1997).

The aetiology of the most common hearing impairment in later life, sensorineural loss (caused by damage to the pathway between the inner ear and the brain), is unclear. A smaller proportion of people may have a conductive hearing problem (caused by anything that stops sound moving from the outer ear to the inner ear). It is helpful to make the distinction to identify any treatable problems. However, in the main, conservative forms of auditory rehabilitations are preferred and may include sound amplification, development of hearing tactics and modification of the listening environment.

The presbycusis syndrome characteristically gives rise to a loss of hearing acuity, meaning that higher volumes are required for sounds to be audible, and impairment is most pronounced at higher sound frequencies. This means that vocal sounds such as 't', 'd', 's' and 'sh' are harder to hear. Laryngeal tones, which are lower and often in the middle of words, such as vowels, remain audible. This why older people can sometimes hear that you are speaking but cannot make out what you are saying. In these situations it is tempting to shout but this further distorts speech. Background noise exacerbates difficulty, so it may be possible to hold a conversation in a quiet area but impossible within noisy group situations such as a busy waiting room.

The functional problem of not being able to hear at volumes comfortable to others, and the impossibility of conversing in group situations, limits opportunities for participation in community and family life. At a personal level older people have reported frustration, embarrassment, irritability, feeling upset and a growing sense of social isolation (Stephens et al., 2001).

Karlsson, Espmark and Scherman's (2003) phenomenological investigation further illuminates the hurt and mixed emotions that can arise when an individual believes that others are deliberately mumbling or excluding them from conversations. Such feelings compound the growing sense of isolation and fuel tensions arising from frustrated communications. People also described feelings indicative of the strong association of hearing problems with a stereotypical view of old age and senility. This association of hearing loss with the state of being old was related to a sense of spoiled identity which seemed to trigger a psychological struggle in response to indisputable signs announcing the arrival of a person's own old age.

The negative impact of hearing difficulties on people's lives and on relationships with others is well documented. Knussen et al. (2005a, 2005b) provide a detailed exploration of the impact of everyday hearing hassles on family members, revealing the fuelling of family tensions and escalation of carer burden. Given the disruptive impact of hearing problems on communication and on the quality of life of both older people and carers there are compelling reasons to intervene.

Auditory rehabilitation approaches

Auditory rehabilitation approaches are multifaceted and include the use of sound amplifying instrumentation, management of the acoustic environment, counselling and the development of hearing tactics (Gatehouse, 2003). Despite the evidence which endorses the benefits of multifaceted approaches, rehabilitation is often confined to the issue of a hearing aid alone. Therefore, it should not be a surprise to learn that the rate of hearing aid rejection remains high. Gianopoulous et al. (2002) found that 8–16 years after hearing aid fitting only 43 per cent of people aged 50–65 years olds were still using their prescribed aid. In a recent Scottish study, the Royal National Institute for the Deaf asked older people who had recently had problems with a hearing aid or were waiting for fitting what changes they thought would help. They emphasized that current services and practitioners did not seem sensitive to the distress and emotional reaction that many experienced as they came to terms with their need for a hearing aid. They were concerned that they lacked access to appropriate information to help them to choose between different types of hearing aid and many were torn between lengthy NHS waiting times, the hard sell of private dispensers and pressures from family members. The key messages from the 240 older people who participated in this study was that they wanted pre- and post-hearing aid fitting support to be provided that recognized the emotions associated with needing a hearing aid.

Scenario 10.1: Hearing loss – the problem is other people – they mumble

Emily Crossan lives with her married daughter and their family. She is 82 years old and because of restricted mobility her main enjoyment seems to be watching TV. They have always been a close family but Emily's deafness is taking its toll with the constant need for repetition, her insistence on turning the TV up excessively and her misunderstandings about plans for the day. Her daughter has a part-time job and on the days that she works has arranged a rota of visitors to pop in and make sure that Emily has some company and everything she needs.

At a recent check up with the practice nurse, attended with her daughter, Emily admitted to being a bit lonely but otherwise said very little, deferring mostly to her daughter. On the few occasions when she spoke she had obviously misunderstood what the nurse had said. Emily fiercely denies difficulties with her hearing, but like her daughter the practice nurse thinks that hearing problems are the source of her low mood. At the end of the check up Emily rejected the suggestion that she should have her hearing checked saying that she would never accept a hearing aid. The problem she reasoned was that others should learn to speak properly and stop mumbling.

- *What strategies would empower Emily to take action to ameliorate her current difficulties?*

Enhancing communication: potential strategies and interventions available to nurses

This section outlines potential strategies for assessment, care planning and person-focused evaluation to support nurses in engaging with older people in ways that are both meaningful and enhance nursing care. It draws on two key documents designed to improve quality of care (Department of Health (DoH), 2003) and to maximize communication with older people who have an age-related hearing disability (NHS Quality Improvement Scotland (NHSQIS), 2005). The essence of care benchmark for communication states that communication needs to be sensitive to individual needs and preferences, promoting high-quality patient care (DoH, 2003). Furthermore, NHS quality improvement has produced evidence-based practice guidance; a strength of this care guidance is its potential achievability and the reassurance that during its development it was implemented within an in-patient and community nursing setting.

In outlining potential strategies, we have also drawn on the experience of older people and asked what they would suggest to support communication with health care professionals. While there is no 'one size fits all' solution to enhancing communication, we hope this section provides a range of strategies that supports the development of communication as a meaningful process for the older person, their families and the staff who support them.

Assessment

Effective communication is vital for the nursing assessment if older people are to be given meaningful choices and be involved in decisions relating to their health care. As a starting point, attention needs to be paid to hearing, vision, physical and cognitive abilities that might influence a person's communication (DoH, 2003). Best practice suggests that if older people use hearing aids, they should be clean, fully functional and well fitted; that if glasses are worn, they are cleaned and being worn during the assessment (NHSQIS, 2005).

Without an appropriate assessment of communication, assessment of other health requirements will not be possible. It has been suggested that registered nurses undertake an initial hearing assessment with older people and record any self-reported hearing deficits in the care plan (NHSQIS, 2005). One older person we consulted, Peter, who has dementia, identifies that all people are able to communicate, even if it is confined to a movement of their head, or tapping of their hands. It is up to the nurse to find out how this is achieved in the initial stages of an admission to a hospital. This might require the support of family members until the nursing staff feel comfortable in understanding the communication strategies used. When completing an assessment of communication, there needs to be sufficient detail for other staff to be able to communicate with this person effectively. For example, documenting that a person is unable to speak is insufficient. This needs to be expanded to identification of how 'yes' and 'no' is communicated, at the very minimum, and regularly re-evaluated as people's needs and abilities change.

If, on assessment, there are key issues in communication, the involvement of the wider multidisciplinary team, including specialists such as a speech and language therapist, would be helpful. Resources like Talking Mats and support to use them may enable older people with reduced speech to be more involved in the assessment process. People with significant communication impairment would also benefit from a communication passport. This document simply and succinctly informs others involved with the person how someone communicates (Millar and Aitken, 2003). Awareness of communication passports ensures consistency of care and safety, particularly when transitions between services occur. Another older person who we consulted, Lydia, finds her communication passport very useful in supporting her communication – it contains family pictures and important pages relating to food and use of the bathroom. It also has an alphabet chart to help her spell out words she might not be able to say.

Assessment of people with dementia

Involving people with dementia in assessment is crucial. However, it is also important to recognize that some people may not always be realistic about what they are still able to do. Peter suggests that people may be reticent to admit they are unable to attend to their own personal hygiene, after all they have done in their lives. While you should give the person with dementia their place in the assessment process, you may also need someone who knows them well to fill in the gaps. However, Peter urges that professionals should continue to include people with dementia in the conversation, and not talk over or around them.

Valuing older people and their contribution is a sign of respect, and the forerunner of ensuring people are treated with dignity in health care environments. Using a biographical approach to the assessment process enables older people to communicate what is important to them through the stories they share. Peter suggests that people should be treated as people first, rather than someone with a disability. As nurses and nursing staff spend the greatest time with older people, they remain in a unique position to identify how this information can be integrated into care planning.

Care planning

Underpinning all care planning are the values of respect and dignity (DoH, 2003), both of which are facilitated through effective communication as older people are supported to make choices and become involved in decision-making (Picker Institute, 2008). What decisions older people wish to be involved in will be personal, and it is important that staff identify these (Davies and Brown Wilson, 2007). The level of involvement may be influenced by the context of care and what level of (ill) health and well-being the person is experiencing. However, it is important that mechanisms are in place to support older people in becoming involved in decisions that affect them. Sufficient time needs to be given for the person to express their needs, choices and concerns. When involving people in care planning, Peter warns about persevering until the task is done and suggests it might be more appropriate to break this into smaller, timed tasks over the course of the day, maintaining an awareness of the time of day and the person's usual routine.

To support effective communication, appropriate environments need to be provided/accessed depending on the purpose of the communication (DoH, 2003). Noise has been identified as a problem for many older people with communication impairment as it prevents people from following or hearing the conversation. Appropriate and acceptable resources need to be accessed to enable older people to communicate as independently as possible (DoH, 2003). Millar and Aitkern (2003) provide a good practice guide for compiling passports as a collaborative process resulting in a concise document written in an accessible way communicating something about who this person is. The ownership of the passport remains with the person and a key worker responsible for working with that person ensures it is kept up to date. Often this may fall to the speech and language therapist but also needs to include other key professionals, such as nurses, who know a lot about a person's life that would be valuable in a communication passport.

Information needs to be accessible and provided in a way that is acceptable to the older person and their supporters. As identified at the beginning of this chapter, it is vital that older people are not overloaded with information and that regular checks on their information needs are made. This might require refining the content to meet an individual's information needs. For example, Parr et al. (2001) suggest that for people with aphasia, it is possible to feel more disabled by the lack of relevant understandable information than by the difficulty of finding a word.

Person-focused evaluation

When an older person has a communication impairment, it is important that interaction is maximized. Older people with hearing impairments do tend to become socially isolated as they struggle to understand what is being communicated (NHSIQS, 2005). In different settings where the older person is being supported, the measures of success for interventions will vary, but still remain individual to that person. Garcia (2008) suggests these could be considered in terms of how somebody's life is enhanced. One example might be that of an older person being able to communicate with others on a ward following a hearing assessment and some simple noise reduction measures. In long-term or community settings, the evaluation might be an improvement in goals or the ability to return to previous activities.

The following section provides three scenarios to support you in considering how you might implement and evaluate how effective communication strategies may be in your own environment and practice. Again, we have developed this information in partnership with people experiencing these conditions.

Communication skills for those with dementia

A person with dementia's ability to produce meaningful speech is often influenced by the interaction. Peter suggests that getting to know how a person communicates is particularly important, along with ensuring they are comfortable and can see your face to read expressions. For example, standing or sitting in front of a window immediately casts your face in shadow. Peter also suggests knowing when people are at their best, and organizing the encounter for a time when it does not adversely impact on their routine. This might include a consideration of when the person with dementia has had medication that could interfere with how they communicate. In conversation, always give way to allow the person with dementia to say what is on their mind, as they might forget later but be aware that they might not be able to orientate you to the change in topic. This might require the use of repair strategies such as attempts to clarify meaning, supporting someone with identification of word through paraphrasing or repeating what has been said, to enable people with dementia to continue to make a meaningful contribution to the conversation. However, doing this over a protracted period of time may have an adverse consequence of exposing a person's lack of competence in this social situation causing them to disengage from the conversational process (Perkins et al., 1998). Peter suggests finishing someone's sentences for them is not a useful strategy.

As dementia progresses, people may have reduced language skills. However, this does not preclude engagement with carers and others in their social environment (Ward et al., 2008). Indeed, when alterations in behaviour are recognized by staff, meaningful interaction often occurs (Brown Wilson and Davies, 2009). There is always the risk that communication with people with limited language revolves around activities of daily living and the support older people require in health care environments. It has been suggested that when this is the only form of interaction between staff and people with dementia, people with dementia may not have the opportunity to express their self-identity through social engagement (Ward et al., 2008). However, using personal routines as an opportunity for conversation about photos, choice of clothing, jewellery or makeup has been found to support older people in expressing their self-identity (Brown Wilson and Davies, 2009).

Scenario 10.2: Dementia – we always ask him

Harold Smith is 78 years old and lives in a care home. He has severe to moderate dementia and has always drunk coffee when he lived at home. There has been a change in staff and at each drinks round he is asked if he would like a cup of tea, to which he always answers yes. The drinks rounds are a busy time in the lounge, with people speaking and joking with each other. The TV or radio is generally on. Harold leaves the cup of tea offered to him and the staff assume he is not thirsty.

- *What might the staff do to facilitate more meaningful conversation with Harold, enabling him to make more effective choice?*

Scenario 10.3: Aphasia – if only I could say

Ann Hardy is a gregarious and outgoing lady aged 85. She is an avid reader and enjoys a busy social life going out with friends. She has two sons who are married and live away. She has recently had a stroke which has left her with a dense hemiplegia on her right side, which is her dominant side. This means she is unable to write. She also has expressive aphasia which means she might say one thing but mean another. She tires easily and is becoming increasingly frustrated at her inability to be understood. The speech and language therapist has encouraged Ann to use Talking Mats but she finds the pictures childish and is refusing to use this communication aid.

- *What strategies might enable Ann to communicate more effectively so she can be more involved in her rehabilitation?*

Lydia's insights into aphasia

Lydia has aphasia and she emphasizes how much she enjoys having conversations, even though she is unable to speak very much. She is happy for people to ask if they do not understand as it does not help her when they pretend to understand her meaning. This underlines how the behaviour of communication partners can impact on how the person with aphasia communicates (Garcia, 2008). For example, collaborative turn taking is very important as people with aphasia might not be able to respond with the right term in time to 'take the floor' (Perkins et al., 1998). Lydia suggests that a conversational partner might support the person with aphasia to express thoughts when they struggle with the use of pictures or objects, or writing down key words as the conversation progresses.

Conclusion

Communication is fundamental to the assessment process and the nurse's approach to support an older person communicate their needs, hopes and aspirations will impact on the involvement the older person has in shaping the decisions made within a health care environment. This chapter has suggested the value of adopting a biographical approach to care planning that values the stories older people or their supporters may share and identifying their relevance to the care planning process.

Effective communication with an older person is an opportunity to strengthen their self-identity and retain what makes them a unique person. Therefore, when other opportunities for self-realization are diminishing, there is a moral and professional responsibility to optimize communication.

Acknowledgements

Lydia has asked that we use her real name. Lydia had her stroke in April 2007 and has been attending Tameside Communication Group, Ashton-under-Lyne since November 2007.

References

Brown Wilson, C. and Davies, S. (2009) Developing relationships in long-term care environments: the contribution of staff, *Journal of Clinical Nursing*, 18: 1746–755.

Brown Wilson, C., Davies, S. and Nolan, M. (2009) Developing personal relationships in care homes: realising the contributions of staff, residents and family members, *Ageing & Society*, 1–23 doi:10.1017/S0144686X0900840X.

Clarke, A. and Ross, H. (2006) Influences on nurses' communication with older people at the end of life: perceptions and experiences of nurse working in palliative care and general medicine, *International Journal of Nursing Older People*, 1: 34–43.

Clarke, A. and Warren, L. (2007) Hopes, fears and expectations about the future: what do older people's stories tell us about active ageing? *Ageing & Society*, 27: 465–88.

Davis, A.C. (1995) *Hearing in Adults* pp. 723–79. London: Whurr Publishers Ltd.

Department of Health (DoH) (2003) *Essence of Care: Patient Focused Benchmarks for Clinical* Governance. London: DoH.

Davies, S. and Brown Wilson, C. (2007) Creating a sense of community, in National Care Homes Research and Development (NCHRBD) Forum *'My Home Life.' Quality of Life in Care Homes: A Review of the Literature.*, London: Help the Aged. Available online at www.//myhomelifemovement.org/down/ocids/mhl_review.pdf; accessed 27 January 2011.

Elman, R., Parr, S. and Moss, R. (2003) The internet and aphasia crossing the digital divide, in S. Parr, J. Duchan and C. Pound (eds) *Aphasia Inside Out* (pp. 103–16) Maidenhead: Open University Press.

Garcia, L. (2008) Focusing on the consequences of aphasia: helping individuals get what they need, in R. Chapey (ed.) *Language Intervention Strategies in Aphasia and Related Neurogenic Communication Disorders* 5th edn (pp. 349–75). Baltimore, MD: Lippincott, Williams & Wilkins.

Gatehouse, S. (2003) Rehabilitation: identification of needs, priorities and expectations, and the evaluation of benefit, *International Journal of Audiology*, 42(2S): 77–83.

Gianopoulous, I., Stephens, D. and Davis, A. (2002) Follow up of people fitted with hearing aids after adult hearing screening: the need for support after fitting, *British Medical Journal*, 325(August): 471.

Gravell, R. (1988) *Communication Problems in Elderly People: Practical Approaches to Management*. London: Croom Helm.

Karlsson Espmark, A.K. and Scherman, M.H. (2003) Hearing confirms existence and identity experiences from persons with presbyacusis, *International Journal of Audiology*, 42: 106–15.

Knussen, C., Tolson, D., Swan, I.R.C., Stott, D.J., Brogan, C.A. and Sullivan, F. (2005a) The social and psychological impact of an older relative's hearing difficulties: factors associated with change, *Psychology, Health and Medicine*, 10(1), 57–63.

Knussen, C., Tolson, D., Swan, I.R.C., Stott, D.J. and Brogan, C.A. (2005b) Stress proliferation in caregivers: the relationships between caregiving stressors and deterioration in family relationships, *Psychology & Health*, 20: 207–21.

Le May, A.C. (2006) Communication challenges and skills, in S J. Redfern and F.M. Ross (eds) *Nursing Older People* (ch. 10). London: Churchill Livingstone Elsevier.

Mental Capacity Act (2005) Available online at www.legislation.gov.uk/ukpga/2005/9/contents.

Millar, S. and Aitken, S. (2003) *Personal Communication Passports. Guidelines for good practice*. Edinburgh Call Centre.

NHS Quality Improvement Scotland (2005) *Best Practice Statement: Maximising Communication with Older People who have Hearing Disability.* Edinburgh: NHSQIS ISBN 1-84404-348-7. Available online at www.nhshealthquality.org.

Parr, S., Moss, R., Newberry, J. and Petheram, B., Byng, S. (2001) *Inclusive Internet Technologies for Those with Communication Impairment.* Available online at www.york.ac.uk/res/iht/projectsl218252051/ParrFindings.pdf; accessed 14 June 2009.

Perkins, L., Whitworth, A. and Lesser, R. (1998) Conversing in dementia: a conversation analytic approach, *Journal of Neurolinguistics*, 11(1–2): 33–53.

Peters, E., Hess, T.M., Vastfjall, D. and Auman, C. (2007) Adult age differences in dual information processes, *Aging and Decision Making*, 2(1): 1–23.

Picker Institute (2008) *On Our Terms: The Challenge of Assessing Dignity in Care*. London: Help the Aged.

Slegers, K., Van boxtel, M. and Jolles. J. (2009) The efficiency of using everyday technological devices by older adults: the role of cognitive functions, *Ageing & Society*, 29: 309–25.

Speros, C. (2005) Health literacy: concept analysis, *Journal of Advance Nursing*, 50: 633–40.

Stephens, D., Gianopoulos, I. and Kerr, P. (2001) Determination and classification of the problems experienced by hearing impaired elderly people, *Audiology*, 40: 294–300.

Tolson, D. (1997) Age related hearing loss: a case for nursing intervention, *Journal of Advanced Nursing*, 26: 1150–57.

Tolson, D. (2008) Health literacy in later life: guest editorial, *International Journal of Nursing Older People*, 3(3): 159.

Tolson, D. and Stephens, D. (1997) Age-related hearing loss in the dependent elderly population: a model for nursing care, *International Journal of Nursing Practice*, 3: 224–30.

Tolson, D. and Swan, I.C.R. (2006) Hearing in S. Redfern and F. Ross (eds) *Nursing Older People* (ch. 1), 3rd edn. London: Churchill Livingstone Elsevier.

Tuckett, A. (2005) The care encounter: pondering caring, honest communication and control, *International Journal of Nursing Practice*, 11: 77–84.

Ward, R., Vass, A., Aggarwal, N., Garfiled, C. and Cybyk, C. (2008) A different story: exploring patterns of communication in residential dementia care, *Ageing and Society*, 28(5): 629–51.

Worrall, L.E. and Hickson, L.M. (2003) *Communication Disability in Aging: From Prevention to Intervention*. New York: Thomson Delmar Learning.

CHAPTER 11

Spirituality, religious practice, beliefs and values

Karen S. Dunn

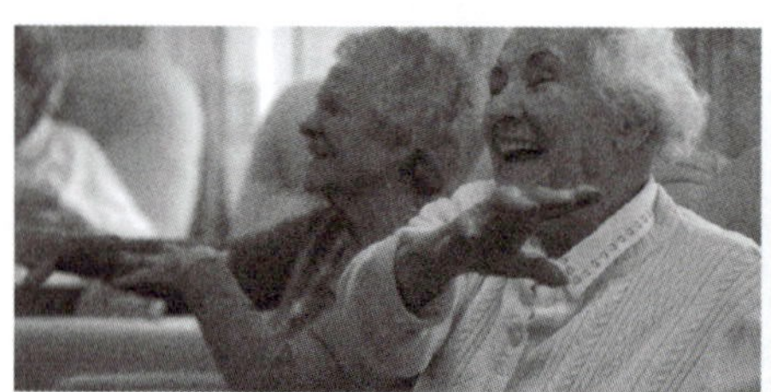
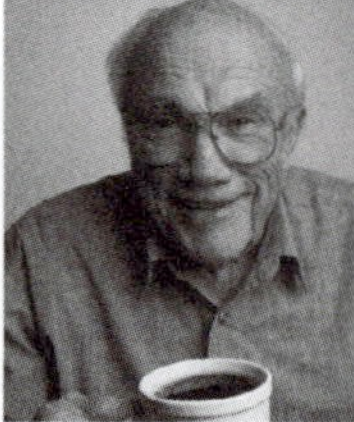
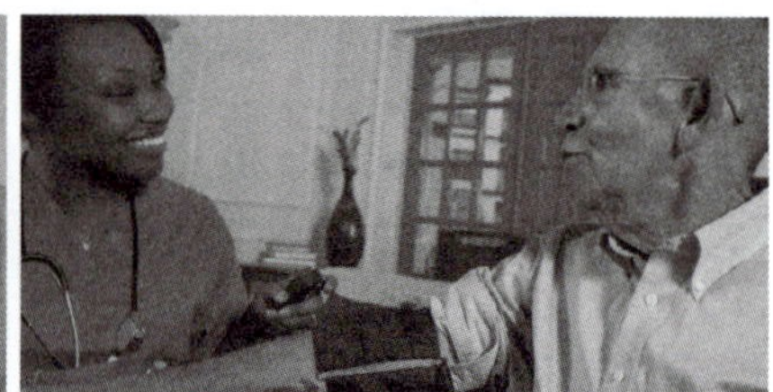

Learning objectives

At the end of this chapter, the reader will be able to:

- delineate the concepts of spirituality, religiosity and spiritual well-being
- discuss spiritual development
- describe how the differing practices and beliefs of Western and Eastern Religions impact on health care
- examine the behavioural cues that may be useful in assessing seven nursing diagnoses related to alterations in spiritual integrity
- identify nursing strategies and interventions that promote and maintain spiritual well-being
- identify available resources that promote and maintain spiritual well-being

When asked why spirituality was important to her, a 66-year-old female responded:

'It helps with the loneliness. I don't feel alone. I always have someone to talk to. I believe in divine healing, which helps me cope with all of the negative things that happen to me, my family, my friends, and in the world. I pray all of the time because I believe it has the power to heal. Praying gives me an inner peace that is calming. I know that some day my prayers will be answered, either in this life or in the life to come. How will God know who I am if I don't pray? Most of my prayers now are thanking God for my health, my life, and my family. I am truly blessed.'

Introduction

This commentary is an example of an older adult who has provided indicators that she is spiritually well, yet what are the indicators or risk factors of spiritual distress or discomfort that nurses should be aware of to warrant further spiritual assessments and support? How do older people grow spiritually with or without religious beliefs? Do all people grow spirituality, and does growing older constitute a relevant context for this?

To address these ageing and spirituality issues, the following topics will be presented in this chapter: spirituality, religion and spiritual well-being, spiritual development, the impact of Western and Eastern Religions on health care, and assessment, outcome planning, nursing strategies and interventions related to alterations in spiritual integrity. Much of the material drawn on in this chapter is material that is based on reflection and debate rather than empirical evidence. Where such evidence is included, it mostly describes evidence of thinking rather than the thinking itself. Unlike other aspects of living, such as eating or sleeping, spirituality does not necessarily have any obvious physical and measurable signs. This means that it is a dimension of life which can go unnoticed, and nurses may not feel comfortable talking about it with patients. This discomfort can come from a feeling that this is a very private matter, and that there is much potential for being intrusive or causing offence. Spirituality is important, however, and we hope that this chapter will provide an overview of the thinking in this field, and support nurses in taking part in conversations with older people.

Spirituality, religion and well-being

According to Haase et al. (1992), spirituality integrates the body, mind and spirit and creates an energy that is life-affirming based on beliefs and feelings of interconnectedness with self, others, nature, the universe or a deity. The spirit enables human beings to seek the supernatural or find some meaning that transcends us, to wonder about where we came from and where we are going, and gives a sense of worth, hope and reason for our existence (Ellison, 1983). Religion is a unified system of beliefs, practices and rituals associated with a specific institutional group centred on some sacred dimension (Musick et al. 2000). Although the terms 'religiosity' and 'spirituality' are often used interchangeably, both are multidimensional and distinct concepts, and must be handled separately.

Within a holistic nursing practice model, spirituality is identified as a major dimension of human beings. However, it is often neglected in nursing practice because it is not always perceived as relevant to the health issues being addressed (Miller, 1999). In addition, the diversity of cultures in the world's global environment challenges nurses to be knowledgeable about different lifestyles, religions, beliefs, values and philosophies (Carson, 1989). Nurses must also be aware of international declines in the belief in deities, and to recognize that atheists and agnostics have spiritual needs that have no religious underpinnings (Altemeyer, 2004; Dunn, 2008). For many older people, however, religiosity or a belief in a deity provides coping mechanisms that allow them to transcend suffering that may result from chronic illnesses, functional disabilities, depression, losses and pain (Dunn and Horgas, 2004). Thus, for a nurse to have knowledge of their own spiritual or religious beliefs and practices as well as those of an older person is essential to promote or maintain spiritual wellness among older people.

> **Key point**
>
> The diversity of cultures in the world's global environment means that nurses need to be knowledgeable about different lifestyles, religions, beliefs, values and philosophies.

Spiritual well-being within the research literature has been conceptualized as an approximate indicator of spirituality and spiritual health (Ellison, 1983; Dunn, 2008). Spiritual perspectives have been found to influence wellness by:

1. providing the motivations to value life with a sense of purpose and meaning
2. influencing perceptions, beliefs and philosophies of living that guide lifestyles and behaviours
3. contributing to a self-transcendence that helps one rise above the context of personal concerns and materialism (Haase et al., 1992).

For example, spiritual beliefs that arise from religious doctrines have been found to decrease the use of alcohol, smoking and consumption of specific types of food, promoting healthier lifestyles (Krause's 1991; Alexander and Duff, 1992; Idler and Kasl, 1997).

Spiritual development

In the following 1873 quote, Florence Nightingale provided an explanation of how one could grow spiritually through a meaningful connection with a higher power or being.

> "For what is Mysticism? Is it not the attempt to draw near to God, not by rites or ceremonies, but by inward disposition? Is it not merely a hard word for 'The Kingdom of Heaven is within'? Heaven is neither a place nor a time.
>
> (Lewis, 1999)"

Nightingale's spiritual development began at the age 17 when she had a mystical revelation that she was called by God to serve (Attewell, 1998). This revelation was the basis for her holistic vision of nursing that included the requirement for nurses to address the spiritual needs of patients along with physical, psychological and social needs (Bradshaw, 1996). According to Carson (1989), spiritual development can occur when one feels connected to self, others and the universe through meaningful relationships, works of art, and music while never developing a relationship with a deity. Therefore, spiritual growth is individualized and an assessment of how persons find meaning and purpose to their existence is essential.

For older people, the spirit contributes to a natural developmental process entitled gerotranscendence. According to Tornstam (1999), gerotranscendence is a 'shift in metaperspective from a materialistic and pragmatic view of the world to a more cosmic and transcendent one, normally accompanied by an increase in life satisfaction' (p. 178). It is a natural progression towards maturation and wisdom that emphasizes change and development to a new stage in life. These changes include decreased self-centeredness, decreased fear of death, longer periods of meditation, decreased interest in material objects, decreased interest in meaningless social interactions, feeling more connected with the cosmos and universe, and increased connectedness with past and future generations (Miller, 1999).

Stages of Faith Development

Fowler's (1981) *Stages of Faith Development* provides a theoretical perspective of how older people develop spiritually over the lifespan towards gerotranscendence. Fowler defined *faith* as a multidimensional concept that represents a way of being, of living, of imagining, and necessary for spiritual growth to occur and for a relationship with an unseen deity to ensue. Faith is a universal phenomenon present in non-religious and religious persons that gives meaning to life through a belief in a deity, self, career paths, country, institutions, family, success and wealth (Carson, 1989). According to Fowler, faith develops chronologically in seven stages. These stages are:

1. **Undifferentiated faith** – *infancy* stage where trust, courage, hope and love are formed through parental–infant bonding.
2. **Intuitive-projective faith** – *early childhood* stage where imagination is stimulated by stories, gestures and symbols not controlled by logical thinking.
3. **Mythic-literal faith** – *childhood and beyond* stage where stories, beliefs and observances are logically categorized to capture life's meaning and/or belong to faith communities.
4. **Synthetic-conventional faith** – *adolescence and beyond* stage where experiences outside the family (at school, with peers, at work, media and religion) build one's identity and self-image.
5. **Individuative-reflective faith** – *young adulthood and beyond* stage where one critically evaluates one's beliefs and values, has a good understanding of self and others as a part of a social system, and assumes the responsibility for making lifestyle choices and commitments to others and vocations.
6. **Conjunctive faith** – *midlife and beyond* stage where an awareness of multiple interpretations of reality are embraced, and symbolization, metaphors and myths are used to define truths.
7. **Universalizing faith** – *midlife and beyond* stage where the work of previous stages is used towards a unifying love for self and others, and the need to overcome division, oppression and brutality among humankind (Fowler, 1981; Carson, 1989; O'Brien, 2003).

Similarities between Tornstam's theory of gerotranscendence and Fowler's last stage of faith are that older people become less self-centred and more connected with the people of the world, bringing them to the pinnacle of their spiritual development. Both also posit that not all older people will achieve these final stages of spiritual development, and that health care providers can intervene to assist individuals' progress through these stages towards spiritual maturity.

Religions and health care

In a global society, knowledge of how religion can impact on health care is vital. Nurses can become more sensitive to the spiritual needs of patients when they have a greater understanding of the beliefs and practices of Western and Eastern religions (Gerardi, 1989). Because of the brevity of this chapter, a table is provided outlining different Western origin (Gerardi, 1989) and Eastern origin religions (Ludwig, 2004) (see Table 11.1) and their impact on health care. Please note that this table is not an exhaustive list of religions, and that the reader should review other resources for more thorough information. It is also useful to remember that a faith may have a particular geographical origin, but with the movement of people and the spread of faiths, beliefs may be evident in many people regardless of their current or past circumstances. People in the West, for example, may have beliefs which have an Eastern origin, and vice versa.

Nursing guidelines

In addition to having knowledge of the various religions, there are standard guidelines that nurses should practise when addressing spiritual issues. The first standard is to be aware of your own feelings regarding spirituality so that you can identify and respond to the spiritual needs of others. Second, to be able to recognize that spiritual needs are universal and uniquely human, and that these needs can lead to spiritual distress and/or spiritual growth. A third standard of practice is to recognize that nursing is a holistic discipline and that the spiritual domain is amenable to nursing care. Finally, that nurses approach spiritual care in a non-judgemental and open-minded manner (Miller, 1999). These standards are foundational for ensuring positive nurse–patient interactions and health outcomes.

Key point

Spiritual needs are universal and uniquely human, and that these needs can lead to spiritual distress and spiritual growth.

Legal issues and religious beliefs

Spiritual dilemmas between religious beliefs and the need for certain types of medical care can cause conflicts in health care providers and clients. Clients that are faced with making a choice between medical treatments and violating religious tenets often experience spiritual distress. Similarly, health care workers can experience confusion, distress and anger because of a desire to respect the client's and family's rights to choose, while trying to provide optimum health care. Jehovah Witnesses, for example, are forbidden to have a blood transfusion because it violates God's laws. When the decision to decline a compulsory blood transfusion is made, hospitals typically petition the local court for guardianship over the adult. The court will look at whether the client is mentally competent, whether minor children will be affected if the client dies, the duty of the state to protect public interests regarding life, and the potential for liability of the hospital and staff before making the decision to mandate or deny transfusions. Medical treatments are also handled in this

Western origin religions	
	Beliefs and practices
Jewish religion (Orthodox)	Babies named by father; males eight days after birth when circumcision is done by a mohel Women are in a state of impurity when bleeding, so men will not touch them. They will bathe in a pool of *mikvah* when complete Kosher dietary laws are followed. Twenty-four-hour fast is required during Yom Kippur except for those excused from illnesses. No leavened products are eaten during Passover. Prayers of thanksgiving and grace before and after meals Sabbath is observed from sunset Friday until sunset Saturday. Laws prohibiting riding in car, smoking, turning lights on or off, handling money, and using telephone and TV Euthanasia is prohibited. Someone needs to be present when the soul leaves the body. After death, the body should not be left alone until burial within 24 hours. Body is untouched for 8–30 minutes after death. Health care personnel should not touch or bathe the body, but routine care with gloves is permitted. If autopsy is performed, all parts must remain in body. No flowers are permitted. Fetuses must be buried. Seven-day mourning without leaving the home except for Sabbath worship is required for immediate family. Organs or amputated limbs must be available for burial Artificial methods of birth control are not encouraged. Vasectomy is not allowed. Abortion is allowed only to save the mother Organ transplants are not allowed except through rabbinical consent Beard is a mark of piety and should not be shaved with a razor but with scissors and electric razor Men wear skull caps at all times and women cover their heads after marriage Praying is directly to God
Roman Catholic	Baptism is mandatory to enter heaven Abstinence from solid food and alcohol is required 15 minutes prior to receiving Holy Eucharist, except for medicine, water and non-alcoholic beverages Anointing of sick with oil when death is imminent or shortly after sudden death is performed by a priest Obligatory fasting is excused while in the hospital and with health restrictions Birth control is prohibited except for abstinence and natural family planning Organ donation and transplantation is acceptable Religious objects such as rosaries, medals and scapulars should be pinned to gowns or pillows
Islam	Babies are bathed immediately after birth, before giving to the mother. A Muslim prayer is whispered in the child's ear as the first sound the baby hears No pork or alcohol is allowed. All meat must be blessed and killed in a special way

Table 11.1 Western and eastern religions and health care (*Continued*)

Western origin religions	
	Beliefs and practices
	Koran is prayed prior to death. Family washes and places body towards Mecca after death. Health care providers must wear gloves when washing. Cremation is forbidden. Autopsy is forbidden, but if legally performed, all body parts remain. Organ donation is not allowed
	Abortion is prohibited. Contraception is allowed but discouraged
	Washing is required during prayer time
	The Koran must not be touched by anyone ritually unclean, and nothing placed on top of it. A taviz (a black string) may be worn and should not be removed
	Husbands sign consent forms. Modesty must be respected with women. Women are exempt from prayer while bleeding
Jehovah Witness	Baptism by complete immersion
	Smoking and alcohol are discouraged
	Autopsy is a private decision. Cremation is acceptable
	Birth control is a private decision. Abortion is opposed
	Organ transplant is a private decision and must be cleansed with a non-blood solution
	Blood transfusions violate God's laws and are not allowed. Will accept alternatives to blood like plasma expanders, careful surgical techniques to decrease blood loss, use of autologous transfusions, and autotransfusions through use of a heart–lung machine
Eastern origin religions	
Hinduism	World view links physical, mental, social and spiritual well-being very closely. Decisions include family
	Issues regarding contaminants are important: contaminants through blood, sickness, death, improper kitchen and food preparation, and polluted water
	May be vegetarian. Should never cut/shave hair or remove any personal items without consent
	Karma plays a key role in their thinking, therefore internal conflicts may arise between the acceptance of disease as a result of karma and the need to fight
	Need to provide opportunities for meditation, prayer, reading of scriptures or devotional material, music and offerings to God. Environment should provide a sense of calm, balance and wholeness
Buddhism	Suffering has spiritual benefits, therefore may not be viewed as something to be cured
	A calm, peaceful mind at death is important. Environment should provide for meditation and other religious rites. Avoidance of analgesics and sedatives at the end of life to maintain wholesomeness and level of awareness
	Abortion and euthanasia are prohibited. Belief that all body systems are interconnected causes concerns regarding issues surrounding brain death and organ donations.

Table 11.1 Western and eastern religions and health care

manner; however, treatment may be mandated in emergency and life-threatening situations regardless of client beliefs (McMullen, 1989).

Scenario 11.1

Andrea, an 88-year-old woman, admitted for a gangrenous left leg, refused to give permission to amputate. The woman was found to be competent based on professional psychiatric testing. The hospital administration petitioned the court for guardianship over the adult. The court found in favour of the woman to refuse amputation because of religious beliefs. The woman died two weeks later from septicaemia secondary to gangrene.

- *Was this a justified ruling by the court and, if so, why?*
- *How could you support other staff and family members who do not share the same religious beliefs as Andrea?*

Spiritual care in nursing

While spirituality is generally perceived to be important to nurses, researchers have found that they often feel unprepared to provide spiritual care, and that there is lack of agreement on what spiritual care should consist of (Tuck et al. 2001; McEwen, 2005). Hence, the purpose of this section is to increase nursing knowledge regarding the provision of spiritual care to patients.

Spiritual care seeks to affirm the value of all people through non-judgemental love (Wright, 2002) and acts of compassion (Greasely et al., 2001). Spiritual care can be implemented on several levels (Narayanasamy and Owens, 2001):

- personal level (use of listening, empathy and reflective techniques);
- procedural level (use of logical and technical approaches to meet spiritual needs);
- culturalistic level (incorporation of cultural sensitivity into care);
- evangelical level (use of prayer and Bible readings).

For this chapter, spiritual care is presented within the context of the nursing process; assessment, diagnosis, outcome planning, implementing and evaluation.

Assessment

According to Massey et al. (2004), there are three levels of inquiry into spiritual health. The first is spiritual screening, where a basic examination is performed to determine if the patient is at a spiritual risk for poor health outcomes as a result of unmet spiritual needs. Spiritual needs are individually defined, although evidence cited in the literature suggests commonalities among all people. These commonalities include the (1) need for meaning and purpose in life, (2) need to give and receive love, (3) need for hope, (4) need to be connected, and (5) need to be productive and successful. Defining behaviours that may suggest that these needs are not being met include expressions of concern or anger with meanings related to self, others, life, death, belief systems, a deity and suffering (Stoll, 1989).

Spiritual history taking

Spiritual history taking, the second level of inquiry, is when more information is needed and so a full history is taken. A good model for spiritual history taking is the **SPIRIT** Model developed by Maugans (1996). The acronym SPIRIT stands for the following:

S = spiritual belief system (may or may not have a religious affiliation);

P = personal spirituality (beliefs and practices of your religion and/or personal spiritual system that individuals accept or do not accept);

I = integration and involvement in a spiritual community;

R = ritualized practices and restrictions (practices, lifestyles and forbidden types of medical care);

I = implications for medical care (how this affects practice);

T = terminal events planning (how this affects end of life care).

The final level of inquiry, spiritual assessment, is an invasive investigation into a patient's spiritual life and history that must be addressed in order to treat the patient's condition more effectively (Massey et al., 2004).

According to Miller (1999), other questions that can be used to assess spiritual needs include:

- What makes your life meaningful and important?
- What do you wish to accomplish in life?
- What gives you pleasure and satisfaction?
- Do you believe in a supreme power or being?
- Do you pray or practise religious rituals or activities?
- What do you do that brings you peace of mind and relieves stress?
- What are your beliefs regarding death and dying?
- Do you need any spiritual objects, like a Bible or rosary beads?
- Would you like a visit from pastoral care or your religious leader?
- Are their any conflicts between the healthcare treatment plan and your beliefs?
- Are there any special religious considerations that need to be addressed, like dietary restrictions or religious observances?

During the interview, listen for evidence of spiritual distress that may include suicidal ideation, anger towards a deity and self, inabilities to forgive self and/or others, feelings of hopelessness, uselessness, loneliness, and abandonment, questions about purpose and meaning to life, losses and suffering.

Spiritual assessment and dementia

Spiritual needs among older people with dementia may not be easily assessed because of communication difficulties, memory problems, and alienation from self and others. Without the assistance of family or significant others, the ability to obtain an accurate spiritual assessment for these patients may not be possible. Thus, it is imperative that health care providers understand that spiritual needs, such as the need to communicate and relate to others, the need to be loved and to love, and the need to stay spiritually connected, still have to be met in people with dementia (Lenshyn, 2004).

Awareness of the degree of cognitive difficulty is also crucial when engaging in conversations about spirituality. Religious behaviours (e.g. praying, listening to gospel music, and reading the Bible) that have been practised every day may still continue whatever cognitive issues may arise. Hence, emotions attached to these religious activities can be assessed by carers as negative or positive within this population (Vance, 2004).

Nursing assessment

According to Carpenito-Moyet (2004), the North American Nursing Diagnosis Association (NANDA) nursing diagnosis of *spiritual distress* is assessed when an individual or group experiences problems related to their belief or value systems that provide strength, hope and meaning to life. Conversely, a NANDA wellness diagnosis of *readiness for enhanced spiritual wellness* is assessed when an individual expresses affirmation of life in relationship to a higher power, self, community and environment that nurtures and celebrates wholeness. O'Brien (1982) identified seven other nursing diagnoses related to alterations in spiritual integrity. These seven nursing diagnoses are:

1 ***Spiritual pain*** – when individuals express discomfort, lack of peace, or suffering related to one's relationship with a deity; feelings of having a void or lack of spiritual fulfilment are voiced.
2 ***Spiritual alienation*** – loneliness or feelings that a deity seems far away; feeling that one has to depend on oneself in difficult times; having a negative attitude that a deity would not be helpful or provide comfort.
3 ***Spiritual anxiety*** – individual expresses fear of a deity's wrath and punishment; a deity is displeased and will not provide for them.
4 ***Spiritual guilt*** – the feelings that one has failed to do what should have been done in one's life; one's lifestyle or behaviours were not pleasing to a deity, self or others.
5 ***Spiritual anger*** – frustrations, anguish or outrage at a deity, self or others are expressed.
6 ***Spiritual loss*** – feeling that a deity has temporarily or permanently taken away love leaving behind a sense of emptiness.
7 ***Spiritual despair*** – no hope of ever having a positive spiritual relationship.

Outcome planning

Outcomes should be individualized and address each nursing diagnosis as it relates to the spiritual care needed to improve the patient's health status. Goal or outcome achievements should be written as subjective, measurable objectives for easy evaluation (Mauk et al.,

2004). Outcome criteria should include expressions of spiritual harmony and wholeness. Indicators can include (a) continued use of spiritual practices and beliefs that are not detrimental to health, (b) verbal reports on a reduction in feelings of guilt and anxiety, (c) verbal reports on an increase in comfort, (d) maintaining previous relationship with a deity or a supreme being (Carpenito-Moyet, 2004).

Spiritual interventions

According to Burkhardt and Nagai-Jacobson (2004), to develop a therapeutic relationship with clients, nurses must master the art of attentive listening and focused presence, which can be used for both assessment and interventions in spiritual care. Being intentionally present with another person means to listen with your whole being and with an open heart, and to recognize that all persons are spiritual beings. Listening in healing ways is to:

- focus on the client as a whole person;
- set aside the need to 'fix,' 'answer,' or 'correct';
- be in silence and interrupt as little as possible;
- hear with all your senses;
- let the conversation flow and hear the meanings and relationships in the story;
- not prematurely diagnose.

Through the sharing of stories, nurses can gain insight into clients' spiritual concerns and needs not being addressed, while the client gains new insights about their own lives, which may lead to affirmations, validations and acceptance. Thus, attentive listening and focused presence are foundational to all spiritual care interventions.

Interventions that aim to instil hope are also important. Hope fosters the belief that the situation will get better and that this situation is temporary and improvement is coming. Behaviours that foster hope in clients include: demonstrating acceptance of the client, accentuating the positive in situations, being honest, promoting self-care, providing accurate information, educating and fostering a healing environment (Mauk et al., 2004). Other interventions used in spiritual care may be classified as complementary and alternative medicine (CAM) therapies. Complementary and alternative medicine is characterized as an unconventional collection of healing systems in the USA. These systems are used to treat illness, and promote health and well-being. In addition, these systems contain their own worldviews, theories, modalities, products and practices (National Institutes of Health (NIH), 2002).

CAM therapies that can be implemented in spiritual care include:

- prayer;
- massage;
- therapeutic touch;
- meditation;
- yoga;
- Tai Chi;
- therapeutic arts (drama, music, art and dance);
- humour;

- pet and/or animal-assisted therapy;
- gardening;
- reminiscence therapy.

Scenario 11.2

During a yearly physical examination, a 78-year-old man began to talk about the death of his wife. They had been married for 50 years and were devout Catholics, attending Mass every Sunday. The man began to cry when he recounted how she had suffered for two years with cancer, and could not understand why God had done this to her. He had stopped going to Mass because it reminded him of her too much, and that remembrances of the dead mentioned often during the Mass would make him break down and cry. He felt embarrassed for his weakness, but missed receiving weekly Eucharist. He complained that he was not sleeping well at night and losing weight.

- *After reviewing the interventions mentioned in this chapter, what spiritual care is needed for this man?*

Evaluation

Evaluation consists of two steps: evaluating goal achievement and reviewing the plan of care. These two steps are foundational for ongoing reassessment, diagnosing, planning and intervention (Mauk et al., 2004). A primary goal in spiritual care is to enhance spiritual well-being. Although numerous spirituality scales exist, to date, there is only one spiritual well-being scale, the Geriatric Spiritual Well-being Scale (GSWB), developed by Dunn (2008) that separates religious items from other scale items. This scale was developed specifically to provide atheists and agnostics a more valid measurement of spiritual well-being. International declines in religious beliefs have been reported although this is not consistent globally, and a large percentage of older people in the USA believe in God and have religious affiliations for example. Therefore, unless religious beliefs are assessed and present, religious items should not be incorporated as scale items.

Four major subscales comprise the GSWB; affirmative self-appraisal, connectedness, altruistic benevolence and faith ways. The affirmative self-appraisal subscale measures the ability of older people to remember and recall past life events as beneficial experiences that provided purpose and meaning to their lives. The connectedness subscale measures one's sense of belonging and feeling connected to self and others. The altruistic benevolence subscale measures one's ability to be helpful or perform altruistic behaviours to assist others. Finally, the faith ways subscale measures one's level of internalized religiosity and/or faith in a deity. This subscale should not be included in the analyses if a belief in a supreme being is not validated (see Table 11.2). To determine whether the faith ways subscale items should be included, a question like 'How important is God in your life?' on a 4-point Likert scale ranging from 1 = 'not at all important' to 4 = 'very important' should be asked prior to addressing the faith way items. If the participant reports that God is not important, they should be prompted to skip over the faith way questions. This eliminates the inherent bias towards those that have religious beliefs.

Affirmative self-appraisal
As I grow older, I find it easier to forgive myself.
*I don't enjoy remembering and talking about my life.
I find meaning and purpose in my life.
I am able to share my past life with others.
Connectedness
I have a good sense of belonging.
*Most people are not friendly to me.
I find it easy to forgive others.
I have somewhere to go almost every day.
Altruistic benevolence
I am still capable of helping others.
*I am not able to give back to my community.
I find volunteering my time and talents rewarding.
I feel better giving rather than receiving from others.
Faith ways
I find peace and comfort in prayer.
*I don't believe God listens to my prayers.
God provides meaning in my life.
My religious beliefs influence my life decisions.

* items to be recoded

Table 11.2 Geriatric spiritual well-being scale with religious items

Conclusion

According to the American Association of Colleges of Nursing (2004), nurse practitioners and clinical nurse specialists must develop cultural and spiritual competences in order to care for older people. This includes 'assessing patients' and caregivers' cultural and spiritual priorities as a part of a holistic assessment and adapting age-specific assessment methods or tools to a culturally diverse population' (p. 14).

In summary, assessing patients' religious beliefs and practice prior to assessing spiritual well-being is essential and nurses need to recognize that agnostics/atheists have spiritual needs that do not include religious beliefs or practices. Having knowledge of an older person's beliefs and practices can open dialogue and enhance nurse–patient relationships through a shared connectedness. Nurses should not be afraid to practise spiritual actions (to pray or read the Bible for example) with older people if they find comfort and peace through these activities. However, nurses should not judge others for their non-belief and/or impose their own beliefs.

References

Alexander, F. and Duff, R.W. (1992) Religion and drinking in the retirement community, *Journal of Religious Gerontology*, 8(4): 27–44.

Altemeyer, B. (2004) The decline of organized religion in western civilization, *The International Journal for the Psychology of Religion*, 14: 77–89.

American Association of Colleges of Nursing (2004) *Nurse Practitioner and Clinical Nurse Specialist Competencies for Older Adult Care*. Washington, DC: American Association of Colleges of Nursing.

Attewell, A. (1998) Florence Nightingale (1820–1910), *Prospects: The Quarterly Review of Comparative Education*, 28: 153–66.

Bradshaw, A. (1996) The legacy of Nightingale, *Nursing Times*, 92(6): 42–43.

Burkhardt, M.A., and Nagai-Jacobson, M.G. (2004) in B.M. Dossey, L. Keegan and C.E. Carpenito-Moyet, L.J. *Nursing Diagnosis: Application to Clinical Practice*, 10th edn. Philadelphia, PA: Lippincott Williams & Wilkins.

Carpenito-Moyet, L.J. (2004) *Nursing Diagnosis: Application to Clinical Practice*, 10th edn. Philadelphia: Lippincott Williams and Wilkins.

Carson, V.B. (1989) Spiritual development across the life span, in V.B. Carson (ed.) *Spiritual Dimensions of Nursing Practice* (pp. 24–52). Philadelphia, PA: W.B. Saunders.

Dunn, K.S. (2008) Development and psychometric testing of a new geriatric spiritual well-being scale, *International Journal of Older People Nursing*, 3: 161–69.

Dunn, K.S. and Horgas, A.L. (2004) Religious and non-religious coping in older adults experiencing chronic pain, *Pain Management in Nursing*, 5(1): 19–28.

Ellison, C.W. (1983) Spiritual well-being: conceptualization and measurement, *Journal of Psychology and Theology*, 11: 330–40.

Fowler, J.W. (1981) *Stages of Faith Development*. New York: HarperCollins.

Gerardi, R. (1989) Western spirituality and health care, in V.B. Carson (ed.) *Spiritual Dimensions of Nursing Practice* (pp. 76–112). Philadelphia, PA: W.B. Saunders.

Greasely, P., Chiu, L.F., and Gartland, M. (2001) The concept of spiritual care in mental health nursing, *Journal of Advanced Nursing*, 33(5): 629–37.

Haase, J.E., Britt, T., Coward, D.D., Leidy, N.K. and Penn, P.E. (1992) Simultaneous concept analysis of spiritual perspective, hope, acceptance and self-transcendance, *Image: Journal of Nursing Scholarship*, 24(2): 141–47.

Idler, E.L. and Kasl, S.V. (1997) Religion among disabled and nondisabled persons II: attendance at religious services as a predictor of the course of disability, *Journal of Gerontology: Social Sciences*, 52B: S306–S16.

Krause, N. (1991) Stress, religiosity, and abstinence from alcohol, *Psychology and Aging*, 6: 134–44.

Lenshyn, J. (2004) Reaching the living echo: a new paradigm for the provision of spiritual care for persons living with Alzheimer's disease, *Alzheimer's Care Quarterly*, 5: 313–23.

Lewis, J.J. (1999) *Florence Nightingale Quotes: Florence Nightingale* (1820–1910). Available online at www.womenhistory.about.com/cs/quotes/a/qu_nightingale.htm (accessed 7 March 2011).

Ludwig, T.M. (2004) South Asian traditions, in K.L. Mauk and N.K. Schmidt (eds) *Spiritual Care in Nursing Practice* (pp. 131–63). New York: Lippincott Williams & Wilkins.

Massey, K., Fitchett, G. and Roberts, P.A. (2004) Assessment and diagnosis in spiritual care, in K.L. Mauk and N.K. Schmidt (eds) *Spiritual Care in Nursing Practice* (pp. 209–42). New York: Lippincott Williams & Wilkins.

Maugans, T.A. (1996) The SPIRITual history, *Archives of Family Medicine*, 5(1): 11–16.

Mauk, K.L., Russell, C.A. and Schmidt, N.A. (2004) Planning, implementing and evaluating spiritual care, in K.L. Mauk and N.K. Schmidt (eds) *Spiritual Care in Nursing Practice* (pp. 243–75). New York: Lippincott Williams & Wilkins.

McEwen, M. (2005) Spiritual nursing care, *Holistic Nursing Practice*, 19(4): 161–68.

McMullen, P.C. (1989) Religious belief, legal issues, and health care, in V.B. Carson (ed.) *Spiritual Dimensions of Nursing Practice* (pp. 76–112). Philadelphia, PA: W.B. Saunders.

Miller, C.A. (1999) *Nursing Care of Older Adults: Theory and practice*, 3rd edn. Philadelphia, PA: J.B. Lippinicott Company.

Musick, M.A., Traphagen, J.W., Koenig, H.G. and Larson, D.B. (2000) Spirituality in physical health and aging, *Journal of Adult Development*, 7: 73–86.

Narayanasamy, A. and Owens, J. (2001) A critical incident study of nurses' responses to the spiritual needs of their patients, *Journal of Advanced Nursing*, 33(4): 446–56.

National Institutes of Health (2002, March) *White House Commission on Complementary and Alternative Medicine Policy: Final Report* (Publication No. 03-5411). Available online at www.whccamp.hhs.gov/finalreport.html (accessed 1 April 2007).

O'Brien, M.E. (1982) The need for spiritual integrity, in H. Yura and M. Walsh (eds) *Human Needs and the Nursing Process* (Vol. 2, pp. 82–115). Norwalk, CT: Appleton Century Crofts.

O'Brien, M.E. (2003) *Spirituality in Nursing: Standing on Holy Ground*, 2nd edn. Boston, MA: Jones and Bartlett.

Stoll, R.E. (1989) The essence of spirituality, in U.B. Calson (ed.) *Spiritual Dimensions of Nursing Practice*. Philadelphia, PA: W.B. Saunders.

Tornstam, L. (1999) Late life transcendence: a new developmental perspective on aging, in L.E. Thomas and S.A. Eisenhandler (eds) *Religion, Belief, and Spirituality in Late Life* (pp. 178–202). New York: Springer.

Tuck, I., Pullen, L. and Wallace, D. (2001) A comparative study of the spiritual perspectives and interventions of mental health and parish nurses, *Issues in Mental Health Nursing*, 22: 593–605.

Vance, D.E. (2004) Spiritual activities for adults with Alzheimer's disease: the cognitive components of dementia and religion, *Journal of Religion, Spirituality & Aging*, 17(1/2): 109–130.

Wright, M.C. (2002) The essence of spiritual care: a phenomenological enquiry, *Palliative Medicine*, 16(2): 125–32.

CHAPTER 12

Sexuality and intimacy

Linda McAuliffe, Rhonda Nay and Michael Bauer

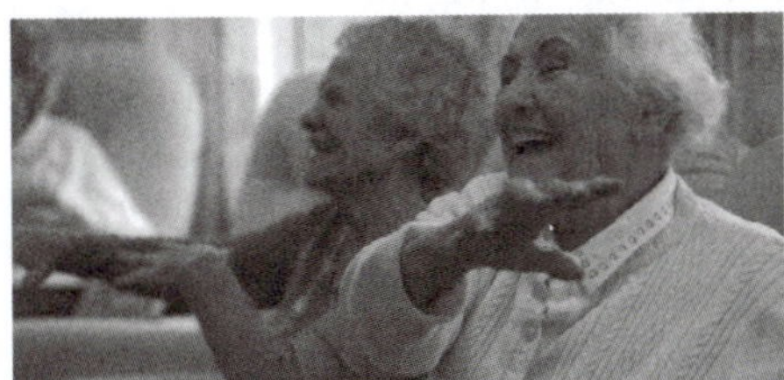 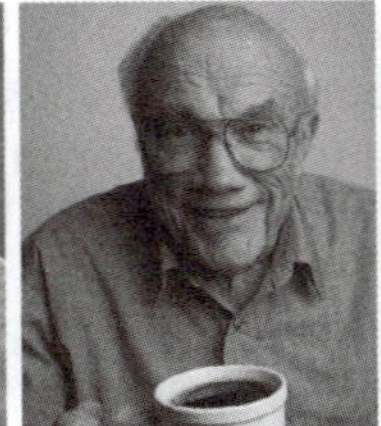 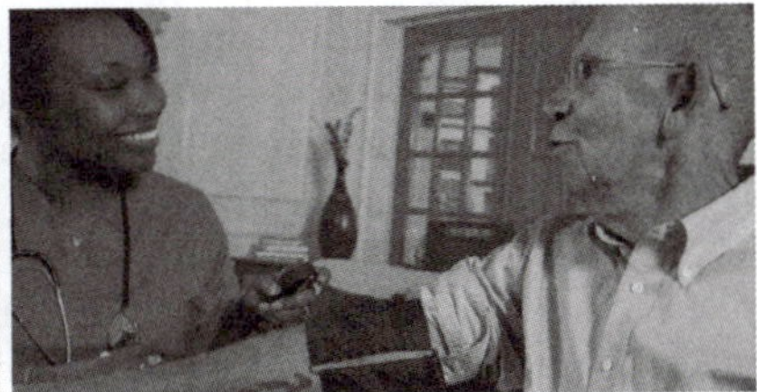

Learning objectives

At the end of this chapter, the reader will be able to:

- understand the multidimensional nature of sexuality
- gain insight into what sexuality means to older people
- appreciate the issues associated with sexuality in older people
- learn strategies such as how to conduct a sexuality assessment

Elaine White (aged 76) comments as follows:

'Societal attitudes regard sexuality as an activity solely for younger people and therefore it becomes a subject of decreasing significance as people age. However, I believe that sexuality is the basis of human existence and maintaining a healthy sexual relationship is very important to me. I have found that if one has had an adult lifetime of intimate physical sexual activity, then this activity will continue to flourish right through older age as long as there is not an overriding medical condition that may cause some loss of libido. Physical sexual activity is just as fulfilling to us older people as it is to the younger generation. Incidentally younger people seem to think that they invented sex, they certainly have got that wrong!

I must admit that the intensiveness and occurrence does slow down a bit. There may be a need to experiment with different positioning and ways of stimulating one's partner, but rest assured the need for intimate contact remains as important as ever. Sometimes it may be worth using, as part of the foreplay, some KY Jelly to increase lubrication. If the arthritis is playing up a bit, one needs to plan ahead by taking pain relief tablets half an hour before any activity and perhaps using pillows to support aching limbs. If the male partner needs pharmaceutical assistance, timing is essential for the best effect. It does take the spontaneity out of the encounter but the end results can be just as rewarding.

(*continued*)

If there are times when libido might be lost temporarily for some medical reason, I believe it is important not to forget to maintain the first levels of intimacy which can be an emotional comfort during a bout of poor health, such as giving and receiving loving warmth and affection, kissing, cuddling, caressing, sharing feelings, holding one another, etc. I would also practise some sensual interventions as well, such as reciprocal massaging one's partner with nice essential oils. The comfort of touch can be very sensuous; a strategy I have learned to prevent passion dying out of the relationship. Maintaining emotional closeness is very important to us older people.

Unfortunately so many of my same aged friends have lost their partners and I always suggest it may be beneficial to purchase an appropriate sexual aid, such as a vibrator. There are many different products available at 'Adult Shops' so it is worth a try.

I have found that keeping involved in active physical sexual activities wards off impotence for the males and certainly can help to keep the vaginal tissue well lubricated. There are other benefits as well! A physical sexual activity with a partner or even self-stimulation, can promote relaxation, as well as improve insomnia. Much better than a sleeping tablet!

Finally, growing old does not put an end to physical sexual activity, despite what younger people think. Keeping sexually active is one of the keys to a successful happier older age. No one wants to 'rust out' due to lack of use!'

Introduction

Sexuality. What does the word conjure up for you? Chances are you associate the word with raunchy images of semi-naked young people on billboards and in the pages of magazines. For this you can be forgiven. Our society does a good job at portraying sexuality as the exclusive domain of the young. But what about the not so young? What role, if any, does sexuality play for the older adult? As Elaine's story illustrates, sexuality can play an important role in later life, and can be just as fulfilling to older people as it is to the younger generation.

Key point

Sexuality can play an important role in later life, and can be just as fulfilling to older people as it is to the younger generation.

Sexuality means much more than just intercourse. A working definition developed on behalf of the World Health Organization (WHO) describes sexuality as encompassing 'sex, gender identities and roles, sexual orientation, eroticism, pleasure, intimacy and reproduction. Sexuality is experienced and expressed in thoughts, fantasies, desires, beliefs, attitudes, values, behaviours, practices, roles and relationships.' (www.who.int/reproductivehealth/topics/gender_rights/sexual_health/html). Our sexuality helps define who we are, and age does not change this.

For older people, sexuality can mean many different things. It can mean engaging in sexual intercourse or masturbation, but it can also encompass the need to convey love and tenderness as well as physical desire (Stausmire, 2004). It can mean kissing and cuddling and sharing private words. It can mean looking and feeling one's best or enjoying the companionship of a close other (Nay, 2004). It can mean expressing oneself when other forms of expression have been taken away.

Expressing sexuality is an act of daily living that is significant for many older adults. Illness, medication, treatment and surgical procedures can all impact on sexual functioning (Hill et al., 2003; Hordern and Currow, 2003; Mott et al., 2005), but this does not necessarily mean sexual interest or desire is diminished. Expressing one's sexuality can even maximize physical and psychological well-being (Trudel et al., 2000) and enhance quality of life (Wang et al., 2008).

Although older adults living in the community can and do enjoy freedom of sexual expression in their own homes, freedom of sexual expression has been found to be denied in both residential (Ward et al., 2005) and rehabilitation (Ali, 2004) settings alike. Unfortunately, this is an area where myths and misperceptions commonly inform clinical practice rather than a sound knowledge base (Gott et al., 2004).

So what are the myths surrounding later life sexuality? What do we really know about sexuality in older people? What does sexuality mean to the older person? And what issues do nurses face in addressing this 'activity of daily living'?

Incidence and type of difficulty

What do we know about older people and sexuality? For over half a century research has consistently shown that older people generally maintain sexual interest and remain sexually capable into their 90s (see Gott, 2005 for an overview of these studies). This is also true in residential aged care facilities, where open displays of an affectionate and sexual nature between residents are not uncommon, and where residents may, as Hubbard et al. (2003) report, engage in intimate touch, kissing, sexual talk, flirting and teasing.

The 'sexless oldie' is clearly then an unwarranted stereotype, as the research indicates that many older adults express interest in and engage in sexual activity. Unfortunately, there are many myths about sexuality and older people that prevent people enjoying this important element of quality of life. These are presented below along with the research that refutes each myth.

Myth: older people do not have sex (and do not want to have sex)

Older people do have sex. Although there may be a decline in sexual activity with age this does not mean sex stops altogether. In a sample of 200 adults aged 80–102 years, Bretschneider and McCoy (1988) found that 62 per cent of men and 32 per cent of women still had intercourse; 26 per cent of men and 10 per cent of women had intercourse 'often'; 72 per cent of men and 40 per cent of women masturbated; 19 per cent of men and 12 per cent of women fantasized about the opposite sex; and 53 per cent of men and 25 per cent of women had a regular sex partner. These results are supported by a more recent study of 3,005 community dwelling adults aged 57–85 years, which found 54 per cent of sexually active adults reported having sex 2–3 times per month; 23 per cent reported having sex at least once a week; and 31 per cent reported participating in oral sex (Lindau et al., 2007).

Not only do older people have sex, they also want more sex. Holden et al. (2005) reported that 27 per cent of men aged 70 years or older desired more frequent sexual activity; some of these men admitted paying for the use of commercial sex services to satisfy this need. A study of older adults living in independent living facilities found that they wanted to maintain a sexual relationship that included touching and kissing and wanted to have more sexual experiences than they currently had accessible (Ginsberg et al., 2005).

Myth: older people who are ill cannot have sex (and do not desire sex)

Just because a person is ill, this does not mean that they are no longer sexually interested or capable. Older people have been found to be sexually interested and active even with numerous health problems and sexual dysfunction (Moreira et al., 2005), and this even extends to older people with fatal illness in the weeks or days prior to death (Lemieux et al., 2004).

Although sexual activity in these cases may have to be modified, and may not allow for penetrative sex, there are numerous ways in which a person can sexually participate. Discussing role changes with one's partner, trying new positions, taking analgesia half an hour before activity to ease the pain from arthritis, and using pillows to support painful body parts (Nay, 2004) are just some ways to help overcome the limitations that illness can impose. The importance of intimacy to well-being cannot be underestimated (Gott and Hinchliff, 2003).

Myth: older people cannot have sex because they experience sexual dysfunction

Older people can have sex despite sexual dysfunction. True, ageing brings with it many changes to the body, and some of these changes can affect both male and female sexual functioning (Trudel et al., 2000; Nusbaum et al., 2005). In men, it may take longer to achieve an erection; in women, vaginal lubrication may be decreased.

However, these changes need not prevent the enjoyment of sexual activity (Brock and Jennings, 2007). Adaptations such as spending more time on stimulating the partner, and using lubricants to facilitate painless intercourse, can help the older adult to maintain their sexual relationship.

Age-related changes such as increased time between erection and ejaculation and the need for stimulation over a longer period may even improve love-making by slowing the experience, and may account for reports by some older people that sex improves with age (Gott and Hinchliff, 2003).

Myth: if older people want to talk about sex or a sexual problem, then they will bring it up

Research suggests otherwise. Treatment-seeking is often inhibited by worrying about how one will be perceived by health professionals when expressing a sexual concern, and shame, fear and embarrassment can also act as barriers to seeking advice (Gott et al., 2004).

Yet, despite any embarrassment older people may feel discussing sexual issues, most older people would welcome the opportunity to discuss sexual concerns with their health professional (Nusbaum et al., 2004; Moreira et al., 2005) and believe that being asked about sexual needs and function should be part of clinical care (Lemieux et al., 2004). The literature, however, suggests that this rarely happens (Lemieux et al., 2004; Moreira et al., 2005) and that sexuality in older people is a topic that is not openly discussed or addressed by health professionals in many cultures (Tsai, 2004).

Myth: older people with dementia cannot have sexual relationships

Older people with dementia can and do have sexual relationships. Some will continue to have an uninterrupted sexual relationship with their spouse; for others, the relationship may change (Kuppuswamy et al., 2007). For others again, new intimate and sexual relationships may be formed in the residential setting. This can happen even when the older person already has a partner. This is hardly surprising, as the need for contact, affection and intimacy is universal and extends beyond cognitive status (Ward et al., 2005).

Key point

Older people with dementia can and do have sexual relationships.

Too often in residential care the sexual behaviour of residents is considered 'problem' behaviour (Hajjar and Kamel, 2003) in need of 'managing' with the use of tranquillizers (Archibald, 2003), or in need of surveying and regulating (Ward et al., 2005). Often this is an attempt to manage 'scary' sexual situations between residents (Archibald, 2003), as consent of both parties needs to be considered. It is possible, however, to protect the right of the person with dementia to freedom of sexual expression by balancing the autonomy of the resident with perceived level of risk (Ward et al., 2005). This is discussed further in the second half of this chapter.

Scenario 12.1

Jean is aged 94 and has been residing with her friend Trudy for many years. They trained together, travelled the world, and shared many of life's experiences. Trudy has dementia and has been admitted to a nursing home as Jean could no longer manage her care. Prior to admission, Trudy spent a lot of time in the garden and fell occasionally but otherwise had no behaviours of concern reported.

Following admission the nurses described Trudy as 'the resident from hell'. She was labelled aggressive, agitated, a wanderer, and was heavily sedated so the nurses could manage and other residents could get some sleep.

Jean was distraught – she had never seen her friend like this – and as an 'old nurse' felt she had to do something. She suggested she too be admitted and share a room to reassure Trudy. This of course was immediately rejected as the 'beds were needed for those assessed as requiring them'. Jean was labelled as difficult and demanding. Eventually Trudy climbed into bed with a 'strange man' who hit her fiercely resulting in head injury and eventual death.

(continued)

Had the staff included sexuality in their assessment they would have discovered that Jean and Trudy had shared a bed for 57 years. Perhaps supporting Jean to continue that tradition would have reduced Trudy's 'aggression, agitation and wandering', allayed Jean's fear and grief, and resulted in a better outcome for all concerned.

- *How can you support the full assessment of older people in your area of work, including sexuality?*
- *If you had been nursing Jean, how would you have been able to manage this situation?*

What are the implications of the above myths? There are many. Such myths deny the older person their right to freedom of sexual expression. This denial can impact on a person's sense of self, their quality of life, and their well-being. It can affect personal relationships and deprive a person of comfort in difficult times. It can pose major health risks, such as undiagnosed sexual health problems. It can cheat a person of the right to exercise choice over their life when many other choices may have already been taken away.

Nursing strategies and interventions

As a health professional, you are in a position to ensure that the rights of the older individual are preserved and that they are able to maintain the same freedom of sexual expression they had prior to entering care. Would you want your right to choose taken away? Probably not. Why would this be any different when you are older? The following section outlines the nursing strategies and interventions one can adopt to overcome barriers to sexual expression and promote health and well-being in the older adult.

Assessment

When older people access health care, we assess many things. We ask about a person's eyesight and whether they wear glasses; we ask about their hearing and if they use a hearing aid; we ask about the person's mobility and how much they are able to do things in their daily life. We even ask about a person's continence, both urinary and faecal. So why then do we not ask about sexual health and needs? Especially when this aspect of a person's life contributes so much to their sense of self and well-being?

Often we avoid things that we find make us uncomfortable. Discussing sexuality with our older patients may be one of those things. Indeed, many health professionals are reluctant to initiate conversation about sexuality and sexual health and needs with their patients due to fear, embarrassment or discomfort (Hordern and Street, 2007). However, we know that many older adults would welcome the opportunity to discuss their sexual concerns with health professionals (Aizenberg et al., 2002; Gott et al., 2004), and the discomfort of the health professional should not prevent a person from doing so or from accessing appropriate intervention where needed.

Discomfort can be reduced by using a number of strategies, such as adopting a professional demeanour; displaying comfort with (and knowledge of) the topic; and being kind, understanding and empathic (Nusbaum et al., 2004). Making sure the discussion takes place where you will not be interrupted, being non-judgemental, using open-ended questions, and using easy to understand language rather than medical jargon can also help the conversation to proceed more smoothly (Hordern and Currow, 2003).

The health professional should approach the assessment with the same sensitivity that is needed when discussing other potentially delicate issues, such as incontinence. Not all older people will want to discuss their sexual health and needs, and this right to choose must be respected. Others will want to participate in a discussion but may feel embarrassed and require reassurance. What is most important is that the person be given the opportunity to discuss their sexual health and needs and receive an appropriate response and follow-up from the health professional, whether this is by referral to a psychosexual medicine specialist or counselling psychologist, arranging for the person to have regular uninterrupted private time, or other appropriate intervention.

Assessment of the older person's sexual health and needs should be comprehensive. It should cover sexual health, history, dysfunction, and preferences of the older person, and should be conducted upon admission and recorded in the care plan, with the topic revisited during regular assessments.

What if the person has dementia? Should an assessment still be conducted? The answer is yes. Having dementia does not extinguish sexual needs. Quality of life should be considered as well as well-being and safety (Hajjar and Kamel, 2003). Capacity to participate in intimate relationships should be assessed, and consideration should be given to the implications associated with progression of dementia and the increased need for supervision and advocacy (Berger, 2000).

The following provides a guide for conducting a sexual health and needs assessment with the older person.

ACEBAC Sexuality and Older People Assessment Guide

Because talking about sex is embarrassing for many people it is good to integrate the assessment into your overall workup – acknowledge it can be embarrassing, advise that it is perfectly normal to be sexually active (or not) in old age, and use a good dose of humour:

- *Okay, we have talked about your bowel function and water works, and have checked your heart and lungs, memory, hearing and eyesight!*
- *Often as we age, things can get in the way of us remaining as sexually active as we might like – things like pain, medications, loss of a partner, and so on. Most people feel a bit embarrassed talking about their sexuality, or having pap smears or prostate exams, and yet all can be very important to our quality of life and relationships, so I just want to check with you if there are areas of your sexual expression causing you any concern.*
- *Ageing can, of course, slow us up a bit and leave us with some concerns and difficulties such as erection or dry vagina problems, so you may find taking more time and using lubricants can be a big help. With the arthritic pain, make sure you have your analgesics regularly and use some pillows to support painful arms or legs.* (How you respond here will depend on issues that may be raised – this could turn into a discussion around impotence, Viagra, vaginal prolapse, aversion

(*continued*)

to masturbation, safe sex, or issues with the partner, and referral may be the most appropriate action.)

- *A lot of people say their sex lives improve with age and we know it is good for reducing pain and depression so we need to keep you active.*
- *There are lots of books and other resources that older people have found useful – I can provide you with a list if you like.*

(Bauer et al., 2009a)

Planning

There is much we as health professionals can do when it comes to planning. We can anticipate what our patients/residents (both current and future) may need; we can make comprehensive assessments routine and ask the older person what is important to them; we can empower older people by ensuring we provide them with clear information that addresses their concerns; we can ensure we have policies in place to guide staff; and we can educate both ourselves and our patients/residents so that we are equipped with accurate knowledge.

Creating the right environment

We all know that intimacy largely depends on the condition of privacy. The residential setting is typically not conducive to this. Often rooms are shared, beds are single-sized, and physical spaces are uninviting (Lemieux et al., 2004), and it is not unusual to have curtain dividers and unlockable doors (Bauer, 1999). Add to this the possibility that any time of the day or night you may be interrupted by a staff member coming to 'check' on you and it is hard to imagine a less private place.

Not being able to live independently in your own home does not mean that you should have to surrender to a lack of privacy and frequent intrusion for the rest of your life. True, the built environment can largely determine whether there are private spaces, and a growing awareness of this has led to facilities factoring this in to renovation plans (e.g. by including more private areas, locks on doors, designing rooms so they can be joined together to form one larger room). However, there are steps that can be taken to promote privacy irrespective of whether any walls are likely to be knocked down in the immediate future. These include providing residents with 'do not disturb' signs and allowing doors to stay closed, providing the option of having a double bed, or allocating a special room for conjugal visits (Mulligan and Palguta, 1991). Creative problem-solving can ensure that the person's right to privacy is respected.

Adopting a person-centred approach

Adopting a person-centred approach to the sexual health and needs of older adults in care can reaffirm that the older person is more than just their age or illness. A person-centred approach respects the older adult's sexual preferences and orientation; recognizes that not all individuals will want to discuss sexual issues or concerns; and acknowledges that priorities will vary for those who are sexually interested (McAuliffe et al., 2007; Nay et al., 2007).

Key point

Adopting a person-centred approach to the sexual health and needs of older adults in care can reaffirm that the older person is more than just their age or illness.

Scenario 12.2

Mrs Green had been a resident of Happy Acres aged care facility for many years. Her husband had died some 10 years previously and she had been living alone prior to moving into the aged care facility. Over the last few months the facility staff had noted that Mrs Green did not appear to be her usual self. She was socializing less with other residents and spent more time in her room alone.

At about this time some final-year students of nursing had commenced their clinical practicum at the facility. The students had attended a few weeks prior to this experience a series of lectures on person-centred care, including sexuality. Two of the students who were attending to Mrs Green's activities of daily living one morning asked whether she would like them to apply some make-up. Mrs Green appeared enthusiastic about this suggestion and the students spent the next hour styling Mrs Green's hair, providing a manicure and applying makeup including lipstick.

Mrs Green thoroughly enjoyed the attention she was receiving and proudly visited the other residents and staff to 'show off' her makeover. The staff commented that the transformation in her mood and behaviour was remarkable. Mrs Green was heard to comment that she had not felt so good about herself in years.

- *What steps could be taken to ensure that Mrs Green's level of personal care is maintained at a level that allows her to 'feel good about herself'?*

Health promotion and education

Nurses are well placed to deliver interventions that promote health, and this is no less true for sexual health. Ageing, illness and surgical interventions can all impact on sexual functioning, and so it is important that the older person is informed that this may be the case. This also applies when prescribing a new medication that may impact on sexual functioning (Nusbaum et al., 2005; Steinke, 2005). Would you want to be prescribed a medication that decreased your libido without being told?

Physiological age-related changes may lead to sexual difficulties, but nurses can normalize these changes and inform the person of possible solutions, such as spending more time on stimulation, using lubricants, or taking medication to enhance erectile function. The impact of impaired sexual functioning on body image and sense of self should not be underestimated. Certain procedures such as hysterectomy, mastectomy, or prostate surgery can also result in changed body image and a loss of femininity or masculinity, and nurses can help normalize these feelings too. When the illness of one partner affects the sexual relationship but sex is still desired, the nurse may suggest the couple consider role changes so that sexual pleasure is possible.

As a society we do not commonly associate HIV or STDs with older people. Educational campaigns are targeted at youth, yet it has been estimated that older people represent

9–11% of AIDS cases (Goodroad, 2003). Most GPs are less likely to consider HIV as a cause of illness in older adults, which is especially alarming given that older adults have less time between diagnosis of HIV to onset of AIDS (Centers for Disease Control and Prevention, 2006). The nurse can also help educate the older person in the area of safe sex practices, such as the use of condoms, which has been found to be less frequent in older people (Holden et al., 2005).

'Problem' behaviour

Sexuality in nursing home residents with dementia is unfortunately all too commonly seen as a behavioural problem (Hajjar and Kamel, 2003) needing to be curtailed, often with the use of tranquillizers (Archibald, 2003). As one researcher so aptly put it, 'What is virility at 25 becomes lechery at 65' (Berezin, 1969).

Inappropriate touching of staff is obviously not acceptable, but it may be understandable. The increased libido sometimes experienced by persons with dementia (Tabak and Shemesh-Kigli, 2006) can lead to such behaviour, as well as other behaviour such as masturbating or disrobing in public spaces. What is needed then is a proactive approach in understanding and preventing or minimizing such behaviour. We ask questions about our patients' behaviour all the time. We ask 'Why is Mrs Smith not finishing her meals? I wonder if she is having trouble with her dentures?' or 'Why is Mr Jones going to the toilet so often? I wonder if he has a UTI (urinary tract infection)?'. Sexual behaviour is no different. We need to ask why the behaviour is occurring and how we can minimize the disruptions the behaviour is causing to others while still respecting that the person has a need. Is Mr Rogers mistaking the neighbour in the next room for his wife? Or is he forming a new relationship with her? Is Mr Johnson masturbating in front of the nurse when she helps him with his morning shower because it has been his lifelong habit to share this shower experience with his wife? An assessment of the person's need is required in order to fully appreciate what is occurring. Options should then be explored as to how best to help the person fulfil their need.

Providing information to prospective nursing home residents

Information provision is one of the easiest ways to reassure the older person that their needs will continue to be met when they enter care. Information leaflets for older people thinking of moving to a residential care setting include information about the number of beds a facility has, but rarely do they address what might be the most important questions for an individual. Can you personally imagine moving into residential aged care? Can you imagine not knowing whether you will ever be able to share a bed with someone again? Whether you will ever be able to have some private time? A recent Australian study investigated the provision of written information by residential aged care facilities in regard to how they cater to sexuality and intimacy needs of residents (Bauer et al., 2009b). The survey of 826 residential aged care facilities found that over two-thirds of respondents did not have any information available on the topic to provide to prospective residents. By simply providing a person with information, we can help reassure them that their rights and preferences will be respected.

Evaluation

Assessing once is not enough. Things change. New medications are prescribed, people develop new illnesses, and new relationships are formed, all of which may impact on a person's sexual interest and activity. We must assess thoroughly and regularly, so that the older person is confident that there will be a forum in which they can discuss any new sexual concerns that may arise. Interventions need to be regularly evaluated to ensure they are the most appropriate for the situation, and if not, then alternatives need to be explored.

Evaluation also applies to staff knowledge and training. We cannot ask nurses to conduct assessments and deliver health promotion interventions and education if we do not ensure they are provided with training that reflects the latest research. Our policies also need to be reviewed and evaluated to ensure that they are consistent with best practice. There are very few policies to guide staff in terms of what organizations expect from staff in relation to sexuality and supporting older people. One such policy developed by Nay (2004; also in McAuliffe et al., 2007) may provide a starting point for your organization to develop a policy and guidelines.

Conclusion

Sexuality is an important part of quality of life for many older people and health professionals can play a pivotal role in debunking the myths relating to later-life sexuality that prevent older adults from freely expressing their sexuality. Older people often want their health professional to initiate conversation about sexuality and needs, and assessment is good way to initiate these conversations.

This chapter has outlined nursing assessment and educational interventions that can help support healthy sexuality among older adults. Conducting a comprehensive assessment of sexual health and needs (and revisiting regularly); planning for the sexual health and needs of older adults in care; and evaluating the interventions we implement to ensure they are effective are all ways we can work towards supporting the older adult's right to sexual expression. Interventions may include examining our own attitudes and practices; creating the right environment; adopting a person-centred approach; delivering health promotion and education; understanding 'problem' behaviour; and providing information to current and prospective older adults in care.

References

Aizenberg, D., Weizman. M. and Barak, Y. (2002) Attitudes toward sexuality among nursing home residents, *Sexuality and Disability*, 20(3): 185–89.

Ali, K.M. (2004) Attitudes among rehabilitation nurses towards love and intimacy in older people, *Geriatrics Today: Journal Canadian Geriatrics Society*, 7(2): 46–48.

Archibald, C. (2003) Sexuality and dementia: the role dementia plays when sexual expression becomes a component of residential care work, *Alzheimer's Care Quarterly*, 4(2): 137–48.

Bauer, M. (1999) Their only privacy is between their sheets: privacy and the sexuality of elderly nursing home residents, *Journal of Gerontological Nursing*, 25(8): 37–41.

Bauer, M., McAuliffe, L. and Nay, R. (2009a) Sexuality and the reluctant health professional, in R. Nay and S. Garratt (eds) *Older People: Issues and Innovations in Care*, 3rd edn (pp. 292–309). Sydney: Elsevier.

Bauer, M., Nay, R. and McAuliffe, L. (2009b) Catering to love, sex and intimacy in residential aged care: what information is provided to consumers? *Sexuality and Disability*, 27(1): 3–9.

Berezin, M.A. (1969) Sex and old age: a review of the literature, *Journal of Geriatric Psychiatry*, 3: 131–49.
Berger, J.T. (2000) Sexuality and intimacy in the nursing home: a romantic couple of mixed cognitive capacities, *The Journal of Clinical Ethics*, 11(4): 309–13.
Bretschneider, J. and McCoy, N. (1988) Sexual interest and behaviour in healthy 80 to 102 year olds, *Archives of Sexual Behaviour*, 17(2): 109–29.
Brock, L.J. and Jennings, G. (2007) Sexuality and intimacy, in J.A. Blackburn and C.N. Dulmus (eds) *Handbook of Gerontology: Evidence-based Approaches to Theory, Practice, and Policy* (pp. 244–68). New Jersey: John Wiley & Sons.
Centers for Disease Control and Prevention (2006) *HIV/AIDS Surveillance Report* (Vol. 18). Atlanta, GA: Department of Human Services.
Ginsberg, T.B., Pomerantz, S.C. and Kramer-Feeley, V. (2005) Sexuality in older adults: behaviours and preferences, *Age and Ageing*, 34(5): 475–80.
Goodroad, B.K. (2003) HIV and AIDS in people older than 50: a continuing concern, *Journal of Gerontological Nursing*, 29(4): 18–24.
Gott, M. (2005) *Sexuality, Sexual Health and Ageing*. Maidenhead: Open University Press.
Gott, M. and Hinchliff, S. (2003) How important is sex in later life? The views of older people, *Social Science and Medicine*, 56: 1617–28.
Gott, M., Hinchliff, S. and Galena, E. (2004) General practitioner attitudes to discussing sexual health issues with older people, *Social Science and Medicine*, 58: 2093–103.
Hajjar, R.R. and Kamel, H.K. (2003) Sexuality in the nursing home part 1: attitudes and barriers to sexual expression, *Journal of the American Medical Directors Association*, 4: 152–56.
Hill, J., Bird, H. and Thorpe, R. (2003) Effects of rheumatoid arthritis on sexual activity and relationships, *Rheumatology*, 42: 280–86.
Holden, C.A., McLachlan, R.I., Cumming, R., et al. (2005) Sexual activity, fertility, and contraceptive use in middle-age and older men: men in Australia, Telephone Survey (MATeS), *Human Reproduction*, 20(12): 3429–34.
Hordern, A.J. and Currow, D.C. (2003) A patient-centred approach to sexuality in the face of life-limiting illness, *The Medical Journal of Australia*, 179(Suppl. 6): S8–S11.
Hordern, A.J. and Street, A.F. (2007) Constructions of sexuality and intimacy after cancer: patient and health professional perspectives, *Social Science and Medicine*, 64: 1704–18.
Hubbard, G., Tester, S. and Downs, M.G. (2003) Meaningful social interactions between older people in institutional care settings, *Ageing and Society*, 23: 99–114.
Kuppuswamy, M., Davies, H.D., Spira, A.P. et al. (2007) Sexuality and intimacy between individuals with Alzheimer's Disease and their partners: caregivers describe their experiences, *Clinical Gerontologist*, 30(3): 75–81.
Lemieux, L., Kaiser, S., Pereira, J. and Meadows, L.M. (2004) Sexuality in palliative care: patient perspectives, *Palliative Medicine*, 18: 630–37.
Lindau, S.T., Schumm, L.P., Olaumann, E.O. et al. (2007) A study of sexuality and health among older adults in the United States, *New England Journal of Medicine*, 357(8): 762–74.
McAuliffe, L., Bauer, M. and Nay, R. (2007) Barriers to the expression of sexuality in the older person: the role of the health professional, *International Journal of Older People Nursing*, 2: 69–75.
Moreira, E.D., Jr., Glasser, D.B. and Gingell, C. (2005) Sexual activity, sexual dysfunction and associated help-seeking behaviours in middle-aged and older adults in Spain: a population survey, *World Journal of Urology*, 23: 422–29.
Mott, S., Kendrick, M., Dixon, M. and Bird, G. (2005) Sexual limitations in people living with Parkinson's disease, *Australasian Journal on Ageing*, 24(4): 196–201.
Mulligan, T. and Palguta, R.F. (1991) Sexual interest, activity and satisfaction among male nursing home residents, *Archives of Sexual Behavior*, 20(2): 199–204.
Nay, R. (2004) Sexuality and older people, in R. Nay and S. Garratt (eds) *Nursing Older People: Issues and Innovations*, 2nd edn (pp. 276–88). New South Wales, Australia: Elsevier.

Nay, R., McAuliffe, L. and Bauer, M. (2007) Sexuality: from stigma, stereotypes and secrecy to coming out, communication and choice, *International Journal of Older People Nursing*, 2: 76–80.

Nusbaum, M.R.H., Singh, A.R. and Pyles, A.A. (2004) Sexual healthcare needs of women aged 65 and older, *Journal of the American Geriatrics Society*, 52: 117–22.

Nusbaum, M.R.H., Lenahan, P. and Sadovsky, R. (2005) Sexual health in aging men and women: addressing the physiological and psychological sexual changes that occur with age, *Geriatrics*, 60(9): 18–23.

Stausmire, J.M. (2004) Sexuality at the end of life, *American Journal of Hospice and Palliative Care*, 21(1): 33–39.

Steinke, E.E. (2005) Intimacy needs and chronic illness: strategies for sexual counselling and self-management, *Journal of Gerontological Nursing*, 31(5): 40–50.

Tabak, N. and Shemesh-Kigli, R. (2006) Sexuality and Alzheimer's disease: can the two go together? *Nursing Forum*, 41: 158–66.

Trudel, G., Turgeon, L. and Piche, L. (2000) Marital and sexual aspects of old age, *Sexual and Relationship Therapy*, 15(4): 381–406.

Tsai, Y-F. (2004) Nurses' facilitators and barriers for taking a sexual history in Taiwan, *Applied Nursing Research*, 17(4): 257–64.

Wang, T., Lu, C., Chen, I. and Yu, S. (2008) Sexual knowledge, attitudes, and activity of older people in Taipei, Taiwan, *Journal of Clinical Nursing*, 17(4): 443–50.

Ward, R., Vass, A.A., Aggarwal, N. et al. (2005) A kiss is still a kiss? The construction of sexuality in dementia care, *Dementia*, 4: 49–72.

World Health Organization, (www.who.int/reproductive health/gender/sexual_health.html).

CHAPTER 13

Risk and safety in nursing older people

Alison Steven, Sheena Blair and Gabriel Telford Steven

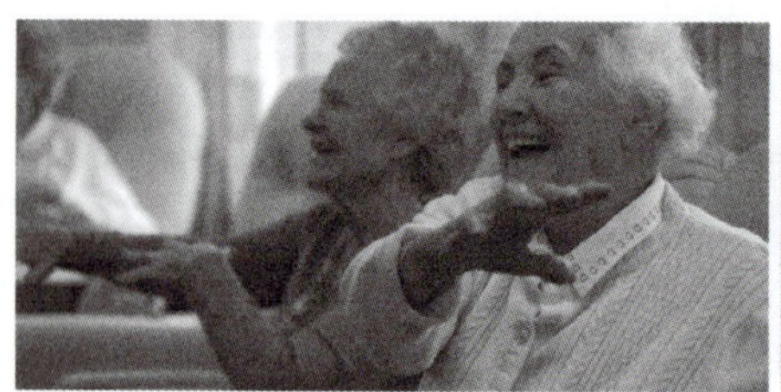
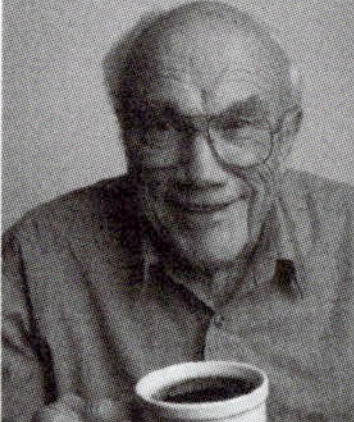
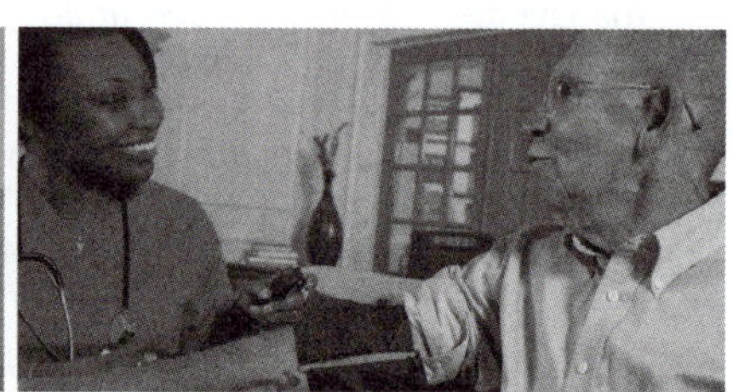

Learning objectives

At the end of this chapter, the reader will be able to:

- identify the different ways in which risk and safety can be viewed and thought about from staff and service user perspectives
- have an understanding of issues linked to the multifaceted and interrelated concepts of risk and safety
- demonstrate insight into the context specific nature of risk and safety in relation to the lives of individual older people
- increase knowledge of risk assessment procedures in relation to older people
- critique a range of resources related to risk assessment and management with older people

Why are the ideas of safety and risk important to me? Mr G. T. Steven comments as follows:

'My first consideration when confronted with the subject of this book and chapter was to ask "who is the older person?" First and foremost, I do not consider myself an old person, and as my wife suggests it is not us who think we are old, but others. We appreciate that as time passes there will inevitably be things that we cannot do so readily, or easily, or agilely due to our ageing bodies, but that should not be allowed to restrict our lives too much as long as we know our own limits and can work out ways around them.

Risk and safety in 'older age' are linked to self awareness of those limitations, choice and independence. It is important that people providing caring services realize these connections and respect them. Although it is inevitable that some people may, for whatever reason, not be able or competent to assess fully the unsafe situations they find themselves in or the risks they face, what is paramount I feel is that care is planned and decided as much as possible with the person and as little as possible "for" them. To take away someone's control and independence to make decisions is a terrible thing.

Another aspect of safe care is related to communication and information. I experienced an episode recently where a new nurse tried to move me in a way which was extremely painful and I screamed. It was not her fault – she did not know of my condition and was very upset. But she should have known. Information about me and my condition should have been passed between staff and there should be systems in place to make sure this happens. That incident has knocked my sense of safety and indeed my trust in the staff, and in order to feel safe one needs to trust those providing care.

Part of being the person I am is being in control, making my own decisions and staying as independent as possible. When I need nursing or other care it is important that I can trust those who provide that care and the systems they work within. I appreciate when staff pass on information and work with me rather than taking away the possibility to decide what risks to take. To do so shows a lack of respect for those you may consider to be "older".'

Mrs Steven's views as an older person and spouse

'You need to let people do things for themselves and take some small risks so that they are forced to maintain or re-gain their independence. If you do it all for them they become helpless – you make them helpless and dependant. That is not caring, that is mollycoddling and over protecting. It is like with children, you have to let them take risks so that they learn, so that they become independent – it's the same for us. You never know what you can do or keep doing if someone else always does it for you!'

Introduction

As we can see from the comments by Mr and Mrs Steven, risk and safety, however we individually define them, are important issues in the lives of those we consider 'older'. In addition, it is evident that the ways in which care is planned, implemented and evaluated in relation to risk and safety can have a major impact on personal feelings of well-being and thus requires careful consideration. Drawing on the comments from Mr and Mrs Steven and other patient scenarios, this chapter considers a number of perspectives on risk and safety in the care of older people.

Is later life more risky and dangerous than any other phase of the life course? The link between growing older and the need for nursing care, which is the topic of this book, suggests that there are particular health-related risks as we grow older. In order to think about risk and safety as it relates to the care of older people, it is necessary to explore the taken-for-granted ways in which these concepts are thought about both on a societal level and within health and social care. We also need to ask if there are different ways of constructing risk and safety when considering them in relation to older people. The notion that risks and safety issues escalate in later life permeates most of lay and professional thinking. This may be compounded by frequent and troubling reports in the press which relate to elder abuse or the poor care of older people with an underlying ageist ethos. The majority of older people negotiate later life uneventfully and take a measured approach to their own management of risk and safety awareness. Nevertheless, positive or successful ageing is reliant upon reciprocal interdependence whereby older people continue to feel involved and see themselves as contributors to family and community life, as discussed by Moyle et al. (2010) in relation to mental health well-being.

A life course approach to the study of later life strives to explain that this stage of life is not homogeneous and that to label all people over 60 as similar in needs and attributes, or more prone to risk, is invidious. In the majority of literature, later life is likely to be characterized by increasing multidimensional health-related issues and the accumulation of possible risk factors. This may well oversimplify the complexity of later life and the contexts which impinge upon experience, but it serves to reveal that there will inevitably be times where risk and safety become important concerns.

Nursing older people covers a wide spectrum of activity involving acute care, rehabilitation and community work. It increasingly also covers health promotion and illness prevention. In all of those areas, the issues related to risk and safety will accompany the reasoning, decision-making ability and practice of nurses. A key concern for practitioners and service users is how to preserve the essential personhood of the older person and avoid the insidious passivity and disempowerment which can be an outcome of the way that people are managed. The transformation of someone from person to patient can happen rapidly. This does not emerge from uncaring or unthinking professionals but rather indicates a difficulty or specific need for critical reflectivity concerning the nature of interaction and communication. This is as important as the clinical observations. Usually, difficulties with this are construed as a feature of problems with resources and that there 'is too little time' to attend to this when there are shortages of staff, heavy nursing commitments and multiple demands. Nevertheless, decision-making is a pivotal attribute in the nursing repertoire and there is a balance to be struck between sensitivity to patient autonomy, careful judgement about risk and risk tolerance and implementation of safe procedures. Ethical guidelines and protocols may not provide the subtlety that is needed, particularly in terms of communication, analysis of subjective constructions of later life and the tension between medical perceptions of frailty in later life and the patient's wish for autonomy. Continued complex and experiential learning is often required to develop professional skills in this respect.

It is also important to consider and explore the prevalence of conditions and issues that affect older people, which increase and change the risks and safety issues they and their carers face. There are particular needs and issues concerning risk and safety for older people who live in residential care but it is out of the scope of this chapter to deal with those systemic and ethical issues. Readers are referred to Marquis (2005) for a sensitive and creative appraisal of the professional communication and human relations required in this area. This chapter focuses primarily on risk and safety in relation to older people who continue to live in their own homes.

For the purposes of this chapter, we conceptualize risk in relation to older people as a concept that needs to be understood in context and that requires careful, holistic judgement and decision-making. As a central tenet, the assessment of risk should involve the person and those closest to them. It is a dynamic concept and decisions about risk and risk tolerance will alter according to circumstances. Safety is meant in this chapter in relation to older people as a concept which is entirely related to the judgement about risk and one that seeks to minimize risks to physical, social, emotional and spiritual well-being. At different points, judgements about the components of safety will be foregrounded such as clinical safety during acute phases of illness.

Background: ideas of risk and safety

Risk and risk-taking is inherent in our everyday lives and formal risk assessment and management is a central part of the practice of all health and social care professionals. Saunders (1998: 72) suggested that 'risk management is the synthesis of the decision-making process, the values of the practitioner (and the organisation) and the needs and aspirations of the service user'. However, the needs and aspirations of the service user should not be last on the list but should be central to any care processes, especially risk assessment which is bound up with concepts of self determination, independence, rights, responsibilities and dignity.

Risk and safety can be seen as concepts that are hand in hand and which involve many related issues. Figure 13.1 illustrates how the concepts of risk and safety interrelate with the processes or actions of risk-taking and maintaining or promoting safety. Each concept and process has a number of associated concerns; for example, the process of risk-taking is concerned with decision-making, choice, self-determination and control; the process of maintaining safety, on the other hand, is concerned with risk assessment, risk management and protectionism. Where there is high risk, safety may be compromised, and where there is complete safety, risk is eliminated – or so it may be easy to assume, yet in fact risk can never be eliminated but is simply moved around such that a physical risk of harm may be reduced by preventing someone 'wandering', for example, but the risk of harm to their sense of

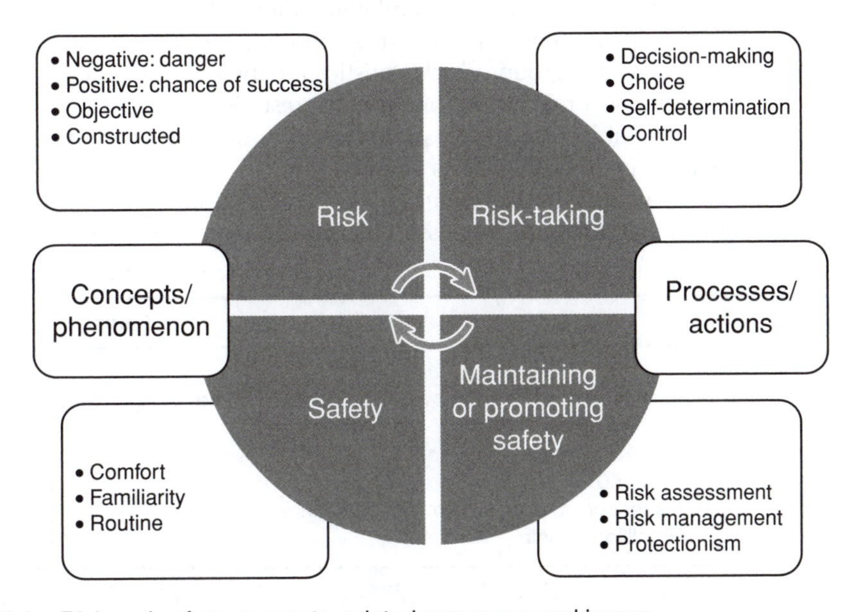

Figure 13.1: Risk and safety: concepts, related processes and issues

self-determination is increased. Given either extreme is not without accompanying philosophical and professional dilemmas (many of which are discussed later), and in the nursing care of older people, risk and safety need to be balanced. Growing older brings with it a number of life changes including social change, ailments and illnesses which require a person to adjust to new and different situations. Such situations may lead to alterations in what is familiar and comfortable, loss of routine and changes in decisions to be made, thus increasing the potential risks (Wade and Wright, 1988). However, much will depend on how risk is viewed both by the older person and those planning and providing care.

The many meanings of risk

Risk is commonly perceived as a negative phenomenon and is associated with words such as danger, jeopardy, hazard or peril (Wynne-Harley, 1991). As Clarke (2003: 14) suggests 'Risk taking is sometimes seen in a negative light, synonymous with danger and needing to be countered by protection and safety'. Indeed, when we care for others, be they children, the ill or infirm, this negative concept of risk tends to promote a protectionist response in which the person at risk needs to be kept safe (Thom and Blair, 1998; Clarke, 2003). It can result in defensive safety behaviours which deny the understanding of an older persons' natural anxiety about changes in their situation and the wish to challenge those restraints.

Nonetheless, risk is a concept which has many meanings and can be viewed from many perspectives. Risk may be seen as something 'actual' or objective which can be measured and calculated; for example, the risk of an 80-year-old sustaining a fracture as a result of a fall, the risk of medication error for an elderly hospital patient with multiple pathologies, or the risk of someone over 65 developing diabetes. This notion of risk as something concrete, external to the observer and potentially measurable, is linked to the concepts of chance and probability and is a common view in medicine and health care (Adams, 1995; NPSA, 2009). Indeed, across the globe, health departments, academic units and organizations such as the World Health Organization (WHO) produce statistics reporting the prevalence of certain injuries and conditions across age groups. Such statistics are then used to calculate the risk or probability of the conditions for particular age groups, resulting in specific groups being deemed at high or low risk. Table 13.1 shows some examples of statistics for older people and representations of associated probabilities and chances.

Without a doubt such calculations are useful for health and social care practice and may assist the practitioner by heightening awareness of the potential for specific health-related

Topic	*Source*
Blindness	
■ 19% of the world's population is aged 50 or over, but over 82% of the world's blind are in that age group	Age Concern (2009)
■ 9% of people over 50 in Africa are blind compared to 0.2% of children and adults under 50	
■ Age-related cataract is responsible for 48% of world blindness, which represents about 17.6 million people	

Table 13.1 Common health risks for older people: statistical prevalences and probabilities (continued over).

Topic	*Source*
Dementia	
■ 1 in 3 people over 65 will die with dementia.	Age Concern (2009)
■ Nearly 700 000 people were estimated to be living with dementia in the UK in 2007 and, by 2025, the number is expected to rise to one million	
■ Dementia affects 1 person in 5 over 80, 1 in 4 over the age of 85 and 1in 3 for people over 90	
Depression	
■ Approximately 10% of people over the age of 60 suffer from depression to the degree that warrants intervention	Wilson et al. (2001)
■ Depression affects 13–15% of people over 65 living in the community and 40% of older people in care homes	Age Concern (2009)
Disease	
■ 44% of all world deaths are due to non-communicable diseases in older people	Age Concern (2009)
■ Throughout the world and particularly in low-income countries, more older people die from malnutrition, respiratory diseases and TB than any other age group, including children 0–14 years	
Falls and related injuries	
■ About 30% of people over 65 years living independently fall each year, and this figure is even higher for people in residential or acute care settings	Towner and Errington (2004)
■ There is an increased risk of falling with age	
■ Population (epidemiological) studies show that hip fractures are the most serious fall-related injury in older people, with 15% dying in hospital and a third not surviving beyond one year afterwards	McClure et al. (2005)
HIV/AIDS	
■ In Southern Africa, the region with the highest HIV/AIDS prevalence, life expectancy across the region as a whole has fallen from 55 years in 1975–1980, to a projected 43 years in 2005–2010	Age Concern (2009)
Long-term illness	
■ Over two thirds (67%) of people aged 85 and over in the UK have a disability or limiting long-standing illness. For those aged 65–74, the figure is 40% and for people aged 75–84, it is 55%	Age Concern (2009)
■ 38% of people in Great Britain aged 65–74 and 50% of those aged 75+ have a limiting longstanding illness	
■ Men in the UK can expect to live their last 6.8 years with a disability. For women, the average is 9.1 years	
Malnutrition	
■ Studies have reported malnutrition in a substantial proportion of hospital patients in the USA, Norway, Ireland, UK, Sweden, The Netherlands and Australia. Data show that elderly patients are more at risk of malnutrition than others	Milne et al.(2009)
Strokes	
There are over 100 000 first strokes every year in the UK, and 90% of these affect people over 65 years	Age Concern (2009)
Every year about 130 000 people in England and Wales suffer a stroke	

Table 13.1 Common health risks for older people: statistical prevalence's and probabilities.

events. However, this type of 'calculated' risk does not take into consideration the meaning of that risk or the risk-taking process for those involved. Furthermore, physical safety aspects of risk (rather than social or psychological aspects) are often privileged in relation to caring for older people (Clarke, 2006; Titterton, 2005) and the emphasis placed by statistics on observable, measurable and recordable events may place greater focus on the physical aspects as they are more amenable to measurement than psychosocial aspects.

Although these views of risk are often taken for granted or seen as common sense, there is a growing acknowledgement that risk may be viewed as a socially, culturally and temporally constructed concept (e.g. Clarke, 2006; Moreira, 2007;). Each of us will have our own idea of what 'risk' means or is, and these ideas may be individual or shared across groups and fuelled by a multitude of factors including personal experience, professional background and dominant political and societal views. It is also important to remember the impact of historical time frames and changes in technology on variations in perceptions of risk and, when thinking globally, to consider the influence of culture on the ways in which risk is conceptualized (Tansey and O'Riordan, 1999). Older people will almost certainly have lived through different eras to those who provide care and they will have experienced many changes in society, technology and lifestyles. These experiences will influence the way they approach decision-making, risk-taking and safety. Although we cannot, and should not, generalize about the ways in which prior experiences may influence risk-taking, it is important that a person's 'history' be acknowledged and taken into account.

Risk as a negative event

At present we live in an era of risk aversion and safety consciousness fuelled by our current 'blame and claim' society. In many parts of the world it is the norm for legal firms to appeal to the public to claim for any accident or injury which was not their fault, and to entice them into doing so through 'no win – no fee' conditions. Accidents no longer happen and everything is someone's fault. In the UK patient litigation is rising in health and social care and it has been suggested that caution and defensiveness are often prioritized over learning in order to avoid further incidents (Pearson and Steven, 2009).

The current socio-political climate has influenced the development of a health and social care system which views the concept of risk as dangerous and negative and tries to reduce risk and promote safety at every possible opportunity. Risks are seen as discreet problems which can be systematically addressed and resolved, and this is what Schön ([1983]1991) termed a technical rationality approach which is found throughout health care literature (Stewart, 2006). Schön also drew attention to the propensity in human service professions to focus on 'problem-solving' without paying attention to 'problem-setting'. In 'problem-solving' solutions are sought and the way in which the problem is framed is taken for granted. Thus, problems (or in this case risks) become seen as something fixed, concrete, definable, stable and independent of context. Consequently, there is the potential for prescriptive progression towards solutions; for example, in the ticking-off list approach in some protocols. Schön suggested that the problems faced by human service professions are messy and uncertain and thus not amenable to straightforward technical solutions. Therefore, an alternative would be to focus on 'problem-setting' and to reflect on and unpick what the problem (or risk) means, how it is framed or thought about and how it is interpreted by those involved (e.g. service users, relatives, carers and professionals). Perhaps a goal which should be aspired to among professionals who work with older people is that risks are acknowledged and shared with the person concerned and mutually explored and appraised, but that there is still encouragement to fulfil potential.

Risk assessments are correctly part of each professional's practice but the overemphasis on the negative concept of risk, a solution-oriented (technical rationality) approach and concern regarding litigation may result in a restricted view of older people's potential. One of the key aims of nursing and other health care professionals is to nurture the return of the service user's internal control mechanisms. Clemens and Hayes (1997) carried out an interesting qualitative study on the dynamics of the decision-making practices of health care professionals in relation to assessing and balancing risk with older people. They found the assessment of risk with older people to be subjective and variable. While autonomy and self-determination were valued, the first priority was safety and they 'operate from their own subjective thresholds for risk tolerance' (Clemens and Hayes, 1997: 17). They identified two ways of approaching decisions about risk; namely, those who were snap decision-makers and those who agonized and weighed up numerous issues. Both styles impacted upon the lengths of time that decisions about older people took and they found that nurses tended towards being 'snap decision-makers' and social workers to be 'agonizers'. However, practitioners were rarely aware of what influenced their decision and this pointed to the need for in-service training.

Scenario 13.1

Alex has dementia and lives with his son with daily support for personal hygiene from a district nurse and support worker. One week, the regular support worker is on leave and a temporary member of staff attends to Alex each day instead. The support worker is alarmed to find on one day that Alex has some scissors and is cutting up the pyjamas he is wearing. She responds by calling the district nurse for advice and suggests that Alex is unable to be left alone while his son is at work in future.

The district nurse is able to contact Alex's son and quickly establish that this is not an infrequent event. Indeed, Alex worked as a tailor prior to retirement and handling scissors and cutting material is something he is very familiar with. With this understanding of Alex's past, the district nurse and support worker are able to reframe Alex's behaviour as something that is meaningful and familiar to him rather than a sign of distress and worsening confusion. The staff now ensure that scissors are out of reach for Alex but that he has a range of fabrics with different textures and patterns available to inspect. This replaces Alex's former activity with something that has a similar meaning to Alex but which is less damaging to his clothes.

- *Identify an older person who you are nursing at present – rather than removing activities that are considered to be too risky, how could these be replaced by activities that are meaningful to the older person?*

Positive aspects of risk

Risk can also be a positive thing, as noted by Mrs Steven in the opening section of this chapter. If no challenges are posed to someone's abilities, whether physical, intellectual or professional in nature, then confidence and skills deteriorate. Indeed, the common English saying of 'nothing ventured nothing gained' which is thought to derive from a Latin proverb, alludes to the positive side of risk-taking (Rees, 1993). Older people are often the experts in dealing with uncertainty and risk, having negotiated many challenging social changes and adapted accordingly throughout their lives. Risk is associated with self-determination and the right to make choices and establish direction for one's own life. This is also linked to the necessity to find ways of accessing the genuine concerns of older people who require nursing care. Risk is part of life and intrinsic to the adjustments that are needed to negotiate the transitions of the life cycle.

Key point

Older people are often the experts in dealing with uncertainty and risk, having negotiated many challenging social changes and adapted accordingly throughout their lives.

Scenario 13.2

Jim is an 85-year-old man who has experienced a haemorrhagic stroke (parietal lobe) three months ago. He is an in-patient in a unit that specializes in caring for people who have experienced a stroke. During his life, Jim has experienced numerous situations which could be termed 'risky'. He was in the Far East during the war, was a seasoned walker and undertook many projects around his home which involved physical risk. He would state that the physical risks that he took are always 'calculated' and 'reasoned'. Three days prior to his stroke he was on the roof of his cottage mending slates; however, any lifting was always undertaken with carefully organized pulley systems.

Although Jim has regained full speech and swallowing ability, the stroke has left him with a moderate degree of right-sided weakness. He remains weak due to a series of complications including: treatment for sepsis; episodes of tachycardia; and elimination problems. Jim has physiotherapy each day but tires quickly. He is able to lift his arm to his face, and move his leg and foot enough to allow him to walk about 3 metres with the aid of a frame.

Jim and his wife live in an isolated cottage in the country six miles from the nearest town and 40 miles from the hospital. He has lots of hobbies and pastimes and remarked that he did not understand how he 'ever had time to work full-time'. Jim has a son who lives in the nearest town and two daughters who live approximately 70 miles away. Over the course of his life, he had very few periods of hospitalization. The concerns Jim voiced were 'what am I going to do now?', 'will I ever drive again?', 'how can I walk down to the bridge again?' and 'I do not want to be a burden'.

- *How could you work with Jim to support him to express his concerns?*
- *What information is available to enable Jim to learn more about his condition and what the future may hold for him?*
- *Are there any peer support groups in your area where Jim could meet other people who have had a stroke?*

Some of the issues which nurses need to consider for Jim are:

- environmental issues;
- complexity of care and multiple pathologies;
- medication and coexistence of medications;
- mobilization (the need to take some risks in order to promote independence and rehabilitation);
- emotional safety – both patient and relatives (spouse) including communication, spirituality, dignity and mental health issues;
- intellectual risk and safety – the need to promote occupation/activities, stimulation, info giving and education, intellectual activity.

This means thinking about Jim's care in relation to ensuring physical safety (such as mobilization, slips, trips, falls) and the safety of carers and partners (considering the physical, psychological and emotional stress) and how to maintain social capital (protecting from isolation), occupation and independence.

Safety

Risk and safety are intrinsically linked. While more positive views of risk tend to associate it with venture and the excitement of gambling (Wynne-Harley, 1991), negative views associate risk with danger which is contrary to ideas of safety. Thus, reductions in risk are frequently equated with an increase in safety. At a global level this link is evidenced, for example, by an online course for risk management and patient safety improvement promoted on the WHO website. Over the past few decades safety has become of paramount concern across health and social care with 'patient safety' developing into a burgeoning area and quickly moving up policy and research agendas around the world (WHO, 2008; NPSA, 2009). For example, the WHO patient safety research team has identified global priorities for patient safety research, ranking them across developing countries, transitional countries and developed nations (WHO, 2008; Bates et al., 2009). In 2003 the UK National Patient Safety Agency (NPSA) launched its *Seven Steps to Patient Safety* (NPSA, 2003) which begin with an emphasis on the construction of an organizational safety culture in which every member of staff feels able to identify *dangers for patients* or colleagues. The following steps focus on the integration of *patient safety, risk management and hazard reporting* in health care organizations, and stress the need for health care workers to involve and communicate effectively with patients and the wider public. While extremely valuable in reducing harm to patients caused by error or mishap, the approach taken by the NPSA embodies a negative view of risk which is associated with hazard and danger, and countered by safety.

Professional and regulatory bodies around the world also emphasize safety. The UK Health Professions Council (HPC) has set generic proficiency standards, which apply to all the 12 professions it regulates. These standards specify that the practitioner must maintain a safe practice environment and select appropriate hazard control and risk management strategies (Health Professions Council (HPC), 2003). The English General Social Care Council (2002) code of practice for social workers states that workers must 'promote the independence of service users while protecting them as far as possible from danger or harm' (para 3).

While the impetus for patient safety comes mainly from a desire to reduce the number of errors, mishaps and incidents arising from interventions that occur during patient care, there is a danger that this emphasis on safety is interpreted as pertaining to all aspects of care and may result in health and social care professionals becoming overcautious when dealing with older people (Wade and Wright, 1988). Furthermore, there is a key difference between protecting patients from the errors and mishaps made by health and social care staff and keeping patients safe from the consequences of what Wynne-Harley (1991) termed their own 'voluntary risk-taking'. It has been suggested that for older people 'a full sense of safety comes from the familiarity and comfort in the environment, which poses no threat to mind or body' (Wade and Wright, 1998: 41).

Therefore, it is paramount that, in order to provide holistic care, nurses explore their own conceptions of risk and safety, those of the older person, and of their family or carers. Otherwise, a desire to promote safety, coupled perhaps with the wish to avoid litigation, may result in nurses and other health and social care professionals becoming overprotective of patients (Wade and Wright, 1988) and may then beg the question 'safety for whom'? These variations of perception of risk and the varying emphases places on maintaining safety can lead to situations where there are tensions between what nurses are trying to achieve in their care and what the older [person and their family wish to achieve too – we saw this in Scenario 13.1 in this chapter to some extent, but see it too in Scenario 13.3. Negotiating the goals of care is essential and establishing a mutually agreed plan of care.

Scenario 13.3

Diane is an 80-year-old lady who has Lewy body dementia. She lives in the family home with her 60-year-old son. Diane's son is a mechanic who owns a small business which necessitates him working fairly long hours. Diane has, over the past six or seven years, become more and more confused and wanders out in the city. The police have returned Diane to her house and called her son on a number of occasions. In order to stop Diane wandering her son now locks her in the house when he goes to work which causes her to become very agitated. Social services have discussed the situation with Diane, the son with whom she lives and his brother who has a family and lives about 20 miles away. Diane's son refuses to allow his mother to go into any kind of nursing or residential home and wishes her to stay at home with him. Social services have implemented a carer scheme so that someone goes to the house to assist Diane three times a day. However, the carer staff change on a regular basis and this causes further confusion at times.

- *What services are available in your area that could be helpful to Diane and her son?*

In assessing and planning Diane's care, nurses need to consider:

- environmental issues;
- complexity of care and multiple agencies/providers;
- medication and coexistence of medications;
- emotional safety – both patient and relatives, including communication, spirituality, dignity and mental health issues;
- maintaining routines, comfort and familiarity.

This means thinking about Diane's care in relation to maintaining her physical safety (avoiding household accidents, use of gas and electrical appliances, slips, trips and falls for example) and the safety of carers/relatives (considering physical, psychological and emotional stress), maintaining social capital (avoiding isolation and maintaining occupation and independence) and ensuring Diane's self-determination.

Approaches to managing risk

So far we have explored a range of ways of thinking about risk and safety and will now cover some of the potential approaches to dealing with risk. The patient scenarios will be used to illustrate and illuminate specific issues.

Just as risk is a concept which forms part of our everyday lives, risk assessment or analysis is a process we all consciously or unconsciously undertake every day. As Lymbery (2005: 138) asserts 'life is risky, and it is neither possible (nor in fact desirable) to eliminate all aspects of life that might carry some element of risk'. Life without risks would be very dull, but risk must be assessed and managed, especially when caring for others. Comprehensive and detailed risk assessment will clarify the issues and assist in the joint decision-making process between an older person and the multidisciplinary carer team. Assessment will not (nor can it) remove the risks (Tanner and Harris, 2008).

Risk assessment is a central feature of all aspects of health and social care. Indeed Saunders (1998: 79) describes risk-taking as 'not external to nursing but is central to its effective practice'. If we take a positive view of risk in relation to the care of older people we can see risk-taking as an opportunity for potential gains (e.g. in the recovery of mobility after stroke – see Scenario 13.2) or the maintenance of situations and states (e.g. maintaining independent living, self-determination and dignity – see Scenario 13.3).

Thus, the assessment and management of risks, and the evaluation of risk management strategies, are necessary parts of a philosophy of care provision which aims to empower and encourage independence and self-determination.

Key point

The assessment and management of risks, and the evaluation of risk management strategies, are necessary parts of a philosophy of care provision which aims to empower and encourage independence and self-determination.

However, a central dilemma for practitioners is maintaining a balance between rights and responsibilities, and the underpinning principles of autonomy and protection (Stevenson, 1999). Nowhere are such dilemmas more heightened than in the care of older people with dementia (as in Scenarios 13.1 and 13.3). The Department of Health (DoH) (2010) have issued guidance specifically on risk management for people with dementia as part of the implementation of the National Dementia Strategy. They urge nurses and other practitioners to weigh up the potential for harm with the potential to contribute to quality of life, highlighting the following domains in particular: physical harm, emotional impact, loss of confidence, relationship changes and loss of financial/independence.

Health and social care provision for older people takes place across a wide range of contexts, including the acute sector, residential and nursing care establishments, rehabilitation and community settings. Each of these contexts will bring particular factors to bear on the risk assessment and management processes which will be further influenced by the national and organizational cultures at play (Tanner and Harris, 2008).

There are a plethora of approaches to the assessment and management of risk which can be applied to supporting older people: some broad or holistic covering a number of principles (see Titterton, 2005; Nolan, 2001), and others focused specifically on conditions (e.g. dementia, stroke) or outcomes which have a high level of morbidity (e.g. through falls, pressure sores, fractures, malnutrition, depression). In addition, health and social care organizations often have their own policies, guidelines and procedures.

Two broad approaches to dealing with risk are compared and contrasted by Titterton (2005: 82). The *safety-first* model incorporates: physical health, disabilities (what the person cannot do), danger, control, and what the assessor thinks is right. While the more holistic *risk–taking* model encompasses: physical, psychological and emotional well-being, rights and responsibilities, abilities and disabilities (what the person can achieve), choices and opportunities, and involvement of the individual and family/carers.

Risk management

Titterton (2005) suggests that risk management should aim to maximize benefits or strengths in any situation and reduce or minimize harm. Using a human service perspective, Saunders (1998: 74) explores factors which may influence definitions of risk and risk management and suggests a series of 'relationships' that the service user may be at risk from:

- his/her own actions;
- the environment;
- the community;
- the actions of the professionals;
- the actions of the significant carer.

These models and relationships may offer useful ideas during risk assessment, planning and management. However, as Tanner and Harris (2008) point out, the identification and management of risk using the above or other approaches raises the question of what processes are used to determine what type and level of risk is acceptable and who is involved. In accordance with Titterton (2005) we suggest that risk management should involve a process of negotiation and compromise, during which the views of all involved are gathered through consultation and then used to inform a plan of action.

Saunders (1998) offers three options for a course of action in relation to risk management:

- to pursue a new or revised activity/course of action;
- to continue with a current activity/course of action;
- to discontinue a current activity/course of action.

The Department of Health (DoH) (2010) add a further very helpful option in their discussion of the importance of substituting activities. For example, in Scenario 13.1, the district nurse substitutes cutting up material with examining the texture of materials – both activities are meaningful to Alex but the latter is agreed by everyone to be safer.

A risk plan then needs to be drawn up and the following are suggested as important components (Titterton, 2005). These are details of:

- who has been consulted;
- who is responsible for developing and implementing the plan;
- steps to minimize potential harm or hazards;
- steps to increase potential benefits;
- agreed time-scales;
- points at which intervention will occur;
- arrangements for record-keeping;
- milestones for evaluating the plan and assessing success or failure.

However, risk management does not stop at the assessment of risks and the development of management strategies. As with any part of the nursing or health care process, such activities need to be regularly and consistently evaluated and revised. Furthermore, revisions need to be made in light of ongoing consultation and negotiation, in order to achieve patient-centred care, as proposed by Nolan (2001), shared decision-making and integrated multidisciplinary teamworking.

Given the immense number of risks and safety issues faced by older people who require health and social care, this chapter has focused on risk assessment and management in this section with the aim of imparting some main principles. There are, however, many specific tools, such as rating scales and questionnaires, available for use in specific situations (e.g. risk of falls, pressure sores, malnutrition, etc.). Such tools are not a substitute for, but an adjunct to person-centred care which aims to empower as much as possible those involved.

Conclusion

Risk assessment and management are processes central to health and social care practice. However, there is a propensity to view risk as a negative phenomenon which must be removed or reduced in order to promote safety. This view is also reinforced by a global emphasis on patient safety which may inadvertently reinforce protectionism by carers. Older people work hard to maintain their independence and autonomy (Nolan, 2001) and therefore key for health and social care providers, family and other carers is finding ways to support them that do not undermine their self-identity and capacity for self-determination (Seale, 1996).

Key point

Older people work hard to maintain their independence and autonomy and therefore key for health and social care providers, family and other carers is finding ways to support them that do not undermine their self-identity and capacity for self-determination.

When involved in risk assessment and management, each situation will require a range of approaches and each older person will view risk differently. Identification of 'objective' risk factors and probabilities in relation to an older person is not enough. The risk assessment and management processes need to engage with the values and biography of the person concerned and their understandings of the risks, potential outcomes and options involved. It is also important that the person is seen in their social context and that those around them are also involved and that a range of 'risk-laden' relationships are considered (Saunders, 1998). Conditions such as dementia, may necessitate the multidisciplinary team adopting a range of approaches in their pursuit of person-centred care. As Nolan (2001: 452) suggests 'issues of personal identity and meaning should figure prominently in debates (considering) the legitimate goals of healthcare interventions' – risk assessment and management being such interventions.

It is essential that nurses work with and communicate honestly with older people to understand their perspectives on what constitutes risk in their lives and what would make them feel safe. This involves learning from older people about how the attention to safety and management of risk is best managed with them. Regular discussion within teams about the nature of risk that may be part of an older persons' ill health and maintaining their well-being will ensure that all team members have a shared understanding of this. Achieving this requires nurses to resist understanding the twin concepts of risk and safety as only a managerial issue but as a key issue in ensuring that the self-determination and the preservation of self-esteem in older adults is high on the nursing agenda.

References

Adams, J. (1995) *Risk*. London: UCL Press.

Age Concern (2009) *Factsheet*. Drawn from various sources. Available online at www.ageconcern.org.uk (accessed 6 July 2009).

Bates, D.W., Larizgoitia, I., Prasopa-Plaizier, N. and Jha,A.K. (2009) Global priorities for patient safety research, *British Medical Journal*, 338(b1775): 1242–44.

Clarke, C.L. (2006) Risk and aging populations: practice development research through and international research network, *International Journal of Older People Nursing*, 1: 169–76.

Clarke, J. (2003) The concept of risk and older people: implications for practice, *Nursing Older People*, 15(7): 14–18.

Clemens, E.L. and Hayes, H.E. (1997) Assessing and balancing elder risk, safety and autonomy: decision-making practices of health care professionals, *Home Health Care Quarterly*, 16(3): 3–20.

Department of Health (DoH) (2010) *'Nothing Ventured, Nothing Gained'. Risk Guidance for People with Dementia*. London: DoH.

General Social Care Council (2002) *Code of Practice for Social Care Workers*. London: General Social Council.

Health Professions Council (HPC) (2003) Generic Standards of Proficiency. London: HPC. Available online at www.hpc-uk.org/assets/documents/10000510Standards_of_Proficiency_generic.pdf; accessed 6 July 2009.

Lymbery, M. (2005) *Social Work with Older People*. London: Sage Publications.

Marquis, T. (2005) *Doing Right in Aged Care: What Will It Take*? Perth, Australia: Curtin University of Technology.

McClure, R.J., Turner, C., Peel, N. et al. (2005) Population-based interventions for the prevention of fall-related injuries in older people, *Cochrane Database of Systematic Review*, Issue No. 1, Art. No. CD004441.

Milne, A.C., Potter, J., Vivanti, A. and Avenell, A. (2009) Protein and energy supplementation in elderly people at risk from malnutrition, *Cochrane Database of Systematic Review*, Issue No. 2, Art. No. CD003288.

Moreira, T. (2007) How to investigate temporalities of health. Forum: Social Research. 8(1) Art 13. ISSN 1438-5627. http://www.qualitative-research.net/fqs/ (accessed 5 July 2009)

Moyle, W., Clarke, C.L., Gracia, N., Reed, J., Cook, G., Klein, B., Marais, S. and Richardson, E. (2010) Older people maintaining mental health well-being through resilience: an appreciative inquiry study in four countries, *Journal of Nursing and Healthcare in Chronic Illness*, 2: 113–21.

Nolan, M. (2001) Successful ageing: keeping the 'person' in person-centred care, *British Journal of Nursing*, 10(7): 450–54.

NPSA (National Patient Safety Agency) (UK) (2009) www.npsa.nhs.uk/; accessed 6 July 2009.

NPSA (National Patient Safety Agency) (2003) *Seven Steps to Patient Safety*. London: NPSA.

Pearson, P.H. and Steven, A. (2009) Patient safety in health care professional educational curricula: examining the learning experience. Final report to the National Patient Safety Research Programme.

Rees, A. (1993) *Dictionary of Phrase and Fable*. Reading: Parragon.

Saunders, M. (1998) Management of risk situations, in S. Pickering and J.S. Thompson (eds) *Promoting Positive Practice in Nursing Older People*. Balliere Tindall, London. p72–89.

Schön, D.A. ([1983]1991) *The Reflective Practitioner*. Aldershot: Arena.

Seale, C. (1996) Living alone towards the end of life, *Ageing and Society*, 16(1): 75–91.

Stevenson, O. (1999) Old people at risk, in P. Parsloe (ed.) *Risk Assessment on Social Care and Social Work*. London: Jessica Kingsley Publishers.

Stewart, J. (2006) Asking for senior intervention: conceptual insights into the judgement of risk by doctors, PhD thesis, Newcastle University.

Tanner, D. and Harris, J. (2008) *Working with Older People*. New York: Routledge.

Tansey, J. and O'Riordan, T. (1999) Cultural theory and risk: a review, *Health, Risk and Society*, 1: 71–90.

Thom, K.M. and Blair, S.E.E. (1998) Risk in dementia – assessment and management, *British Journal of Occupational Therapy*, 61(10): 441–47.

Titterton, M. (2005) *Risk and Risk-taking in Health and Social Welfare*. London: Jessica Kingsley Publishers.

Towner, E. and Errington, G. (2004) *How Can Injuries in Children and Older People be Prevented?* Copenhagen: WHO Regional Office for Europe Health Evidence Network report. Available online at www.euro.who.int/Document/E84938.pdf; accessed 17 July 2009.

Wade, L. and Wright, S. (1988) Promoting safety and comfort, in S.G. Wright (ed.) *Nursing the Older Patient* (pp. 40–60) London: Lippincott.

Wilson, K., Mottram, P.G., Sivananthan, A. and Nightingale, A. (2001) Antidepressants versus placebo for the depressed elderly, *Cochrane Database of Systematic Reviews*, Issue No. 1, Art. No. CD000561. DOI: 10.1002/14651858.CD000561.

World Health Organization (WHO) Patient Safety (2008) *Global Priorities for Research in Patient Safety*. Research priority setting workgroup. Available online at www.who.int/patientsafety/research/priorities/global_priorities_patient_safety_research.pdf; accessed 6 July 2009.

Wynne-Harley, D. (1991) Living dangerously: risk taking, safety and older people. Report 16, Centre for Policy on Aging, London.

CHAPTER 14

Social participation and social networks

Soong-nang Jang

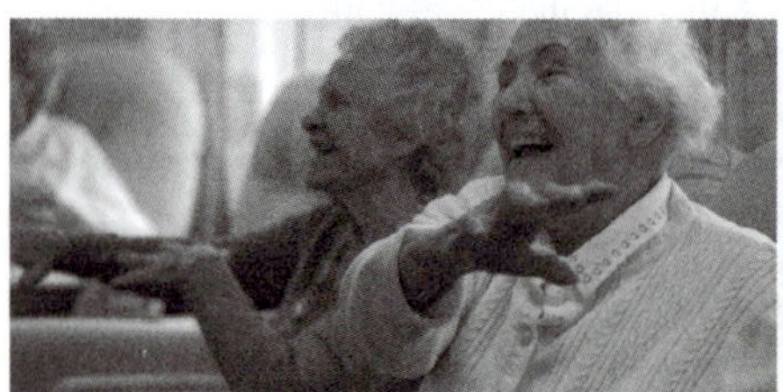
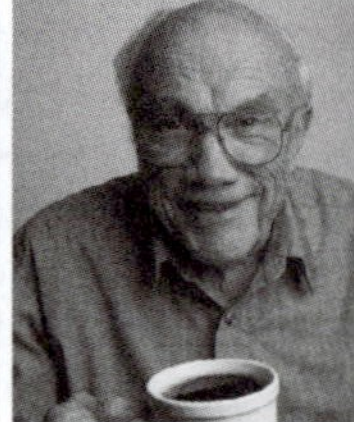
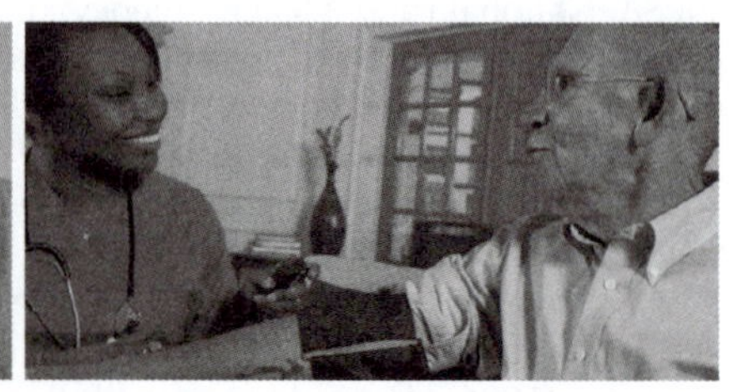

Learning objectives

At the end of this chapter, the reader will be able to:

- understand the concepts of social participation, social networks and social support, and why they are so important to older people
- explain the effect that social participation, social networks and social support have on health in later life
- identify community health resources that are available for social participation, social networks and social support in later life

Elizabeth commented:

'Never before in my life have I had any unlimited time, as I have now in old age, to make a coffee break last an hour or lunch with a friend for half the afternoon. Time has offered me the great opportunity to pursue hobbies, revive old friendships and meet new people. Joining clubs, classes and charity organizations has given a framework to each day, each week, my life, and prevented the state of aloneness becoming loneliness, for I, like many old people, now live alone for the first time in my life. Sometimes it has taken courage to seek new experiences, embrace change and look for opportunities to be useful but this is how I meet the people that make my life interesting and bring me contentment.'

Phoebe commented:

'Going to the club gets us out of the house – you get sick of looking at the four walls all the time. It keeps you going, meeting up with people and having a chat. We girls are very respectable, mind, we don't misbehave. We could if we wanted to, mind you.'

Introduction

Social participation, social networks and social support are vital for successful and active ageing. A large body of evidence from ageing research has highlighted the importance of social engagement, including social participation and social support via networks for overall health in later life (e.g. Hyppä and Mäki, 2001; Anderson and Stevens, 1993; Lindström et al., 2004). In recent years there has been growing consensus regarding the limited role of individual risk factors in determining health status and the importance of social factors, such as socio-economic status, social participation, social networks and social support. This is particularly the case in relation to physical disability, cognitive function, depression and chronic disease, including cardiovascular disease in the older population (e.g. Berkman et al., 1992; Seeman, 2000).

The effect of social engagement is significant for all age groups. However, the influence of social participation on health status increases with age (Desrosiers et al., 2004). Why is social participation more important for health and more strongly indicative of quality of life for older people than for young adults, even though social participation decreases significantly as people age? This is because social engagement may be a potential mediator of worsening health and functional status as people age. Promoting social participation would lead to better health, and thus the time has come to develop practical community nursing interventions as an effective strategy for enhancing community integration and citizenship of the older population. Concerns about the social integration and social participation of older people do not relate only to the issue of individual survival and quality of life, but are also social issues with implications for health policy and public service. These factors should be considered in developing nursing care plans with older people to enhance their functional capacity, manage chronic diseases, and improve quality of life. Most developed and developing countries adopted promoting volunteering as a policy priority for 'active ageing'. However, there are some debates that government views of social participation among older people are discordant with the views of older volunteers. Government approaches have focused on pressures and constraints so that the older people could be discouraged from formal volunteering because the volunteerism is more likely to be an expression of 'citizenship' rather than 'work-like' (Lie et al., 2009).

This chapter begins with a discussion of the concepts of social participation, social support and social networks, which together comprise the basic elements of social engagement. We then explore how these factors influence physical and mental health among older people and consider strategies for nursing action. The last section of this chapter reviews community resources and community-based interventions for promoting the health of the older population and draws in particular on an example of good practice from Korea.

Defining the concept of social participation

Social participation is generally defined as social sharing of individual resources and is related to how actively a person takes part in social activities, such as activities associated with religious organizations, hobbies, volunteer work and political groups. People take part in both collective and productive participation: collective participation is defined as taking part in group activities; for example, activities associated with religious organizations or hobby groups. Productive participation is defined as the rendering of services, goods and benefits for others, as in volunteer work (Bukov et al., 2002).

Scenario 14.1

Ahmed and his wife Careen are both in their 70s and have had a busy working life running their own business and raising their family. In retirement, Ahmed is enjoying 'collective participation' by joining woodwork classes and is making some toys for his grandchildren. Careen is more involved in 'productive participation', teaching older women about business skills through the University of the Third Age.

- *How might Ahmed and Careen have found out that these activities were available?*
- *Do older people in your own area always know what opportunities are available in their community? How could you promote this?*

The quality of social participation often appears to be more important than the amount of participation in social activities in later life. However, we would not anticipate a beneficial effect from infrequent participation in various activities. The frequency, intensity level and social value of activities should be considered when we measure social participation, because active responsible activities have a different impact on social intimacy, attachment and health.

Social participation, ageing and health

The influence of social participation on health can be explained from various points of view. Social activities promote good health by protecting against the negative effects of social isolation (Kawachi and Berkman, 2000). A person living in an area where there is little opportunity for social participation may have few chances to establish social solidarity and may become isolated from society. Low social support and low social anchorage have been negatively associated with mental health, both directly and indirectly (Araya et al., 2006). Kawachi et al. (1999) indicated that low social participation may be a pathway through which relative deprivation may influence health. For instance, social participation will lead to greater emotional support and community involvement, which can lead to even broader emotional support. Social activities may transmit messages that promote health more effectively via information channels, and can provide a supportive environment in which negative health behaviours are exchanged for positive ones. Thus, this supportive environment can make it easier for individuals to choose healthy behaviours (Ganster and Victor, 1988). For example, Christine was gaining weight as she found it harder to exercise and had little incentive to do so. Talking one day with the local shopkeeper, she found out about a walking group for older people. She joined this group and now walks each week and has enjoyed meeting several new people.

The influences of social participation on health may differ by age and sex; in this case, social participation may be a critical factor for health promotion in population segments in which health is more influenced by social participation. Men and women play different social roles. Women in particular may become socially isolated due to childrearing and family responsibilities (Cheng et al., 2000). Consequently, women may have different patterns of social participation and associated health impacts. Older adults generally have limited opportunities to participate in social activities compared with young adults and may experience relative deprivation. Each social activity may influence one's health status, whereby those who participate in more social activities may have better health status than those who participate in fewer social activities.

Social participation and self-rated health

Lee et al. (2008) confirmed that the relationship between social participation and self-rated health became stronger with age and was greater in women than in men. This study concluded that the influence of social participation on women was greater than on men in all age groups and was greatest for older women. Those who participated in more than two activities were more than twice as likely to self-rate their health as good. Men and women play different social roles, which in turn shape their lifestyles in different ways (Szaflarski, 2001). Lower social participation may limit the motivation to improve health, and women may more easily become socially isolated because of household and family responsibilities such as housework and caring for small children. Women are also more likely than men to report lower levels of functional status, a finding in keeping with reports of poorer overall health (Fried and Guralnik, 1997).

The gender difference in the way that social participation affects health can also be explained from the perspective of differences in men's and women's educational levels and occupations. In many societies, women typically have lower educational attainment and more limited occupational opportunities than men. Therefore, social participation may provide more benefits to women than to men.

Scenario 14.2

Jane is a former teacher who now has a diagnosis of dementia. She attends a day centre twice a week which she loves. She says she no longer feels alone and realizes that there are other people like her. The staff notice that she enjoys the company of a small group of other women and together they spend hours putting the world to rights and laughing. Without the day centre, Jane would spend all of her time with her husband and she says she would miss the company of other women.

- *How would you support Jane to do activities that she wants to do?*
- *How could you express Jane's need for company in her care plans so that it is seen as important and maintained?*

Social roles and activities decrease as a function of age, but other factors are more important than age in contributing to an individual's level of social participation. Advancing age cannot wholly explain the reduction in social activities (Lefrancois et al., 1998). Factors other than age also shape a person's health status. Accordingly, we can expect that the influence of social participation is a consequence of major changes related to ageing, such as changes in job status or the loss of a spouse. Education, gender and marital status are contributing factors to greater interest in and opportunities for social activities. For instance, Anderson and Stevens (1993) reported that low social participation negatively affected health status among older people as they experienced diminished health when they lost their partner. Social activities may challenge participants to develop abilities and skills, which may have a stimulating effect on their physical health. This result is also in accord with psychosocial theories of ageing. Ebersole and Hess (1994) documented major psychosocial theories of ageing that are considered universal and applicable to the aged in all cultures. These theories propose that ageing is influenced by how successfully one manages one's later life, by the maintenance of activities in middle age, and by the reinforcement of personal continuity. They also suggest that adaptation patterns in the lives of older people vary from person to person, sometimes with unpredictable psychological outcomes, and that for satisfaction in old age, it is necessary to maintain regular activities, roles (formal and informal) and social solidarity, as well as social pursuits. That is, satisfaction in old age mostly results from maintaining the activities of middle age.

If social participation influences an individual's health, health in turn may influence an individual's social participation. If this feedback occurs, the relationship between social participation and health will become stronger, and the two factors will influence each other. As a result, if one condition is improved, the other will improve correspondingly. In other words, social participation may help to delay or interrupt the cycle of poorer health that occurs as people age.

Defining the concept of social network and social support

Social networks are defined as structural characteristics, such as the number of social linkages and the frequency of contacts as mediators for the distribution and exchange of social support (Antonucci and Akiyama, 1987). Networks focus on the patterns of ties between persons in a social system rather than on the characteristics of individuals. Individuals exchange their self-perceptions, attachment and support via social networks in daily life (Litwin, 1996). In addition, individuals maintain their social identity and receive information through their network. People begin to construct their own social network from birth and continue until death, surrounding themselves with various others. This network may change continuously, as relationships with network members are added or lost. Members of social networks reciprocate social support.

Social support can be defined as the perceived caring, esteem and assistance that people receive from others. Support can come from spouses, family members, friends, neighbours, colleagues, health professionals or pets. Basic types of social support are emotional support, instrumental support and informational support. Emotional support provides people with a sense of love, reassurance and belonging. When individuals feel they are being listened to and valued, they develop a healthy sense of self-worth. Emotional support has a strong and consistent relationship to health status (Israel and Schurman, 1990). Instrumental support refers to the provision of tangible aid and services that directly assist people who are in need. Examples are financial help and household maintenance. Good instrumental support has been correlated with a decrease in psychosomatic and emotional distress, and with greater life satisfaction (Revicki and Mitchell, 1990). Informational support is the provision of advice, feedback and suggestions to help a person address problems. This type of support underpins one of the recommendations of the National Dementia Strategy in England (Department of Health (2009, DoH)) to provide dementia adviser services to ensure that people with dementia and their families have easy access to information about dementia and about the services that are available.

Key point

Basic types of social support are emotional support, instrumental support and informational support.

Social networks, social support and health

According to the longitudinal study of ageing by Bassuk et al. (1999), older people who have a social network including about five or six individuals may be protected from severe cognitive decline compared to those who lack such a network. This indicates that deficits of social networks and support are a major factor driving the decrease in cognitive function that occurs in old age. In addition, social networks, and especially relationships with family and relatives, prevent declining mobility and disability among older people (Giles et al., 2004). The psychosocial mechanisms affecting health, including hypertension, cardiovascular diseases, depression and mortality in later life, have been explained by the existence of positive social support via a network of others; for example, adult children, spouses and friends.

Older people can avoid social isolation and loneliness through social networks and support, and, more actively, they can achieve successful ageing: ageing that is healthy and happy.

The effect of social support on health can be summarized in terms of three main mechanisms (Ganster and Victor, 1988). The first consists of behavioural mediators by which social support promotes healthy behaviours to improve health and/or prevent negative influences from stress-inducing factors. Supportive others can give information including advice about responding to stress, such as seeking psychological treatment for emotional problems, and can also provide instrumental support by helping with household chores and transportation, providing financial assistance, and so on. Such support from others can also act as a psychological mediator, so that the perception of support from others may promote and maintain a positive mental state that might influence mental and physical health. This is described as the 'general perceived affiliation benefit'. Lastly, as a physiological mediator, social support can buffer against excessive stimulation or depression of immunologic responses, including increase in blood pressure, cardiac output or catecholamine.

Although older people can now live longer than ever, they experience increasing difficulty in interacting with their neighbours and family. Thus, social isolation, disintegration and disconnectedness may influence mortality and therefore longevity or life expectancy by influencing the rate of ageing of the organism. Although there is much evidence suggesting the influence of social networks and social support on health in old age, there have been few studies on nursing intervention with regard to this. Connecting community resources to provide social networks and support for the older population would be an important role for community health nursing and public health nursing.

Key point

Connecting community resources to the older population to provide social networks and support is an important role for community health nursing and public health nursing.

Nursing for social participation, social networks and social support

Older people live in communities with various community resources, community-based programmes for promoting health, and available services. Centres for older people are available in almost every community, and these provide various health education programmes and opportunities to make and meet with friends, and most have links to medical resources (Leanse, 1986). The programmes offered by centres for older people might include exercise, dancing and health education. For example, the Senior Wellness Project of Senior Services of Seattle/King County in 1997 at the North Shore Senior Center in Bothell, Washington was a research-based health promotion programme that included a chronic care self-management programme (Lorig et al., 1999). The ancient Chinese martial arts, Tai Chi, programmes are currently taught at many community centres. Leadership programmes for older people, carers programmes, health screening, and support group programmes are also offered at many community centres.

Medical institutions are also an important community resource for social support, social networks and social participation for older people in the community. Many hospitals have health programmes for older patients and their families. Hospital-based programmes might include various types of health education, health promotion programmes and medical screening, including chronic disease self-management programmes in collaboration with centres for older people or other community resources. Most hospital volunteer programmes are open to older people, which is helpful for enhancing the social participation of older people.

Educational institutions also offer low-cost education and health promotion programmes for older people. Shopping-centre based educational programmes, web-based programmes and religious institutions are potentially important resources for health programmes in the community. Voluntary organizations such as AARP in the USA have community service programmes including education, leadership and health education volunteer programmes. Social networking through the Internet has also come to be considered an important resource for providing information to older people.

Social engagement in later life involves positive adaptation to a changing environment, efforts at self-development through creative work, and an attitude contributing to social development in old age (Yoon, 1994). Increased connections between older individuals and society would be a key factor leading to enhancement of the human rights of older people and social development in an ageing society.

Key point

Increased connections between older people and society is a key factor in enhancing the human rights of older people and social development in an ageing society.

An example of good practice – community-based rehabilitation (CBR) in Korea

The example of good practice described here is based in Korea, a health system quite different from western Europe. This is very helpful in encouraging us to think 'outside the box' and understand how things may be done in a different way.

Korea launched a nationwide community-based rehabilitation (CBR) programme in 2000, and assigned CBR to public health centres (PHCs) evenly throughout rural, mixed and urban areas. The programme chairs of CBR are community health nurses in PHCs. Mid-level rehabilitation workers are also community nurses who play a key role in planning, co-ordinating, education efforts and the management of CBR in each community.

The main components of CBR are:

- the assessment of the health care needs of people with disabilities and older people in communities, assessment of community resources and planning of the CBR programme;
- the registration and enrolment of the older population and disabled individuals who experience barriers to receiving care;
- the provision of a wide range of care, such as primary health care, rehabilitative care, family support care, and information regarding social networks and participation;
- the construction of a community network and social support system using various community resources;
- education, an advertising campaign, research and evaluation.

A total of 475 sub-programmes were developed in 16 CBR programmes for three years in PHCs (2000–2002) on a pilot basis, and almost 50 PHCs had CBR programmes in 2009 (see Table 14.1) (Jang, 2004).

Domains	*Goals*
1 Maximizing potentials	Functional independence Health education Economic independence Social participation in community/family Leadership in the community Participating in self-help groups
2 Service delivery	Programme planning and management of community resources Funding and human resource management Training and education of workers Continuity of programme services
3 Modifying environment	Physical environment modification Perception, attitude modification and integration of community and family

Table 14.1 Domains and goals of community-based rehabilitation in Korea

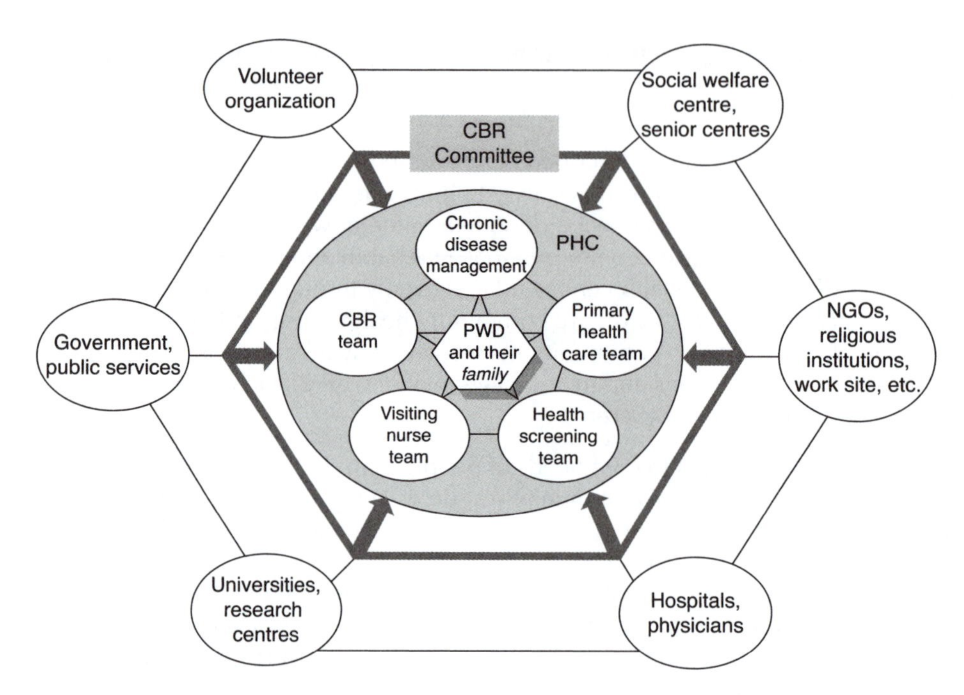

Figure 14.1: Intersectoral collaboration model of community-based rehabilitation for social networks, social support and social participation of people with disabilities (PWD) in Korea

In a study evaluating Korean CBR (Jang, 2004), the social support of people with disabilities was significantly improved. The quality of life of people with disabilities, especially in the mental domain, also improved greatly after the programme. Community-based rehabilitation workers such as community health nurses suggested that the motivation of the CBR chair had a positive effect on the success of CBR. However, less financial support and frequent replacement of the CBR workers were negative influences on the CBR process. The most difficult factor in establishing the comprehensiveness of the CBR was structuring interactions with other community resources.

The comprehensive care model developed through networking and constructing a support system with community resources significantly influenced the promotion of health and quality of life of people with disabilities and older people. An interdisciplinary service team, a single programme co-ordinator and a community committee for care were suggested to optimize communication, information-sharing, and collaboration between services based on theories of social networks, social support, and social participation. The comprehensive care model is focused on the functions of public health centres, so it may diffuse across the country through the public health system (see Figure 14.1).

Conclusion

Sharing individual resources with society is the goal of social participation, networks and support. In old age, an individual's opportunities to share his or her accumulated resources decline rapidly. Communication via social networks, exchanging support and active participation in society make individuals healthy, which in turn may work to make society healthy. Community resources should be developed to support and promote the social engagement of the older population in their communities. Social participation, social networks and support should also be a basic consideration in the field of community nursing intervention, especially for promoting the health of older people. We should consider the perspectives of older people on social participation in order to adopt realistic and practical nursing practice for social engagement in later life.

References

Antonucci, T. and Akiyama, H. (1987) Social networks in adult life and a preliminary examination if the convoy model, *Journal of Gerontology*, 42: 519–27.

Anderson, L. and Stevens, N. (1993) Associations between early experiences with parents and well-being in old age, *Journal of Gerontology: Psychological Sciences*, 48: 109–16.

Araya, R., Dunstan, F., Playle, R., Thomas, H., Palmer, S. and Lewis, G. (2006) Perceptions of social capital and the built environment and mental health, *Social Science & Medicine*, 62(12): 3072–83.

Bassuk, S.S., Glass, T.A. and Berkman, L.F. (1999) Social disengagement and incident cognitive decline in community-dwelling elderly persons, *Annal of Internal Medicine*, 131: 165–73.

Berkman, L.F., Oxman, T.E. and Seeman, T.E. (1992) Social network and social support among the elderly: assessment issue, in R.F. Woolson and R.B. Wallace (eds) *The Epidemiologic Study of the Elderly*, New York: Oxford University Press.

Bukov, A., Maas, I. and Lampert, T. (2002) Social participation in very old age: cross-sectional and longitudinal findings from BASE, Berlin Aging Study, *The Journals of Gerontology B: Psychological Sciences and Social Sciences*, 57(6): 510–17.

Cheng, Y., Kawachi, I., Coakley, E.H., Schwartz, J. and Colditz, G. (2000) Association between psychosocial work characteristics and health functioning in American women: prospective study, *British Medical Journal*, 320: 1432–36.

Department of Health (DoH) (2009) *National Dementia Strategy*. London: Her Majesty's Stationery Office (HMSO).

Desrosiers, J., Noreau, L. and Rochette, A. (2004) Social participation of older adults in Quebec, *Aging Clinical and Experimental Research*, 16(5): 406–12.

Ebersole, P. and Hess, P. (1994) *Toward Healthy Aging: Human Needs and Nursing Aging*, 4th edn. St. Louis, MO: Mosby-Year Book, Inc.

Fried, L.P. and Guralnik, J.M. (1997) Disability in older adults: evidence regarding significance, etiology, and risk, *Journal of the American Geriatric Society*, 45: 92–100.

Ganster, D.C. and Victor B. (1988) The impact of social support on mental and physical health, *British Journal of Medical Psychology*, 61: 17–36.

Ganster and Victor (1988) The impact of social support on mental and physical health, *British Journal of Medical Psychology*, 61: 17–36.

Giles, L.C., Metcalf, P.A., Glonek, G.F., Luszcz, M.A. and Andrew, G.R. (2004) The effects of social network on disability in older Australians, *Journal of Aging Health*, 16(4): 517–38.

Hyppä, M.T. and Mäki, J. (2001) Individual-level relationships between social capital and self-rated health in a bilingual community, *Preventive Medicine*, 32: 148–55.

Israel, B. and Schurman, S. (1990) Social support, control, and the stress process, in K. Glanz et al. (eds) *Health Behaviour and Health Education: Theory, Research and Practice* (pp. 196–210). San Francisco, CA: Jossey-Bass Publishers.

Jang S.N. (2004) A development of comprehensive care model for people with disability in community in Korea. Doctoral dissertation, Seoul National University (in Korean).

Kawachi, I. and Berkman, L. (2000) Social cohesion, social capital, and health, in L. Berkman and I. Kawachi (eds) *Social Epidemiology* (pp. 175–90). New York: Oxford University Press.

Kawachi, I., Kennedy, B.P. and Glass, R. (1999) Social capital and self-rated health: a contextual analysis, *American Journal of Public Health*, 89(8): 1187–93.

Leanse, J. (1986) The senior center as a wellness center, in K. Dychtwald (ed.) *Wellness and Health Promotion for the Elderly* (pp 105–18). Rockville, MD: Aspen.

Lee, H.Y., Jang, S.N., Cho, S.I., Rhee, S.J. and Park, S.O. (2008) The relationship between social participation and self-rated health by sex and age: a cross-sectional survey, *International Nursing Studies*, 45(7): 1042–54.

Lefrancois, R., Leelere, G. and Poulin, N. (1998) Predictors of activity involvement among older adults, *Activities, Adaptation, and Aging*, 22(4): 15–29.

Lie, M., Baines, S. and Wheelock, J. (2009) Citizenship, volunteering and active ageing, *Social Policy & Administration*, 43(7): 702–18.

Litwin, H. (2001) Social network type and morale in old age, *Gerontologist*, 41(4): 516–24.

Lorig, K. et al. (1999) Evidence suggesting that a chronic disease self-management program can improve health status while reducing hospitalization: a randomized trial, *Medical Care*, 37: 5–14.

Revicki, D.A. and Mitchell, J.P. (1990) Strain, social support, and mental health in rural elderly individuals, *Journal of Gerontology*, 45(6): S267–74.

Seeman, T.E. (2000) Health promoting effects of friends and family on health outcomes in older adults, *American Journal of Health Promotion*, 14(6): 362–70.

Szaflarski, M.A. (2001) Gender, self-rated health, and health-related lifestyles in Poland, *Health Care for Women International*, 22: 207–27.

Yoon J.J. (1994) Social participation and older people, *Korean Journal of Gerontology*, 14(1): 169–78.

CHAPTER 15

Dying

Amanda Clarke and Paula Smith

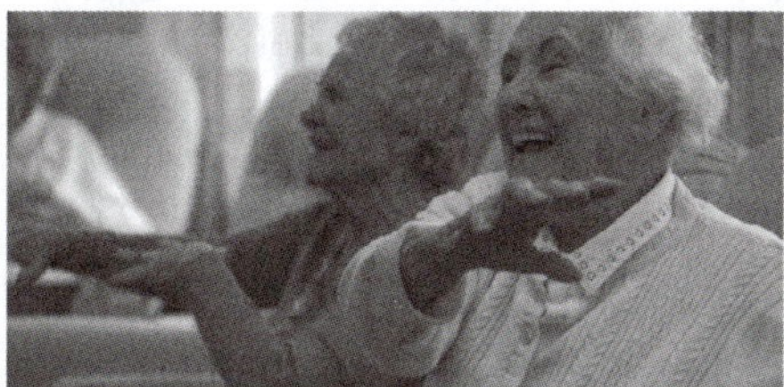
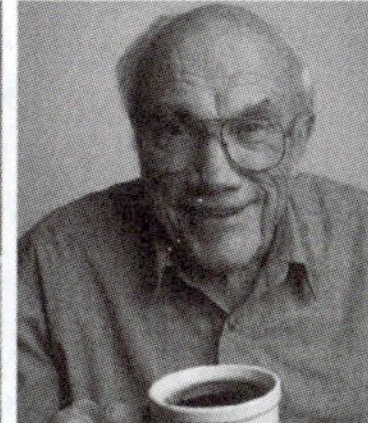
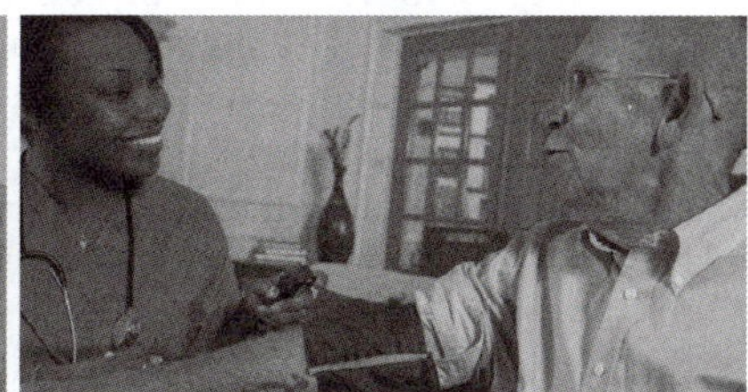

Learning objectives

At the end of this chapter, the reader will be able to:

- demonstrate a holistic understanding of older people's needs and nursing care as they approach the end of their lives; one that takes into account the differing disease trajectories that older people are likely to experience
- critically examine contemporary policy and initiatives concerning the end-of-life care of older people in the context of person-centred care
- reflect on approaches to caring for older people (and their carers) at the end of their lives. In particular, the extent to which the older person's choices, needs and concerns about death and dying are considered and the way in which approaches to end-of-life care will be influenced by staff's personal life experiences and attitudes
- identify how changes may be made in your practice and demonstrate strategies to improve the delivery of end-of-life care to ensure that it is person-centred. This means considering the individual's needs and their personal and social resources, as well as the wider organizational resources available

Ivy Sharpe comments as follows:

'Old age passed me by until I was almost eighty and, despite being a widow, I seldom thought about my future in terms of possible illness or death. I kept busy with several projects – a local pensioners' group – working towards being a peer educator involving older people – and helping at our local Hospice. Then I noticed that my eyesight was not as good as it was and my optician referred me to the local hospital for cataract treatment. I had the left eye done first and a few weeks later, the right eye. This was a wonderful experience and well worth the few little set-backs.

I then became more aware of problems with my knee and legs which I had experienced for a few years. At first, I thought this was only to be expected in later

(*continued*)

life – in my head I would think 'it's my age' – until one leg let me down several times. I was once again referred to hospital where both knees were x-rayed and the result was not good. I had a complete left knee replacement in June 2008. My family and partner gave me full support and, six months after, I felt the benefit of my new knee. I am now on a waiting list for my right knee to be replaced; before this can be done, I have to have an operation on my right foot to remove a bunion to make two straight toes.

At eighty-four, it could be asked whether all this surgery is worth weeks of struggle to get my balance, avoid steps, walking with a stick, giving in to needing help from people? My answer is a resounding 'YES'! I can be mended and let people pamper me. Older people still have a lot to give the world today. Despite knowing that I still have a lot to contribute and do, I have reached the point in my life where I feel that I must talk with my family. It may be a few years ahead before the end of my time on earth, but for them to know my wishes may help. I don't want my life to be prolonged with drugs – I would like to go as peacefully as possible – hopefully, in my own home or with my family around me.

I have had a happy and fulfilled life and life on earth doesn't go on forever. I am a Christian and, following my death, would wish to have my funeral in church, have my favourite hymns sung, and a priest who knows me to lead the service. I would then like to be cremated and, having lived all my life in the country-side, have my ashes scattered somewhere peaceful: I don't want sadness!'

Introduction

We have commenced this chapter with a commentary from Ivy Sharpe since care for older people as they near the end of their lives should be centred on the experiences and views of older people themselves. Despite having views on what she wants to be done (and not done) at the end of her life, Ivy is not 'waiting' to die; rather, she is determined to die as she has lived her life; in a self-determined and forward-thinking way. Ivy's account illustrates that in late old age there are perceived opportunities for living, enjoying activities and looking forward to the future (Owen, 2005; Clarke and Warren, 2007). Despite being in her 80s, Ivy concedes that she did not consider death and dying until the cumulative effect of illness became apparent. Many of us, however, are not comfortable thinking about death. The death of someone close to us, particularly someone who is of a similar age to ourselves or someone in the public eye (such as Jade Goody, Michael Jackson or Stephen Gately), may pull us up sharp and focus our attention on aspects of our existence which we usually keep well away from our thoughts. Often this is momentary; we can reassure ourselves in the belief that 'it won't happen to us' – not yet anyway. However, such denial is more problematic for those who, with increasing age, may become ever more conscious that they are nearing the end of their lives.

It is in old age that most of us will die and with 'problems caused by great old age and its troubles as well as any final illness' (Davies and Higginson, 2004: 15). As one woman in a research study confided, 'the older you get, the nearer to the front of the church you get' (Clarke, 2001); and, as Ivy Sharpe comments, it is often illness and disability that causes older individuals to begin to consider death and dying. Ivy describes the surgery she has had over the last few years and empathizes with an American surgeon's older patient who told him 'death keeps taking little bits of me' (Kafetz, 2002). The fact that we are living longer is a cause for celebration but this has implications for health and social care; the population requiring care in the twenty-first century is much older and increasingly likely to be living their last days affected by some type of disability (Davies and Higginson, 2004).

Everyone, whatever their age, should be able to expect a death that involves privacy, dignity, good quality care in comfortable surroundings, adequate pain relief and appropriate support (General Medical Council, 2006). In the UK, however, evidence suggests that for older people, the experience of living in the last year of life has been marked by extreme disadvantage in terms of health and social care provision, particularly specialist palliative care (George and Sykes, 1997; Grande et al., 1998; British Geriatrics Society, 2009). Perhaps this is because of the negative attitudes towards death and older age *per se* that have predominated the twentieth century – the disproportionate focus on the more 'heroic' deaths of younger people and also because it is assumed that older people do not want to, or are incapable of, engaging in discussions about their care (Seymour et al., 2005).

It is also suggested that the disease-focused models of palliative care policy, provision and delivery, while appropriate for cancer patients, may not meet the complex health and social needs of older people as they near the end of their lives (Seymour, 2007). In older people, the processes of dying tend to be more ambiguous than in younger people, particularly those with cancer (Kafetz, 2002). Hospice care is primarily directed towards persons with cancer who usually have a well-defined course of illness, making it possible to accurately determine their diagnosis and prognosis (Seale and Cartwright, 1994; Addington-Hall and McCarthy, 1995). In terms of place of death, while many older people would like to die at home, younger people are more likely to be given the opportunity (Seymour et al., 2005). Supporting older people to die at home needs to be assessed in the light of the individual's experiences and circumstances; for example, older people may have less support from family and friends than their younger counterparts and may find themselves isolated. In other words, where people live and die needs to be based on an informed choice, shaped by the person's individual circumstances. Nonetheless, it must also be a *realistic* choice; the resources available – health and social, as well as personal – must also be taken into account.

Care delivery tends to neglect the heterogeneity of views held by older people on death and dying and the way in which these will be influenced by cultural attitudes and their life experiences. It is therefore important that nurses should consider the provision and care for older people as they near the end of their lives within a framework that is centred on the older individual's views and biography (Clarke and Hanson, 2001). Although many older people remain in good health well into late old age, some may worry about future illness and the end of life, particularly if they know they have a serious illness, have experienced bereavement or live alone and are unsure where to seek help (Sanders et al., 2006). Nurses are in the privileged position of being able to spend time listening to and caring for older people towards the end of their lives, so better understanding and meeting the needs of older dying individuals is a nursing priority.

Where appropriate throughout the remainder of this chapter, we draw on the views of older people themselves – their hopes and concerns – as expressed in discussion groups held across the UK which sought to listen to the experiences and views of older people about death and dying (see the next boxed section). A fuller account of the events and findings have been published elsewhere (Clarke et al., 2006; Clarke and Seymour, 2010).

Listening to older people's views and experiences about death and dying

All comments from older people in this chapter are from four listening events delivered across the UK as part of a collaborative venture between Help the Aged (who funded the events) and researchers from universities in England.

The aim of the events (held in the north and south of England, Wales and Scotland) was to increase understanding of the concerns many older people have around end-of-life issues and to provide advice and information to address these concerns. Using the principles of focus group conduct, the research team, including five older volunteers, facilitated discussions among small groups of older people (n = 74) in four workshops. In the morning, participants talked about their feelings, experiences and concerns about the end of life. In the afternoon, discussion was guided using a booklet *Planning for Choice in End-of-life Care* (Seymour et al., 2006) piloted in an earlier study (Sanders et al., 2006).

Following framework analysis, six main themes arose:

- perspectives on talking about the end of life;
- raising concerns about death and dying with family members;
- spirituality;
- after death;
- end-of-life care;
- and concerns about death and dying.

Participants' reported apprehension about discussing the topic was overridden by their desire to know more about the decisions and choices available to them at the end of their lives. Many had not been given the opportunity to discuss the subject before – either with their families, friends or health professionals – or in a public forum. The heterogeneity of stories told illustrated how people's responses and needs at the end of life vary tremendously, but also revealed shared reactions and experiences from which nurses can learn.

(Clarke et al., 2006; Clarke and Seymour, 2010).

Dying in older age: causes

As preventive health care reduces disease-related death at a younger age, more people can expect to die eventually in older age: the majority of deaths in European and other developed countries occur in people aged over 65 (Davies and Higginson, 2004). In the UK, at the beginning of the twentieth century, more than 50 per cent of all deaths occurred under the age of 45. In 2007, only 4 per cent of deaths occurred at ages under 45. Deaths at the age of 75 and over comprised only 12 per cent of all deaths in 1901, rising to 39 per cent in 1951 and 66 per cent in 2007 (www.statistics.gov.uk/cci/nugget.asp?id=952). There is little data on the patterns of decline due to age-related causes of death although disability, frailty and dementia become increasingly common in later life. We do know, however, that people who die from long-term, degenerative conditions other than cancer tend to be aged over 65 years and to have a long-term illness trajectory that ends, in the majority of cases, in death within the acute hospital setting (Seymour et al., 2005). Hospital-based staff (usually nurses) caring for older people are the practitioners providing end-of-life care for the majority of those who are dying.

Terminology

Nurses have always cared for people who are dying (Payne, 2008); yet, determining the point at which someone moves from living to dying is increasingly complex. As a result, the terminology around 'dying', particularly in relation to health care delivery, has grown. Palliative care, end-of-life care, terminal care, hospice care and specialist palliative care are all terms that are used – sometimes interchangeably – to focus on the area of care surrounding dying. The increase in use of these terms reflects a growing understanding that dying is not just about the last days or hours of life but rather something that patients and their families become aware of sometimes weeks, months or even years before the actual physical death occurs. Our understanding of the complexity of the topic area has led to the development of more specific terminology that, in turn, has influenced the delivery of service to people who may or may not be aware that their disease process may shorten their anticipated life span.

Palliative care

The World Health Organization (WHO) defines palliative care as the following:

> “Palliative care is an approach that improves the quality of life of patients and their families facing the problem associated with life-threatening illness, through the prevention and relief of suffering by means of early identification and impeccable assessment and treatment of pain and other problems, physical, psychosocial and spiritual.
>
> (Sepulveda et al., 2002)”

Palliative care:

- provides relief from pain and other distressing symptoms;
- affirms life and regards dying as a normal process;
- intends neither to hasten or postpone death;
- integrates the psychological and spiritual aspects of patient care;
- offers a support system to help patients live as actively as possible until death;
- offers a support system to help the family cope during the patient's illness and in their own bereavement;
- uses a team approach to address the needs of patients and their families, including bereavement counselling, if indicated;
- will enhance quality of life, and may also positively influence the course of illness;
- is applicable early in the course of illness, in conjunction with other therapies that are intended to prolong life, such as chemotherapy or radiation therapy, and includes those investigations needed to better understand and manage distressing clinical complications.

(WHO, 2009)”

Across the world, 56 million people die annually; most of these deaths (approximately 40 million) take place in resource-poor countries; for example, sub-Saharan Africa. It has been estimated that about 60 per cent of people (33 million) who die would benefit from palliative care support at the end of their lives. When the close friends or family members of each of these 33 million people are included, this figure increases to 100 million people who might benefit from palliative care in its most basic form (Stjernswärd and Clark, 2005: 1199).

Clark and Seymour (1999) describe the philosophy of palliative care as a vital part of all clinical practice: it is defined as promoting patients' physical and psychological well-being while also including family carers and where decision-making is guided by patients' concerns and anxieties, rather than medical/physical considerations alone. It is argued that this culture needs to be disseminated to general medical settings if the care of all dying patients, including older people, is to be improved throughout services (Department of Health (DoH), 2000).

The WHO definition of palliative care refers to the point of diagnosis of death, with increasing levels of support as death approaches. Within Western societies, palliative care has become aligned with specialist palliative care services and the hospice movement. These services developed with an emphasis and focus on cancer care and, in particular, the care of younger cancer patients such that older adults with cancer are much less likely to access these specialist services than younger people (Seymour et al., 2005).

End-of-life care

The term 'end-of-life care' is now often preferred in connection to discussing death and dying in older age since this encompasses a broader approach that is applicable in a variety of care settings and, potentially, over a longer period of time (Seymour and Ingleton, 2008). This is reflected in the following definition from Canada:

> “(End-of-life care) requires an active, compassionate approach that treats, comforts and supports older individuals who are living with, or dying from, progressive or chronic life-threatening conditions. Such care is sensitive to personal, cultural, and spiritual values, beliefs and practices and encompasses support for families and friends up to and including the period of bereavement.
>
> (Ross and Fisher, 2000: 9)”

The terms 'palliative care' and 'end-of-life care' are broader than the more traditional 'terminal care' that in nursing is used to refer to the final few weeks or hours of someone's life. Both terms share in common an ongoing holistic and person-centred approach to care throughout the disease trajectory. In the UK, it is mainly health care professionals who use the term end-of-life care; patients and their families more often refer to terminal illness and terminal care, which focus on the dying phase of an illness. Within this chapter, we refer to the broader term end-of-life care since this is important in the longer-term care of older people.

Policies and initiative to improve palliative and end-of-life care

With an ageing population, palliative and end-of-life care are recognized as key factors in the delivery of quality health care in the twenty-first century. In the UK, ensuring that services are prepared and available at the point of need is the responsibility of government and local health care providers. To facilitate this process, strategic aims are set in the form of national policies outlining minimum standards of care that can be expected by the population. The delivery of these goals at a local level is then implemented by the local health and social care organizations within set guidelines. This ensures that the national policy is implemented locally and that local factors are taken into account when organizing and planning the care that will be required. Currently, key policy documents in end-of-life care in the UK are the NICE (2004) guidelines *Improving Supportive and Palliative Care for Adults with Cancer, The End-of-Life Care Strategy* (DoH, 2008) and *Living and Dying Well* (Scottish Government, 2008).

While there are currently no national polices which relate specifically to the care of older people at the end of life, the following section outlines initiatives which can be drawn on to support the nursing care of older people.

The national end-of-life care strategy

The national *End of Life Care Strategy* is a strategic document published in England in 2008 (DoH, 2008). Similar initiatives are being taken forward in Wales, Scotland and Northern Ireland in holding the aim of improving end-of-life care and providing people approaching the end of life with more choice about where they would like to live and die. Its key points focus on the development of care pathways that are facilitated by the identification and rapid response to people with end-of-life care needs in all locations, which include the home and institutional care settings. The strategy comprises the following sections: raising the profile of end of life; strategic commissioning; identifying people approaching the end of life; care planning; co-ordination of care; rapid access to care; delivery of high-quality services in all locations; last days of life and care after death; involving and supporting carers; education and training and continuing professional development.

Once strategic decisions have been made about the level of care that can be expected to be delivered, then initiatives need to be put in place to ensure that this work is actualized. In the case of palliative and end-of-life care, this can be found in initiatives such as the Liverpool Care Pathway, the Gold Standards Framework, and so on.

The Liverpool Care Pathway

The Liverpool Care Pathway is not actually a policy but grew out of a need to address end-of-life issues in an acute hospital setting in a more systematic and appropriate manner. Increasingly, it is being used to assist in improving care for patients dying both in hospital and at home, mainly for the last week or hours of life. The pathway is designed for people with a known diagnosis who have deteriorated to such an extent that death appears inevitable. Symptoms are monitored and treated expectantly with an emphasis on comfort, communication and preparation for death with spiritual support.

Gold Standard Framework

The Gold Standard Framework is primarily a primary care-based initiative developed in conjunction with Macmillan UK and offers primary care practitioners a number of areas to consider and discuss with their patients and families when thinking about

(*continued*)

future care and dying needs. The documentation provides a toolkit for nurses and other health practitioners for initiating these discussions.

Gold Standards for Care Homes
Within a community setting, tools such as Gold Standards for Care Homes may be used. Homes that wish to use this tool to enhance their care of dying patients are also provided with training. The aim of this work (led by the DoH's Gold Standard Framework group) is to aid high-quality end-of-life-care for care home residents with the aim of helping residents to 'live well until you die'. The use of such tools prompts preferences for place of care (see also *Preferred Priorities for Care*, DoH, 2007) and other aspects of end-of-life care.

Limitations of initiatives

While these policies and initiatives may be helpful in assisting health practitioners to systematically review and provide appropriate services, they should not be taken as a prescriptive solution to all situations and evidence is needed regarding their use in the care and treatment of older people. Nurses need to consider the individual's needs and personal resources, as well as the wider organizational resources available when implementing these initiatives. This is particularly the case when planning the end of life of older individuals, given that they are likely to experience multiple pathologies and differing disease trajectories.

Further, while there are a number of policies and initiatives being suggested to encourage a systematic approach to end-of-life care, there are few that focus specifically on the carer. Family carers are increasingly recognized by the government and other organizations as being essential in enabling the older person to continue to be cared for in his or her own home if this is what the individual wants; however, identification of carers' needs are not always acknowledged, either by the health care professional or the carer themselves. This is especially true when working in the end-of-life care setting, since the focus of care and activity here is on delivering the patient's wishes. Within the *Improving Supportive and Palliative Care for Adults with Cancer* guidelines (National Institute for Clinical Excellence (NICE), 2004) and the *End-of-Life Care Strategy* (DoH, 2008), carers' contributions and the effect that their role may have on their own physical and psychological well-being should be acknowledged and highlighted as an area of need. The National Council for Palliative Care (NCPC and NCI, 2009), in collaboration with the NHS National Centre for Involvement, has produced a useful guide to involve patients, carers and the public in the planning and delivery of palliative care and end-of-life care services.

Key issues in nursing older people at the end of life

Nursing older people at the end of life, therefore, has a number of challenges; not least of which is being able to prognosticate when the last year of life may be. Individuals are living longer but their extended years of life are not necessarily better quality (Brown 2008). Dying in older age is likely to be complicated by multiple pathologies and generalized decline that make identification of the final 'dying' phase difficult. What is more, some disease trajectories have an unpredictable course with periods of crisis, remission and relapse. Traditional specialist palliative care has been developed largely around the cancer disease trajectory that has a fairly well-defined dying phase. One reason that specialist palliative care services may be reluctant to take on large numbers of older people is that older individuals may be seen to require an unpredictable and long-term need for care, as a result of the types of disease with which they commonly present.

According to the British Geriatrics Society (2009), the following are important factors in enabling older people to live comfortably until they die:

- comprehensive assessment (especially the frailest with complex co-morbidity);
- enhanced communication and honest prognostication to identify treatment priorities as part of effective clinical decision-making;
- adopting principles of palliative care, including pain and symptom management;
- advanced planning and integrated care pathways to enhance the quality of end-of-life care;
- giving older people access to specialist palliative care teams, where appropriate, regardless of diagnosis or place of care.

The following section embraces these factors in outlining the key issues to be considered for nurses caring for older dying people, which are multiple pathologies, care settings and communication issues, each of which should be addressed in nursing assessment, implementation and evaluation.

Multiple pathologies

As people age, there is increasing likelihood that they will experience multiple pathologies. This complicates health care delivery as one illness management treatment may impact adversely on another disease process, or create additional challenges for the older person. For example, opiates, which are commonly prescribed for cancer pain, have different absorption rates in older people and can cause increased toxicity or side-effects – such as constipation – which may be viewed by the older person as more distressing than the original pain (Smith, 2001). When supporting people with these difficulties, the focus of medical and nursing care often becomes centred around symptom control which fails to take the psychological, social and spiritual dimensions of the older person's everyday life into account.

Care settings

Older people live and die in a variety of care settings, including their own homes, care homes and assisted living facilities. The challenge for nurses (working alongside other health and social care practitioners) in assessing and planning care is to facilitate the older person's wishes to die in the setting of his or her choice. For many, this will be their own home (or the setting which they consider to be home). Although most people state that they would prefer to die at home, relatively few currently do so; death in hospital remains common in many countries (Davies and Higginson, 2004). Evidence from the UK suggests that older people are less likely than younger people to receive care at home (British Geriatrics Society, 2009). There are also discrepancies among those with cancer: in the UK, 8.5 per cent of older people who die from cancer do so in a hospice, compared with 20 per cent of all cancer sufferers (Seymour et al., 2005).

Key point

Most people state that they would prefer to die at home but relatively few currently do so and death in hospital remains common in many countries.

Davies and Higginson (2004) point out that variation in place of death suggests that the organization of services is significant in determining the options that people can consider. They support their view by describing studies in the USA, which indicate that the proportion of people dying at home ranges from 18 per cent to 32 per cent and seems to vary primarily according to the availability of hospital beds per head of population (Davies and Higginson, 2004). Davies and Higginson (2004) also emphasize the importance of cultural values, citing the examples of Italy and the Netherlands. In Italy, death in hospital is more common in the north of the country while families in the south prefer to care for people at home. The Netherlands is citied as successful in providing a range of palliative care services in different settings and giving people the resources to die at home if they wish (Davies and Higginson, 2004). The need to provide a range of palliative services in a variety of care settings is illustrated by the following comments from participants in listening events about end-of-life care in the UK. These show the heterogeneity of views concerning place of care at the end of life:

> I just want to close my eyes and drift away.
>
> I want to be in a home not cared for by my family; I want my family to live their lives – I don't want to be a burden.
>
> I want to die in my own home, but it depends if I can cope.
>
> I want to go into our local hospice.
>
> (Clarke et al., 2006)

Some participants questioned whether older people really had a choice in deciding where they died:

Scenario 15.1

'My uncle spent his life in the RAF then went to Australia. He came back to Wales when he retired and he got ill. I was his only relative here. He had a stroke and went into a Community Hospital and then into a residential home, but he didn't like it in there. He wanted to go home but he couldn't.'

- *Do older people you are nursing have choices about where they die?*
- *Do you know what their choices are?*

They recognized that this choice had an effect on family relationships but felt that the choice of the dying person should be central (see Scenario 15.2).

Scenario 15.2

'My sister became very ill with cancer, she couldn't eat and was allowed to go home. My other two sisters were very against her going home and it became very difficult between us. It is the person themselves who matters. We all gathered round her bed and she had a peaceful death. Every person has the right to a dignified death. We need to ask people, not just have young people legislating for them.'

- *Reflect on a situation you have been in when there has not been agreement about someone going home at the end of their life – did the older person themselves have a voice in decision-making?*
- *How could you have supported them?*

While dying at home may be seen as a desirable aim in many countries, and is in line with UK government policy (see *Preferred Priorities of Care*, DoH, 2007), the practicalities of achieving this may mitigate against these actions. In addition, by suggesting that everyone has a choice of where they die, we may in fact be raising expectations that might not be met; it could be argued that neither control, nor choice, are things that are readily available to a wider population of older people as they reach the end of their lives (Seymour et al., 2005). Although many people – whatever their age – value choice and control, research suggests that many older people also recognize that practical and other issues may take priority over their own preferences (Gott et al., 2004; Arber et al., 2008), such as the desire not to 'burden' their families (Gott et al., 2004). In care homes, some research has suggested that end-of-life care may be impeded by inadequate staff training, poor symptom control and lack of psychological and emotional support (British Geriatrics Society, 2009); however, where training and support is in place, a nursing home may be a more appropriate setting for an older person to die than an acute care setting.

Communication issues

Older people are not usually fully involved in discussions concerning the options available to them at the end of life (Seymour et al., 2005) and many nurses feel unprepared to discuss end-of-life issues with older people (Clarke and Ross, 2006). Communication with older people about end-of-life care may be affected by common negative stereotyping of older people as 'slowing down', 'stupid' or 'dependant' (Seymour et al., 2005) as seen by the comment in Scenario 15.3 from a participant in the listening events:

Scenario 15.3

'I went into hospital with pneumonia recently. I noticed after a few days they had put the wrong name above my bed. I asked them and they said, "Oh don't fuss. Old ladies fuss more than old men."'

- *Select an hour at work tomorrow and listen hard to the words spoken to older people.*
- *In what ways could older people be more respected?*

These stereotypes may mean that older people are less likely to be listened to by nurses and others with whom they come into contact. Further, May's (1990) study found that physical tasks were seen by nurses as 'work', whereas verbal communication was not. Costello (2001, 2004) described nurses' care of dying patients as focused on meeting physical, rather than psychosocial needs. Similarly, McDonnell et al. (2002) found that where time was short, nurses gave priority to physical care at the expense of patients' psychosocial needs. In Clarke and Ross's (2006) study, one student's comment about 'emotional exhaustion' echoed McDonnell et al.'s (2002) assertion that nurses' own psychological needs were unmet. This highlights the need for further training and support of nurses and other health practitioners in this area.

Implications for practice: assessment and implementation of a person-centred approach to end-of-life care for older people

For older people, the dominance of the medical model in end-of-life care can result in less attention being paid to other issues which may be of greater importance to the individual than his or her physical health. This is not to suggest that the relief of physical symptoms is not important but rather to emphasize that nursing assessment of the dying individual must go beyond disease or symptom processes.

Research studies have identified inadequacies in the end-of-life care of older patients; including that dying patients, frequently, do not receive essential nursing care, adequate pain relief or assistance with eating and drinking (Edmonds and Rogers, 2003; Kite, 2006). Neglect of assistance with eating and drinking is reflected in the following comment by an older man in the listening events (Clarke et al., 2006):

> " I was on a hospital ward and the guy next door kept leaving his food. The nurses would come along and ask if he wasn't hungry. I noticed that he couldn't hold a spoon and was giving up, so I ended up feeding him. The nurses didn't stop to ask why he wasn't eating. It went on for days! They moved him to a geriatric ward. His daughter came up and thanked me for helping and said she wished he'd stayed on my ward because he was deteriorating now. "

Alternatively, staff may focus on meeting physical needs at the expense of psychological and spiritual care (Clarke and Ross, 2006). Carmen Franklin, an older peer educator in end-of-life care, stresses the importance for nurses to consider the spiritual needs of older people:

> " People nearing the end of life tend to look beyond the everyday concerns to what lies beyond – towards the spiritual dimension of things. Whatever their religious beliefs, many people hope for a better life after death. For those who have no religion or faith, the word spirituality, though commonly used, has a more practical meaning. Those who care for the sick and dying, particularly for older people, may be required to aid the spiritual as well as physical needs. For example, a person may ask for permission to have short daily bedside prayers as a comfort and/or a short reading of verse from a holy book. "

Clearly, there is a need for nurses to approach the assessment, implementation and evaluation of care of older people at the end of life in a way that takes into account their potentially complex needs; this includes medical, social, psychological and spiritual concerns as encompassed in the term 'end-of-life care'. This embraces a person-centred approach; 'treating older people as individuals and enabling them to make choices about their care' (DoH, 2001: 12) at the end of life that are centred on the person's needs and life perspectives (McCormack, 1996).

In the following section, we suggest practical ways, once more illustrated by older adults' comments at the listening events, for nurses to implement a person-centred approach in caring for older people as they approach the end of their lives.

Suggestions to improve person-centred care from older people

- Staff should call you by your surname until you say that you want to be called by your first name.
- Simply by asking people what they want, asking their permission to do something; for example, the consultant's ward round at the bottom of your bed... it's as if you're not there.
- Listen to older people about life.
- Engage with us as human beings with individual values; we're not just patients.
- Having more respectful attitudes.
- By not patronising us.

(Clarke et al., 2006)

The above suggestions, which may be applied to all care situations, show the need for nurses to respect the older person, their values and beliefs; taking into account their life experiences and how this might influence the decisions they may take about their own end-of-life care needs.

Although there were many illustrations about poor care in the listening events, some participants pointed out that they had witnessed or received good care in hospital and in the community. Caring for older people as persons, taking into account their biography, rather than seeing them solely as patients, was appreciated, as these comments demonstrate:

> “ When my husband went into hospital, they asked me to make a diary of his life. Things he liked, things he didn't. Pictures of important people and all the nurses looked at it and said 'oh, hasn't he had an interesting life? ”

> “ My mother-in-law is in care, with dementia. I agree with the concerns about low pay and also rapid staff turnover. But all the clients in her establishment are addressed by name, all have a Memory Box and there is a potted history of everyone for new staff. ”

These comments reflect research which has found that some older people desire to have their personal biographies recognized and valued as the basis for individualized care (Nolan et al., 2001).

Given the challenges outlined above regarding individuals' choices as they approach the end of life, one of the nurse's roles may be to present a realistic account of the options available in facilitating the ideal place and approach to death for the individual and their family. This will enable them to make an informed and realistic decision about care choices.

Nurses should also recognize that decisions about care choices may change over time with an individual's altering or deteriorating health and their social or economic circumstances. A statement of wishes and preferences as part of advance care planning (ACP) is one approach that may help nurses ascertain the personal goals, values and everyday preferences of individuals (Henry and Seymour, 2007). Clearly, giving people the opportunity to express their wishes and preferences needs to occur before an individual is at the end of their life.

Initiating a discussion

Below are examples of questions to initiate discussion about care choices:

- Can you tell me about your current illness and how you are feeling?
- Could you tell me what are the most important things to you at the moment?
- Who is the person most important to you right now?
- Is there anything worrying or frightening you about the future?
- Have you thought about where you would prefer to be cared for as your illness gets worse?
- What would give you the most comfort when your life draws to a close?

(Based on Horne et al., 2006: 172–78)

The time at the end of life is unique for each person; each person has specific needs for information, for support and for care. It is important that nurses supporting older adults at the end of life allow for individual exploration of each unique older person's viewpoint. Although people's readiness to talk about death and dying is likely to be influenced by personal circumstances, it is not necessarily the case that these are subjects that older people will find distressing, as our experience in research with older people about death and dying has shown (Clarke et al., 2006; Sanders et al., 2006; Seymour et al., 2006). Some people may find it helpful to have the chance to discuss their concerns and fears; others may prefer not to: this should be approached with sensitivity and their viewpoint respected. The Dying Matters coalition set up by the National Council for Palliative Care (NCPC) encourages people to talk about their wishes towards the end of their lives. Useful information for laypeople can be found on their website: www.dyingmatters.org/site/about-us. Advance care planning can assist nurses with this communication process since it facilitates a dialogue between the older person, their family and/or close companions and the health professional.

Advance care planning (ACP)[1]

Advance care planning (ACP) interventions have been described in the North American literature (Hammes, 1994) where there has been a state-sponsored emphasis on increasing the completion of advance statements. In the UK, these issues have come under policy and media attention due to new legislation in the form of the Mental Capacity Act (Department of Constitutional Affairs, 2005).

[1] It is important for nurses to be aware of the main ethical and legal issues concerning the end of life; however, it is also important to be aware that they are subject to rapid change. More specific details about ACP can be found at www.endoflifecare.nhs.uk/eolc.

The guide to ACP for health and social care professionals (Henry and Seymour, 2007) published under the auspices of the NHS End-of-life Care Programme, points out that one of the key aspects of the nurse's role is to discuss with individuals (if the individual so desires) their preferences about the type of care they would wish to receive and how they wish to receive it. If the individual wishes, their family and friends may be included. The outcomes of such discussions then need to be documented, regularly reviewed and communicated to other relevant people, subject to the individual's agreement. This is the process of ACP. The importance of considering ACP is summed up by this comment by an older woman in the listening events:

> “Everyone needs to be prepared, especially those engaged in the caring professions, since no-one knows what lies in the future.”

Advance care planning discussion might include an individual's:

- concerns;
- values or personal goals for care;
- understanding about illness prognosis;
- preferences for care or treatment that may be beneficial in the future.

The outcomes of ACP are outlined in detail in Henry and Seymour (2007).

Many of the principles involved in ACP are ones which will be familiar to all nurses: skills of listening and reflecting, of summarizing and of unconditional regard for the point of view of the patient and their family. Communicating with older people about sensitive issues does not necessarily require protected time, but, as nurses in Clarke and Ross's (2006) study indicated, could be integrated into everyday care activities to encourage older people to feel actively involved in decision-making. In this study, nurses described how they learnt to feel more comfortable about approaching and talking to older people about end-of-life issues through a combination of learning from others and experience (Clarke and Ross, 2006). Students and new staff (registered nurses and support workers), however, felt unprepared for their experiences with dying people (Kiger, 1994; Hopkinson et al., 2003; Clarke and Ross, 2006). In England, the National End of Life Care Programme (DoH, 2009), in collaboration with *Skills for Health and Skills for Care*, outlined the core skills and principles for all staff across care homes, hospitals and other settings, not just specialists in end-of-life or palliative care working with people approaching the end of their lives. These are designed to achieve a 'cultural shift in attitudes and behaviour related to end of life care'. The principles are that:

- Choices and priorities of the individual are at the centre of planning and delivery.
- Effective, straightforward, sensitive and open communication with individuals and their families underpins all planning and activity.
- Delivery is through multidisciplinary and inter-agency working.
- Individuals, families and friends are well informed about the range of options and resources available to be involved in care planning.
- Care is delivered in a sensitive, person-centred way, taking account of the circumstances, wishes and priorities of the individual, family and friends.
- Care and support are available to anyone affected by the end of life and death of an individual.

- Workers are supported to develop knowledge, skills and attitudes and take responsibility for their continuing professional development.

(DoH, 2009)

When planning care that is likely to be required in the future, it is important that nurses include the older person and their family members and/or close companions, if that is what they wish. Such open communication will help reduce the unexpectedness of the dying process as the death of a relative in difficult circumstances can have a significant impact on the psychological well-being of the family and may also impact on their bereavement experience (Chaplin, 2003). In the listening events, some people recalled how, as the relatives of a dying person (often their spouse), they felt they were given insufficient information (Clarke et al., 2006). Consequently, they felt unprepared for the person's death as this woman explained:

> “I was totally unprepared. My husband's experiences of dying were appalling. It took 18 weeks for a cancer diagnosis. We were then introduced to a Macmillan nurse who we never saw again. . . .The cancer specialist only said four words to me to say that he was incurable. In the end, I was unable to say goodbye. Everything that happened convinced me there was ageism in the Health Service.”

Key point

When planning care that is likely to be required in the future, it is important that nurses include the older person and their family members and/or close companions, if that is what they wish.

Advance care statements: a study

Seymour et al.'s study (2004) which explored older people's views about advance care statements found that the benefits of advanced statements were seen primarily in terms of the potential they have for providing a guide for family members or in terms of ensuring that their 'burden' of decision-making was lessened.

Many participants in the listening events also felt that they were given insufficient information about their own or their relatives' condition as they approached the end of life (Clarke et al., 2006). A variety of reasons were offered for staff's reluctance to share information, including ageism. One participant commented, 'I want the dignity of being able to decide these things for myself – not to be treated like a baby.' Indeed, some participants felt that older people – by virtue of their age and experience – should not only be given more information but also consulted more about their condition and care:

> "You've lived with your body for 70 years, so they should listen to what you say. You know when it's not working."
>
> "Health professionals assume they know the level of information that you can absorb about your condition (in hospital), in the old days we would never question the doctor, but you are entitled to know as much as possible."

A person-centred nursing assessment of an older person *approaching* the end of his or her life should therefore:

- provide opportunities to learn more about the individual, their current situation, past experiences, present attitudes, values and beliefs, as well as their hopes and concerns for the future;
- place the older person at the centre of the assessment and should enable them to feel empowered by the process. Any other significant person in their life should be involved, if that is what they want;
- facilitate the building of a relationship, to offer a professional and realistic view on challenges and to plan with the individual and family or other carers what sort of support or services would best meet their needs within social, cultural and organizational boundaries.

(Clarke, 2000; Heath, 2000; Henry and Seymour, 2007).

Conclusion

Within the context of an ageing population, end-of-life care will be increasingly dependent on the availability, effectiveness and flexibility of general social and health care to the needs of the older person, with support from, and for, those close to them, although some people will also need access to specialist services (Kite, 2006). Therefore, generalist nurses need to become more familiar and comfortable with discussions about death and dying with older people and their families; this includes high-quality symptom management and treatment, psychological, spiritual and social support and variety of care settings in which older people live and die. One way for all nurses to achieve this is to take a person-centred approach to care decisions and provision, including that at the end of life. Research suggests that older people want to be cared for as individuals, to be included in discussions about their care needs and preferences and to be able to take control – when they wish to – over how they live their lives and how they die. Nurses will not be comfortable with what older people say they want as they approach the end of their lives until they have explored the issues for themselves and understand what is helpful and supportive for older people, rather than adopting a somewhat paternalistic approach to care.

Key point

Nurses will not be comfortable with what older people say they want as they approach the end of their lives until they have explored the issues for themselves and understand what is helpful and supportive for older people, rather than adopting a somewhat paternalistic approach to care.

Acknowledgements

The authors would like to thank the Peer Education Project team led by Jane Seymour Sue Ryder Professor in Palliative and End of Life Care at the University of Nottingham and Help the Aged (funders of the Listening Events drawn on here).

References

Addington-Hall, J. and McCarthy, M. (1995) Dying from cancer: results of a national population based investigation, *Palliative Medicine,* 9: 295–305.

Arber, S., Vandrevala, T., Daly, T. and Hampson, S. (2008) Understanding gender differences in older people's attitudes towards life-prolonging medical technologies, *Journal of Aging Studies*, 22(4): 366–75.

British Geriatrics Society (2009) Palliative and End of Life Care of Older People. *BGS Best Practice Guide 4.8*. Available online at www.bgs.org.uk/Publications/Compendium/compend_4-8.htm; accessed June 2009.

Brown, G. (2008) *The Living End: The Future of Death, Aging and Immortality*. Basingstoke: Palgrave Macmillan.

Chaplin, D. (2003) A bereavement care service to address multicultural user needs, *Nursing Times*, 99(39): 26–29.

Clark, D. and Seymour, J. (1999) *Reflections on Palliative Care: Sociological and Policy Perspectives*. Maidenhead: Open University Press.

Clarke, A. (2001) Looking back and moving forward: a biographical approach to ageing. Unpublished PhD thesis, Department of Sociological Studies, University of Sheffield, Sheffield, Yorkshire.

Clarke, A. (2000) Using biography to enhance the nursing care of older people, *British Journal of Nursing*, 9(7): 429–33.

Clarke, A. and Ross, H. (2006) Influences on nurses' communications with older people at the end-of-life: perceptions and experiences of nurses working in palliative care and general medicine, *International Journal of Nursing Older People*, 1: 34–43.

Clarke, A. and Seymour, J. (2010) At the foot of a very long ladder: discussing the end of life with older people and their carers, *Journal of Pain and Symptom Management* 40(6): 857–69.

Clarke, A., Seymour, J.E, Welton, M., Sanders, C., Gott, M., Cock, M., Franklin, C., Richards, M., Sharpe, I. and Thompson, D. (2006) *Listening to Older People: Opening the Door for Older People to Explore End of Life Issues*. London: Help the Aged.

Clarke, A. and Hanson, S. (2001) Death and dying: changing the culture of care, in A. Warnes, L. Wavren and M. Nolan (eds) *Care Services for Later Life: Transformations and Critiques*, (pp. 204–18). London: Jessica Kingsley.

Clarke, A. and Warren, L. (2007) Hopes, fears and expectations about the future: what do older people's stories tell us about active ageing? *Ageing and Society*, 27: 465–88.

Costello, J. (2001) Nursing older dying patients: findings from an ethnographic study of death and dying in elderly care wards, *Journal of Advanced Nursing*, 35: 59–68.

Costello, J. (2004) *Nursing the Dying Patient.* Basingstoke: Palgrave Macmillan.

Davies, E. and Higginson, I. (2004) *The Solid Facts: Palliative Care*. Copenhagen: World Health Organisation.

Department of Health (DoH) (2008) *End of Life Care Strategy: Promoting High-quality Care for all Adults at the End of Life*. London: DoH.

Department of Health (DoH) (2007) *Preferred Priorities for Care* (formerly *Preferred Place of Care*). Available online at www.endoflifecareforadults.nhs.uk/eolc/CS310.htm; accessed October 2009.

Department of Health (DoH) (2009) *National Health Service. End of the Life Programme-Preferred Priorities for Care (Formerly Preferred Place Care)*. Available online from www.endoflifecareforadults.nhs.uk/assets/downloads/ppc_guidance.pdf.

Department of Health (DoH) (2000) *The NHS Plan: A Plan for Investment, a Plan for Reform*. London. DoH.

Department of Health (DoH) (2001) *National Standards Framework for Older People*. London. DoH.

Department of Constitutional Affairs (2005) *Mental Capacity Act 2005: Code of Practice*. London: The Stationery Office.

Edmonds, P. and Rogers, A. (2003) If only someone had told me: a review of patients dying in hospital, *Clinical Medicine,* 3: 149–52.

General Medical Council (2006) *Withholding and Withdrawing Life-prolonging Treatments: Good Practice in Decision-making. Guidance from the Standards Committee of the General Medical Council.* London: GMC. Available onle at www.gmc.org.uk; accessed October 2009.

George, R. and Sykes, J. (1997) Beyond cancer? In D. Clark, S. Ahmedzai and J. M. Hockley (eds) *New Themes in Palliative Care* (pp. 239–54). Maidenhead: Open University Press.

Gott, M., Seymour, J., Bellamy, G., Clark, D. and Ahmedzai, S.H. (2004) Older people's views about home as a place of care at the end of life, *Palliative Medicine*, 18(5): 460–67.

Grande, G., Addington-Hall, J. and Todd, C. (1998) Place of death and access to home care services: are certain patient groups at a disadvantage? *Social Science & Medicine,* 47(5): 565–79.

Hammes, B. (1994) *Respecting Your Choices. Training Manual.* Lacrosse, WI: Lutheran Hospital Press.

Heath, H. (2000) Assessing older people, *Elderly Care*, 11(10): 27–28.

Henry, C. and Seymour, J.E. (2007) Advance Care Planning: A Guide for Health and Social Care Professionals. London: NHS End of Life Care Programme.

Hopkinson, J., Hallet, C. and Luker, K. (2003) Caring for dying people in hospital, *Journal of Advanced Nursing*, 44: 525–33.

Horne, G., Seymour, J.E. and Shepherd, K. (2006) Advance care planning for patients with inoperable lung cancer, *International Journal of Palliative Nursing,* 12(4): 172–78.

Kafetz, K. (2002) What happens when elderly people die? *Journal of the Royal Society of Medicine*, 95: 536–38.

Kiger, A. (1994) Student nurses' involvement with death: the image and the experience, *Journal of Advanced Nursing*, 20: 679–86.

Kite, S. (2006) Palliative care for older people, *Age and Ageing,* 35: 459–60.

May, C. (1990) Research on nurse–patient relationship: problems of theory, problems of practice, *Journal of Advanced Nursing*, 15: 307–15.

McCormack, B. (1996) Life transitions, in P. Ford and H. Heath (eds) *Older People and Nursing* (pp. 71–86). London: Butterworth.

McDonnell, M., Johnson, G., Gallagher, A. and McGlade, K. (2002) Palliative care in district general hospitals: the nurse's perspective, *International Journal of Palliative Nursing*, 8: 169–75.

National Council of Palliative Care (NCPC) and NHS Centre for Involvement (NCI) (2009) *Guide to Involving Patients, Carers and the Public in Palliative Care and End of Life Care Services.* London: NCPC.

National Institute for Clinical Excellence (NICE) (2004) *Improving Supportive and Palliative Care for Adults with Cancer*. London: NICE. Available online at www.nice.org.uk/csgsp; accessed June 2009.

Nolan, M., Davies, S. and Grant, G. (2001) Integrating perspectives, in M. Nolan, S. Davies and G. Grant (eds) *Working with Older People and Their Families: Key Issues in Policy and Practice* (pp. 160–78). Maidenhead: Open University Press.

Owen, T. (2005) *Dying in Older Age: Reflections and Experiences from an Older Person's Perspective.* London: Help the Aged.

Payne, S. (2008) Introduction, in S. Payne, J. Seymour and C. Ingleton (eds) *Palliative Care Nursing: Principles and Evidence for Practice*, 2nd edn. (pp.1–15). Maidenhead: Open University Press.

Ross, M. and Fisher, R. (2000) *A Guide to End-of-life Care for Seniors*. Ottawa: Health Canada.

Sanders, C., Seymour, J.E., Clarke, A., Gott, M. and Welton, M. (2006) Development of a peer education programme for advance end-of-life care planning: an action research project with older adults, *International Journal of Palliative Nursing*, 12(5): 216–23.

Scottish Government (2008) *Living and Dying Well: A National Action Plan for Palliative and End of Life Care in Scotland.* Edinburgh: Scottish Government.

Seale, C. and Cartwright, A. (1994) *The Year Before Death.* Aldershot: Avebury.

Sepulveda, C., Marlin, A., Yoshida, T. et al. (2002) Palliative care: the World Health Organization's global perspective, *Journal of Pain and Symptom Management*, 24(2): 91–6.

Seymour, J. (2007) Windows on suffering: sociological perspectives on end of life care. Plenary address to the Annual BSA Medical Sociology Group Conference, Liverpool, 8 September. Available online at www.medicalsociologyonline.org/archives/issue22/jseymour.html; accessed October 20009.

Seymour, J. and Ingleton, C. (2008) Overview: Chapter 10, in S. Payne, J. Seymour and C. Ingleton (eds) *Palliative Care Nursing: Principles and Evidence for Practice*, 2nd edn (pp.181–11). Maidenhead: Open University Press.

Seymour, J., Gott, M., Bellamy, G., Ahmedzai, S.H. and Clark, D. (2004) Planning for the end of life: the views of older people about advance care statements, *Social Science and Medicine*, 59: 57–68.

Seymour, J., Witherspoon, R., Gott, M., Ross, H., Payne, S. and Owen, T. (2005) *End-of-life Care*. Bristol: The Policy Press in association with Help the Aged.

Seymour, J.E., Sanders, C., Clarke, A., Welton, M. and Gott, M. (2006) *Planning for Choice in End of Life Care: An Educational Guide*. London: Help the Aged.

Smith, S. (2001) Evidence-based management of constipation in the oncology patient, *European Journal Oncology Nursing*, 5(1): 18–25.

Stjernswärd, J. and Clark, D. (2005) Palliative medicine: a global perspective, in D. Doyle, G. Hanks, N. Cherny and K. Calman (eds) *Oxford Textbook of Palliative Medicine,* 3rd edn (pp 1199–224). Oxford: Oxford University Press.

World Health Organization (WHO) (2009) *Palliative Care*. Available online at www.who.int/cancer/palliative/definition/en; accessed June 2009.

CHAPTER 16

Mental health issues for older people

Mima Cattan

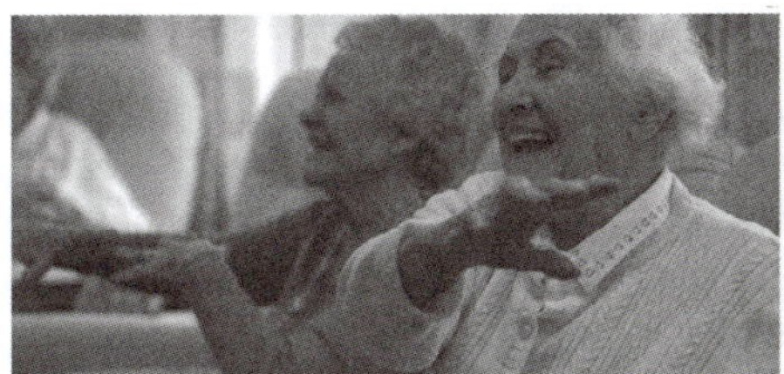
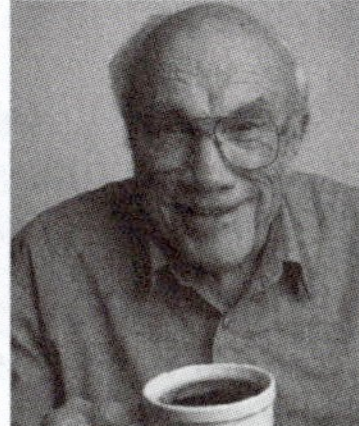
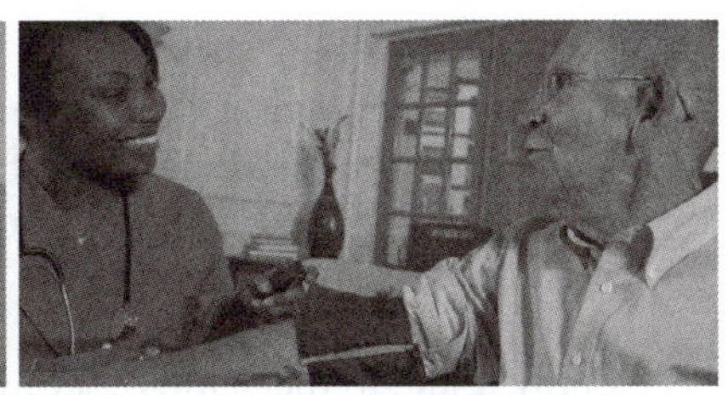

Learning objectives

At the end of this chapter, the reader will be able to:

- describe the factors that influence the mental health of an older person
- describe the socio-economic, environmental, biological, personal factors and health behaviours that are the determinants of mental health in later life
- understand the impact of events such as bereavement and the influence of loneliness of mental health
- describe ways in which the mental health of older people can be supported

Two older people comment on their experience of their mental health:

'I will sit here and sometimes I don't know what to do . . . if it wasn't for people ringing in the mornings I'd go in there and just lie on the bed.'

'I became extremely lonely and depressed when I had to give up work. I didn't know what to do with all the time I had. That's what made me turn to volunteering.'

Introduction

Ask a younger person what mental health means in later life and the most likely answer is 'dementia'. Ask an older person the same question and the response will probably be different. A survey of older people in Scotland found that keeping active, maintaining independence and having a role in life, physical health, attitudes and values, and coping with loss were key factors in mental health (Bostock and Millar, 2003). The survey suggested that for many older people mental health and well-being is not about illness, but rather something that enables them to look forward to the day and enjoy life. The European Community consultative Green Paper states:

> "An ageing EU-population, with its associated mental health consequences, calls for effective action. Old age brings many stressors that may increase mental ill health, such as decreasing functional capacity and social isolation. Late life-depression and age-related neuro-psychiatric conditions, such as dementia, will increase the burden of mental disorders. Support interventions have shown to improve mental well-being in older populations.
>
> (Commission of the European Communities, 2005: 9)"

Although this chapter deals with mental health issues in the chronologically defined population group of 'older people', it is obvious that mental health issues and mental health promotion are not 'fixed' to older people as a homogeneous group. First, 'old age' can span a large part of a person's life and, clearly, an individual's physical capacity and health status will change over that period. Second, mental health issues explored under 'old age' may not necessarily relate to the same older age group everywhere as they will be influenced by a range of environmental, cultural and social factors.

Some facts are as follows:

- It is estimated that about 10 per cent of older people have some form of mental health problem.
- Generally, older people in the UK have a lower prevalence of mental health disorder than other age groups.
- Older women are more likely than men to suffer from depression and anxiety, but single women have the lowest prevalence of mental health problems over all.
- The prevalence of mental health problems decreases with age from the age of 60 (Evans et al., 2003).

What are the issues?

Although many mental health issues span all age groups, there are a number of issues that are of greater relevance in older people's lives. Retirement, for example, is a major life transition which impacts on people's mental health and well-being. For some people retirement may mean a positive release from the 'daily slog' and other responsibilities, while for others it may mean the loss of important social networks and meaningful activities. In addition, a gradual deterioration in physical health, changing environments (e.g. moving home), and the sense of loss of social, physical or psychological factors, may impact on the individual's mental health.

For people aged 80 years and over the sense of loss may become increasingly chronic through the loss of their companions or close friends, their functional ability and the fear of losing their independence. In addition, if people's mobility decreases and their access to the outside world as a consequence becomes more restricted, they may become socially isolated and lose their sense of belonging with their previously familiar environment (Cattan, 2010). Loneliness, although not restricted to old age, becomes more prevalent among 'older old' people (Victor, 1989), which is discussed later. Caring for someone who is frail or in the early stages of dementia may contribute to an older person's social isolation and feelings of loneliness. Finally, at this stage in life people are facing the end of life and develop different strategies for dealing with dying and death.

Thus, some of the main factors that influence the mental health of older people include (Cattan and Tilford, 2006; Windle et al., 2007; Windle, 2009; Department of Health (DoH), 2010):

- retirement; positive active ageing or loss of social networks and meaningful activities;
- discrimination;
- quality/availability of relationships;
- deterioration in physical capability and physical health;
- changing environments; moving home;
- lack of money;
- sense of loss; of social networks, 'significant others', physical capability, or perceived belonging;
- sense of loss more chronic; loss of 'significant others', sense of purpose and loss of independence;
- loneliness and social isolation;
- grandparenting;
- caring for someone with dementia or someone who is becoming increasingly frail;
- cognitive decline;
- facing end of life; dealing with dying and death.

The list above provides some issues that may affect older people's mental health and well-being. These factors do not carry equal risk or weighting, nor are they necessarily negative (e.g. grandparenting can be both positive and negative). However, the list illustrates that mental health and well-being is influenced by a range of factors at different times in our lives.

Determinants of mental health in later life

It is now widely accepted that the determinants of health fall into four main categories: socio-economic factors, environment, health behaviours, and biological and personal factors (EUPHIX, 2009). The World Health Organization's (WHO) Active Ageing framework (2002),which is based on the determinants of health, can be adapted to help us understand the factors and processes involved in maintaining older people's mental health and well-being. The framework suggests four interdependent levels: micro-, meso-, macro and global (see Figure 16.1). The Active Ageing framework does not differentiate between the levels, nor does it include a global level. Instead, it assumes equal value to the determinants because it is currently not possible to attribute direct causation to any one determinant (WHO, 2002), and in addition suggests that culture and gender are cross-cutting determinants, which influence all other determinants of active ageing.

The first thing to note is that most of the determinants in the framework are factors that traditionally would not have been dealt with by the health services. However, nurses have a key role in assessing older people and need to draw on all of these factors to understand the well-being of individuals and explore the ways in which they can support them. The figure also suggests that the determinants of mental health are placed on a continuum of levels of control, which

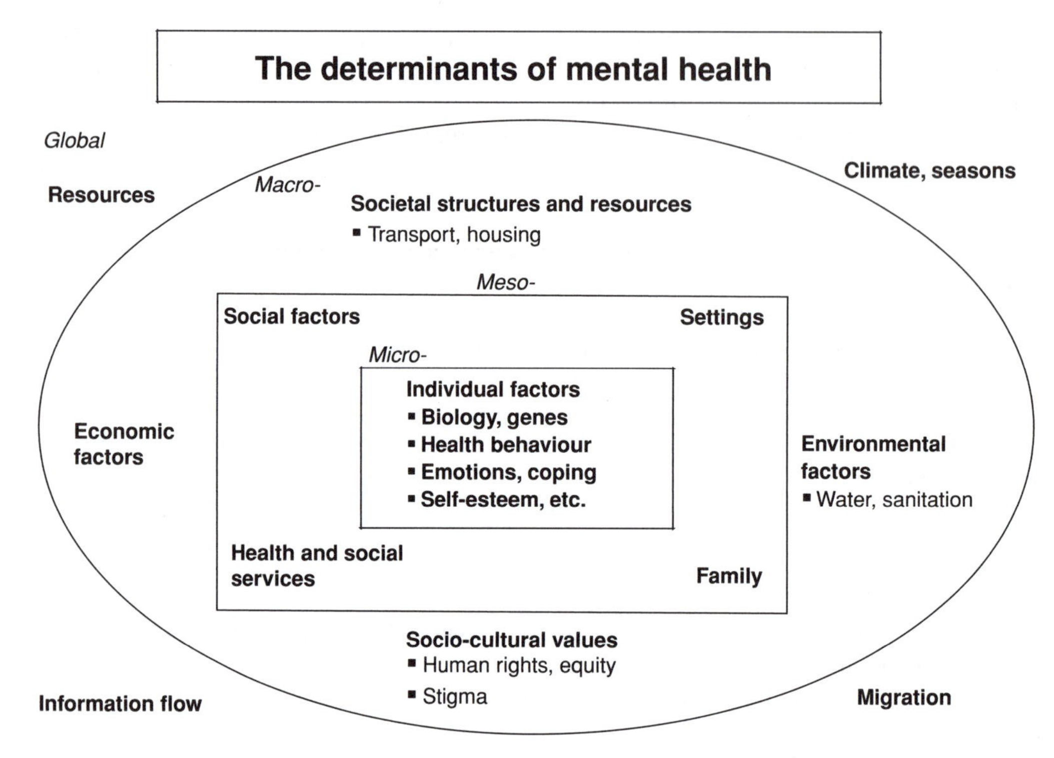

Figure 16.1: The determinants of mental health
Source: Adapted from World Health Organization (WHO), *Active Ageing* (2002)

we return to later in the chapter. Before discussing the main determinants of mental health and well-being in relation to older people, there follows a brief comment on culture and gender.

Culture

Cultural values and norms determine how a society views older people and how mental health and mental illness are conceptualized. Culture influences how we respond to the world around us, how mental illness symptoms are manifested, and the level of stigma attached to mental illness (Abrahamson et al., 2002). Importantly, as Windle (2009) points out, we need to bear in mind that most concepts of mental health reflect theoretical developments in Western cultures, which are based on individual and personal qualities. In many other countries, mental health reflects a collectivist perspective, drawing on religions such as Buddhism or Taoism (Windle, 2009).

Gender

Although it is well known that women are recorded more frequently than men with mental health problems, particularly depression, the association between gender, mental health and ageing can easily be oversimplified. A study of 14 European countries reported an excess of depression among older women in 13 of the 14 countries (Evans et al., 2003). However, a survey of ethnic minority psychiatric illness rates found a considerable variation in prevalence among women across ethnic groups (Sproston and Nazroo, 2002). In many societies, women have lower social status than men and consequently less access to services, education, food and employment. Women's traditional role in the family can be a factor in women experiencing increased poverty and deprivation in old age and as a consequence poorer mental health. Women also tend to live longer and are more likely than men to live alone in later life. This may lead to isolation linked to inadequate pension, lack of affordable and accessible transport, loss of property and status and real or perceived threats of violence in the external environment. For an older person the loss of what is seen as traditional gender roles, whether male or female, with associated loss of status, respect and independence is likely to have an impact on their mental health.

Scenario 16.1

Fred and Mary are in their early 60s and both physically well. They have three children who have settled nearby with their own young families. Fred is preparing to retire from his job. The practice nurse met Mary after she visited the GP with complaints of poor sleeping and weight gain. The nurse assessed Mary and established that Mary was feeling quite lonely. She rarely saw her children and grandchildren, stating that they were too busy with their own lives to be bothered having her around. Mary was also worried about Fred and what he would do when he retired.

With the nurse's support, Mary talked with Fred about his retirement. They both decided that they wanted to do something together and got an allotment where they could grow vegetables. This became a focus point for the whole family and in time the grandchildren loved to come there to spend time with Mary. Mary's poor sleeping and weight gain had resolved itself within months.

- *Think of an older person you are supporting at the moment – what could you suggest they might do to improve their overall level of well-being?*

Micro-level individual determinants

The process of ageing is determined by many factors; biology, genetics and how well the individual adapts to changing circumstances. Physical performance will gradually change as people get older and the decline may impact on older people's mental health, although the association is not clear. Studies suggest however, that *self-reported health* is associated with depression in later life (Herman et al., 2001; Alpass and Neville, 2003). Ageist attitudes in society and loss of control over the personal environment are thought to have detrimental effects on older people's cognitive functioning (Coleman, 1996; Bengtson et al., 1997). In addition, negative attitudes towards age can be compounded by discrimination on the grounds of race, disability, sexual identity, gender or religion (Social Exclusion Unit, 2006). But, ageism is the most common form of discrimination. One of the consequences of ageism can be a sense of not being in control and social isolation, which in turn are associated with loneliness and mental health problems.

Coping

One of the most important recent areas of study and intervention regarding older people's mental health is how older people adapt to and cope with 'old age'. One of the myths about old age is the assumption that ageing is a long negative experience of having to cope with ill health, loss and loneliness. However, we know that many older people despite experiencing significant life events such as bereavement, impairment and chronic ill health, are in fact able to adjust to and cope with the negative effects of these life changes. The *Berlin Aging Study* found that the 'younger old' (aged 70–84 years) who tended to be cognitively fit, extraverted, not lonely, with high social embeddedness for most part demonstrated higher subjective well-being. However, some of the 'oldest old' (aged 85–103 years), many of whom were cognitively impaired, with high external control, high social loneliness, and high levels of anxiety and fearfulness also expressed moderate levels of well-being (Smith and Baltes, 1997).

Coping skills could be explained by a number of psychological theories or models, including salutogenesis. According to the salutogenic theory of health, there is a range of factors that play a role in helping the people cope and survive. These factors have been called generalized resistive resources (Antonovsky, 1987). These are the properties of a person, (or a collective) which facilitate successful coping with the inherent stressors of human existence. The generalized resistive resources foster repeated life experiences that help someone to see the world as *making sense* cognitively, instrumentally or emotionally, and contribute to or create a sense of coherence. Antonovsky defined sense of coherence as:

> “a global orientation that expresses the extent to which one has a pervasive, enduring though dynamic, feeling of confidence that one's internal and external environments are predictable and that there is a high probability that things will work out as well as can reasonably be expected.
>
> (1987: xiii)”

Community-living older people often describe a range of different coping strategies to deal with changes in life. The strategies they use can provide useful clues as to where interventions are needed.

Another important personal determinant is the desirability to retain control over life events (Francis and Allgar, 2005). For older people having a sense of control is linked to feeling valued and having a purpose in life. Several studies of older people moving into residential care have shown that the perception of control and self-esteem are critical components in adjusting to institutional living (Antonelli et al., 2000; Shyam and Yadav, 2002).

Key point

Having a sense of control is linked to feeling valued and having a purpose in life. For older people moving into residential care, the perception of control and self-esteem are critical components in adjusting to institutional living.

Falls

Having a fall is seen by many older people as a threat to independence. Older people who have experienced a falls-related injury are more at risk of depression if improvement in physical function slows down (Scaf-Klomp et al., 2003). In an Australian study older women declared that they 'would rather be dead than experience the loss of independence and quality of life that results from a bad hip fracture and subsequent admission to a nursing home' (Salkeld et al., 2000: 344).

Lifestyle factors

Lifestyle factors are also associated with mental health, although the association is probably quite complex (van Gool et al., 2003). There is a clear association between positive effects of physical activity and mental well-being and a significant association between depression and low levels of physical activity. This suggests that participation in regular physical activity promotes mental well-being. However, in activities such as gardening and walking, it is likely that it is not just the exercise component which impacts on mental health, but a range of other factors as well (Windle et al., 2007; DoH, 2010). Importantly, psychological well-being also seems to be a predictor for staying physically active in later life (Ruuskanen and Ruoppila, 1995; Satariano et al., 2000), whereas being lonely has been found to reduce physical activity among adults aged 50 and over (Hawkley et al., 2009). It is perhaps therefore not surprising that the main reasons older people give for remaining physically active are the social aspects of exercise and physical activity (Stathi et al., 2002), self-acceptance and a sense of purpose (Crone et al., 2005).

The association between nutrition and mental health is complex and not particularly well documented with regard to older people. Older people at risk of malnutrition have been found to have significantly lower levels of social support and higher depression scores than those not at risk (Johnson, 2005). Johnson suggests that there may be a two-way interaction between nutrition and depression in that older people may be at risk of poor nutrition because they are unable to acquire and eat nutritious food without social support. Therefore, the perceived quality of social support may have a direct impact on malnutrition.

Social control

As health professionals it is important to consider the possible psychological distress caused by social control of health risk behaviour in addition to individual behaviour and mental health (Rook et al., 1990). Social control in health refers to the social regulations we impose on others in our social network (direct control), or the feelings of responsibility and obligations we have towards others (indirect control), in order to promote compliance with group norms and to encourage engagement in healthy lifestyles. This could, for example, be prompting an older patient to engage in sound health practices and to avoid risky behaviours. It has been suggested that social control through its perceived regulatory action may lead to psychological distress even though it simultaneously leads to reduced risky behaviour. This hypothesis has not been borne out by recent studies. Instead, findings indicate that social control in the health domain is associated with both positive and negative responses depending on the type of social control and level of relationship satisfaction (Tucker, 2002). Positive health regulatory action is in the main associated with less psychological distress (Rook et al., 1990). There may be several reasons for this. One possibility is that social control may provoke psychological distress only when there is some form of ambiguity in the health regulatory message. Another possibility is that social control may be perceived as an indication of care and concern rather than as an intrusion.

Bereavement

Bereavement is associated with a range of physical and mental health risk factors. Although the causes are not fully understood, studies have suggested that there are some important links between depression, loss, older age and perceived health, which may be more salient for older men (Tijhuis et al., 1999; Alpass and Neville, 2003). Here, we need to distinguish between awareness of death and dying and the experience of bereavement and grief. For anyone who is particularly interested in mental health in relation to dying and death in later life there are several books available (see, for example, Dickenson et al., 2000; Hockey et al., 2001; Owen, 2005; Resnick, 2005).

We know that there are differences in the grieving process depending on if the death has been sudden and unexpected or anticipated after a long illness, or if the widow(er) was present at the time of death. Older widow(er)s can also 'rekindle' their grief after many years of acceptance if their personal circumstances deteriorate (Sidell, 1996), which is important to understand when supporting older people towards the end of their lives. One of the serious problems linked to bereavement and grief in later life is loneliness, which in turn is linked to depression. The association between widowhood and loneliness is multifaceted through the interaction of many factors such as the ones mentioned above, health, gender or having to move into a care home (Tijhuis et al., 1999; Costello and Kendrick, 2000). Lopata (1980), in a well-known study of widows, suggested that widows can be grouped into three main categories depending on the type of loneliness they express; missing the partner, missing the lifestyle, or a sense of inadequacy in relationships with other people. Clearly, if this is the case different actions would be required depending on the type of loneliness identified. This is only partially borne out by research with most intervention studies focusing on self-help, education and skills training.

Key point

Nurses need to support older people towards the end of their lives and understand that older widow(er)s can also 'rekindle' their grief after many years of acceptance if their personal circumstances deteriorate.

Meso-level social determinants

Low levels of education and literacy are associated with increased risk of physical and mental health problems in old age. Basic education in childhood combined with opportunities for lifelong learning may help increase older people's confidence, provide them with the skills to adapt to a changing world and improve their quality of life (HelpAge International, 2002; WHO, 2002).

Elder abuse

Elder abuse takes the form of physical abuse, psychological abuse, financial abuse, sexual abuse or neglect. Studies have shown that the person being subjected to the abuse is not necessarily a frail older person being cared for at home, but may be an older carer (Penhale and Kingston, 1997). Dixon et al. (2010) found that older people define different levels of trust to indicate the personal impact of the abuse. Nurses and care staff in care homes are often uncertain about what constitutes 'abuse' reflecting the complexities of detecting abuse or the circumstances leading to abuse in care institutions (Daly and Coffey, 2010).

Family, friends and loneliness

The role of family and friends in maintaining mental well-being in later life has been investigated in a large number of studies (see, for example, Bowling, 1991; Reinhardt, 1996; Phillipson et al., 1998; Seeman, 2000). The association between the different dimensions of mental well-being and social contact with family and friends is dependent on several factors, with both cultural and geographical differences in how older people perceive social contacts. Research suggests that while adult children are the main source of instrumental support, they are not necessarily the main source of emotional support, but the availability of a companion or confidante is linked to the perceived adequacy of instrumental and emotional support (Matt and Dean, 1993). In an overview of the health-promoting effects of close social interactions in older people Seeman (2000) notes that negative and/or non-supportive social interactions between close social relations are probably main sources of stress, suggesting that negative relationships may have a greater impact on affect and mental health than positive ones!

In Europe, there seems to be a north–south divide regarding older people's experiences of loneliness, with more older adults in northern Europe living alone, but a greater proportion of older people in the south feeling lonely (Jylhä and Jokela, 1990; van Tilburg et al., 1998). Jylhä and Jokela (1990) hypothesized that this was due to different value systems between the north and the south, while van Tilburg et al. (1998) suggested that the variance was mainly due to differences in individuals' social integration.

Social isolation and loneliness

Loneliness is a subjective, negative and unwelcome feeling of not having a close companion, desirable friends or social contacts. It is characterized by negative feelings such as not belonging, being left out, boredom, sadness, depression and anxiety. Loneliness and social isolation are closely associated but also distinct, with social isolation defined as an objective state that can be measured by the number of contacts and the number of interactions between individuals and their wider social network (Cattan, 2009; Victor et al., 2009). We can distinguish between three types of loneliness in terms of the duration of the experience. Transient loneliness relates to the common everyday swings of mood, unlikely to require intervention. Situational loneliness follows a change in life circumstances, such as becoming widowed or moving to an unfamiliar area. Chronic loneliness is an ongoing enduring experience of loneliness where the nature and quality of the individual's social networks affect their ability to deal with their loneliness. Research in the UK suggests that there has been an increase in the number of older people who report being lonely sometimes (Victor et al., 2009) but not in the number of those who are often lonely. However admitting to being lonely may be seen as a social failure and not being able to cope and therefore the stigma of loneliness may lead to underreporting of loneliness.

In later life social networks change and reduce in size. With increasing numbers of older people living alone, older women are particularly vulnerable to social isolation as a result of living longer, increasing population mobility and the likelihood of living in poverty (see for example research by Vanessa Burholt, Thomas Scharf and Clare Wenger). This may be compounded by widowhood, the loss of family members and friends, which in turn is associated with an increased risk of loneliness (Victor et al., 2005) and depression. Interviews with older people suggest that deteriorating general health, loss of mobility and fear of being burgled or mugged could lead to social isolation (Cattan, 2010; Cattan et al., 2003). There are several know risk factors (direct and indirect) that relate to social isolation and loneliness. These include: demographic characteristics such as very old age, gender, culture and living alone; people's perceptions of personal control, coping and feelings of dependency; the experience of major life events, such as retirement, loss of friends, relatives and companions, moving home and health problems; personal resources, such as mental health (particularly depression), disability and decreased mobility.

Preventing and reducing isolation

The prevention and reduction of social isolation and loneliness have received increasing attention because of the profound impact on older people's mental health and quality of life and life satisfaction. Research evidence is still limited to a few types of interventions (mainly group activities). Increasingly, however, policy-makers are showing interest in 'good practice': community-based interventions that have not (yet) been evaluated. One example is the promotion of peer support networks in the form of activities such as Dementia Cafes in the National Dementia Strategy (DoH, 2009).

Factors in the physical environment

It almost goes without saying that a safe and accessible environment is conducive to mental well-being. Older people mention transport, housing and the quality of the external environment as particular barriers to social participation (Cattan et al., 2003) and contributing to the loss of independence. In other words, costly or inaccessible transport, inadequate or unsafe housing, and unsafe external environments may lead to social isolation, increased mobility problems and associated mental health problems such as depression. Moving into supported housing of some type can have both a positive and negative impact on an older person's mental health. Positive effects can include feeling safe and increased social contact, while negative effects might be sense of loss of independence and control and depression (Cattan et al., 2010a).

Access to transport is frequently linked to the opportunity to stay active. Access to reliable public transport is linked to elevated quality of life, and older people report that improvements in public transport would improve their quality of life, mental and emotional well-being and social engagement (Gilhooly et al., 2005; Marsden et al., 2010). With regard to older drivers, several studies have found that driving cessation is linked to an increased risk of depression (Fonda et al., 2001; Siren et al., 2004).

Key point

Improvements in public transport would improve the quality of life of older people, their mental and emotional well-being and social engagement.

Environmental disasters

In some parts of the UK floods occur regularly, with both a short- and long-term mental health impact on older people. HelpAge International points out that many of the implications of natural disasters are similar to all 'vulnerable' groups, but that some, such as staying behind, are specific to older people (HelpAge International, 2009). They suggest that by supporting older people to develop resilience to such impacts, communities will also be supported to adapt to rapid environmental changes. The experience of loss is a major contributor to mental health problems in disaster situations. Loss can refer to family, close neighbours and friends, physical possessions, including the home and 'memories', such as family photographs and other irreplaceable 'things'. Not all older people are vulnerable and some surveys show that older people who have experienced natural disasters want their past experiences and their independence to take decisions to be recognized (HelpAge International, 2005; Duggan et al., 2010). Rather than being treated as 'in need' older people are frequently able to support their communities and act as resources in disaster situations.

Economic determinants

Retirement and mental health

It is often assumed that retirement has an inevitable adverse effect on health and in particular on mental well-being. Not having enough income or old age pension may of course affect older people's mental health. However, Moffatt (2009) suggests that it is the circumstances which lead to retirement and in which retirement is experienced that influence mental health. The type of pension system, societal norms regarding retirement, whether retirement is entered into voluntarily, the individual's physical and mental health, financial circumstances, family and friends, and the interaction with social class, gender, ethnicity and place all play a part. Multiple, overlapping problems of low income, poor housing and limiting illness are particularly common among the very old, older women living alone and those living in rural areas (Social Exclusion Unit, 2006).

Increasingly, retirement is not determined by old age, but is viewed as a period of transition, rather than as entry into old age. As Johnson (2004: 40–41) puts it:

> “Indeed, when the population of seventy-year-olds includes both the physically fit and active and the bedridden, the very wealthy and the abjectly poor, the socially connected and the socially excluded, the family figurehead and the isolated singleton, then it is no longer evident that age should be regarded as a meaningful social or economic category.”

According to Moffatt (2009: 71): 'What really appears to matter to individuals is having control over when and how to retire. The evidence from British studies is that having a strong financial position and high occupational status leads to a high degree of choice and control over the transition to retirement and that those with low to average earnings have restricted options' (see for example: Arthur, 2002; Mein et al., 2003).

Health and social services

Older people's mental well-being is also dependent on appropriate, accessible and affordable social and health services being available (see, for example, WHO, 2002; European Union, 2010), which is covered by other chapters. For these services to be meaningful, it is important that older people are not treated as one homogeneous group, but that we recognize the diversity among older people and ensure that health and social services meet the individual mental health needs of these diverse groups. Groups to consider include: Black and minority ethnic older people; older lesbians, gay men and bisexual men and women; older prisoners; older homeless people; and grandparents. Because of the 'invisibility' of these groups very little research has been conducted about their specific mental health or mental health promotion needs, although it has been suggested that it is because they are invisible that their mental health needs are not recognized or addressed, rather than because of what they are. In other words, it is the combination of being older and, for example, homeless or a care that shapes their vulnerability and resilience in relation to mental health.

The special issue of care givers/informal carers

Worldwide older people are frequently the primary informal carers of family members, friends or neighbours. Over 15 per cent of older people aged 65 and over provide care, which means that a quarter of all carers in England are over 65 years old (GfK Social Research, 2010). Even among people aged 85 and over 5 per cent provide some form of care in the home. Women tend to be the main carers but among people aged 65 and over, men are more likely to provide care for a family member. Added to this, a substantial number of these carers are themselves permanently sick or disabled (Soule et al., 2005), with 14 per cent of older carers suffering from some form of mental health problems (Singleton et al., 2002). Mickus and Owen (2009) suggest that supporting older carers' coping strategies in stressful situations may help them to retain control and manage the caring situation These figures do not take into account the substantial contribution grandparents make. Studies have found that around 25 per cent of grandparents look after their grandchildren on a regular basis (Soule et al., 2005), which can be either a positive, uplifting experience or a negative demanding role depending on the circumstances (Forte, 2009).

Key point

Around 25 per cent of grandparents look after their grandchildren on a regular basis.

Older people's perceptions of mental health and mental ill health

Older people's descriptions of their perceptions of mental health may help us to develop individually appropriate and acceptable interventions to support their mental well-being. In a Scottish survey most older people found it quite difficult to define 'mental well-being' as they felt that it encapsulated everything that contributed to feeling mentally well, such as family and friends, leading active lives, good health, maintaining independence, having a positive attitude to old age, financial security and a continued role in retirement (Bostock and Millar, 2003). It demonstrates how broad and complex the notion of mental health is for most people. However, it may also be that older people are unaccustomed (and reluctant) to discuss issues around their personal mental health and avoid the subject by describing it in very general terms.

Inquiry into mental health and well-being in later life

A survey conducted in the UK as part of the 'Inquiry into Mental Health and Well-being in Later Life' showed that almost half the respondents took the phrase 'mental health and well-being' to be negative and more about mental ill health. Dementia was cited frequently, as was 'being fearful', 'being thankful for their own good mental health and well-being' and 'feeling sorry for people suffering mental ill health' (Third Sector First, 2005: 14). However, phrases that were also used included 'healthy mind', 'healthy body' and 'happiness'. Happiness was described as contentment, having a sense of self-esteem, having a balanced outlook and being positive and cheerful. Some of the interviewees considered mental health to be able to cope with life and to be in control. Although the survey did not find any significant gender differences, there were significant differences between age groups regarding mentioning 'happiness'. Far more people aged 60–69 years cited happiness than those aged 80–89 years, and no one over the age of 90 said that mental health was about feeling happy.

When older people are asked about what worries them and upsets their mental well-being, the main issues they list are: their own physical health, losing capability and independence, social isolation from family and friends, finances and retirement, not being respected as individuals, not being able to maintain physical or mental activity, and world affairs (Bostock and Millar, 2003; Third Sector First, 2005). The main worry for the 'young old' (50–59 age group) is finance, while those aged 90 and over are mostly concerned about the possibility of having to go into a care home, and consequently losing their independence. Poor physical health, not being able to do the things they used to do and not being able to get out and about were said to make things worse. Not being able to cope, being alone and having no one to share their problems with were frequently mentioned as contributing to poor mental health. The four most commonly given answers to what makes them feel good and motivated focused on being with others and getting out of the house for reasons such as 'interests', 'friends', 'outings' and 'family'. These findings are similar to issues raised by older people about combating social isolation and loneliness; the ability to stay physically and mentally active, to maintain a role in life, social activities with family and friends and the fear of losing their independence (Cattan, 2002).

Environmental resources	*Attitudes*	*Individual characteristics*
Community support	To keep busy and involved	Good health
Family support	Positive outlook	Education
Companionship	Independence	Gender
Happy family relationships	Control over one's life	Cultural background
Stress	To keep going	Resilience
Worries and fear	Use of humour	Self-esteem
Bullying and peer pressure	Lifestyle choices	Self-efficacy

Figure 16.2: Factors suggested by older people regarding the promotion and maintenance of mental well-being in later life

Source: Reproduced with permission from Giuntoli and Cattan, 2010

What helps older people to retain their mental well-being

In a series of focus groups older people suggested that [environmental] resources, attitudes and personality were the three main, interacting factors that promoted and maintained mental well-being in later life (see Figure 16.2) (Giuntoli and Cattan, 2010).

Group-based social support interventions for specific groups of older people, such as those with mental health problems, widows, women living alone and carers have been found to reduce distress, stress, social isolation and loneliness, and increase self-esteem, morale and social activity (Tilford et al., 1997; Cattan et al., 2005). Most such interventions include some form of structured activity, such as a negotiated and agreed peer and professionally led educational programme, self-help support, directed group discussion or supported social activation. Participant planned and led activities also seem to improve effectiveness. The use of the Internet to reduce social isolation has also been investigated. Despite the interventions not leading to significant reductions in perceived social isolation or loneliness, there was an indication that education groups set up in congregate housing (White et al., 2002) and an Internet forum for carers (Brennan et al., 1995) were used for social contact and social support.

Older people who are housebound with mobility or sensory problems are at serious risk of social isolation, loneliness and depression (Cattan et al., 2010b). Many housebound older people respond favourably to befriending services (face-to-face visiting or telephone calls), stating that 'the volunteer gives them a reason to get up', 'is someone to share interests and worries with', 'offers both practical help and companionship', 'is a true friend', and 'alleviates the fear of being alone should "something" happen' (Dean and Goodlad, 1998; Cattan et al., 2010b). Older people also emphasize the importance of reciprocity, which may be more likely if there is a shared culture and common interests (Cattan et al., 2003).

The Internet

The Internet is increasingly being used as a tool to improve older people's mental well-being and reduce social isolation and loneliness. Although research is still rather patchy, studies have demonstrated that email and the Internet are used for different purposes: email is mostly used for social contact to reduce loneliness, whereas the Internet is used for practical purposes such as information or simply to pass the time. It would also seem that mobile technology such as cell phones or videoconferencing and social networking sites might help to decrease feelings of loneliness. However, little is currently known about *how* different groups utilize cell phones or websites for this purpose.

Exercise and music

The value of exercise and music to improve mental well-being is increasingly being recognized. Music is used to express emotions, communicate feelings and ultimately to improve and maintain a sense of well-being (Hays and Minichiello, 2005). Hays and Minichiello (2005) argue that music can provide a cultural and normative 'bridge' between individuals, and can be used to form contacts and social links with others, which can be observed in a number of therapeutic interventions with older people with dementia.

Scenario 16.2

Rani has dementia and finds it increasingly hard to communicate verbally with staff and other residents in her residential home. This is compounded by her difficulty using English as it is not her first language. Her isolation as a result of poor verbal communication is leading to Rani becoming increasingly distressed and agitated. The residential home started weekly dance sessions which the staff find Rani loves. It is at these times that she is most animated and looks most happy. With the support of staff, Rani is able to stand and be supported to move with the music, or while sitting Rani claps in time with the music and watches others dance. This encourages the staff to think carefully about the sounds in Rani's environment and they notice that she is much more relaxed with music playing than if people are talking on the TV, so they now limit the amount of time that the TV is left on in the room.

- *Are there any changes that you could make in your work environment that might better support older people to feel relaxed and able to interact with others more?*

Several evaluation studies show the benefits of exercise for older people's mental health. In the UK, low-intensity exercise to music has been shown to result in significant improvements in happiness and well-being, enjoyment and other social and psychological benefits (Paulson, 2005). Tai chi and moderate intensity exercise in particular seem to be beneficial for older people's mental well-being, while the combination of health education and exercise has been shown to reduce loneliness in later life (Hopman-Rock and Westhoff, 2002). It may not necessarily be just exercise *per se* that improves mental health but also the social activity effects of group participation (Helbostad et al., 2004). The positive impact of walking and gardening on mental well-being, for example, is thought to be associated with a range of additional factors such as the social contact element (see, for example, Milligan et al., 2005).

Reminiscence

Reminiscence has become an almost natural part of activities in care work to enable older people to recall past events and life experiences. It is used for a variety of reasons; for example, to find meaning and purpose in life, to reduce boredom, and to teach and inform. It has been used therapeutically to deal with depression and traumatic memories with residents in sheltered housing to improve well-being, and with demented older people. Interestingly, it would seem that some ethnic groups utilize reminiscence more than others, although as Coleman and O'Hanlon (2004) point out, it is not clear whether this is because some cultures have a stronger oral tradition or because these groups have a greater need to promote self-understanding, preserve identity and educate ensuing generations. Reminiscence has been criticized at times for focusing too much on upsetting memories and loss, without supporting the individual to reflect on the positives of 'here and now'.

Volunteering

Volunteering is seen by many as an effective way of maintaining mental well-being (Seymour and Gale, 2004; Social Exclusion Unit, 2006). Volunteering undoubtedly has beneficial effects in terms of mental health, mainly because of the social aspects of the activity and because it can give a sense of worth. It may also be that the reciprocity of volunteering could add to a sense of well-being in that the mutual benefits of providing and receiving support are effective in giving a sense of social support. Most of our research evidence comes from the USA where perspectives on volunteering are quite different from many European countries, including the UK (Wheeler et al., 1998; van Willigen, 2000 in Seymour and Gale 2004: 56). It would be wrong to suggest that volunteering is not beneficial for older people's mental well-being, but we cannot assume that older people's attitudes to and experiences of volunteering are identical in all cultures. There are indications, at least in the UK, that the number of older people volunteering is actually dropping.

Adult learning

Although adult learning (lifelong learning) and the acquisition of new skills are frequently put forward as an effective means of maintaining older people's mental well-being and alertness, and even in preventing Alzheimer's Disease the 'jury is still out' because of the lack of evidence. Reported improvements in self-esteem, social and self-confidence and a sense of purpose are probably dependent on several other factors, which are not well understood. We should not forget as Hammond (2004) points out that the experience of education can be extremely negative for some!

Better Government for Older People programme

The *Better Government for Older People (BGOP)* programme was established in 1998 to address ageism and improve public services for older people by better meeting their needs, listening to their views and encouraging and recognizing their contributions (Hayden and Boaz, 2000). The main focus was on: housing and the home;

neighbourhoods; social activities, fun, social networks, learning and leisure; getting out and about; income; information; health and healthy living; employment; lifelong learning; mental health services; black and minority ethnic older people; age diversity (Better Government for Older People, 2005). Although not initially set up specifically to improve and maintain older people's mental health, the programme seems to have affected participants' mental well-being simply through its ethos of participation and policy influence and the types of activities that have evolved as a result.

Summary of effectiveness of mental health promotion interventions with older people

- There is good evidence that group-based social support activities are effective in reducing social distress, social isolation and loneliness.
- There is increasing evidence that exercise promotes self-esteem, happiness and well-being, and reduces depression.
- There is conflicting evidence regarding the effectiveness of befriending and home visiting schemes for older people. Qualitative research suggests that they are acceptable and helpful.
- Despite a significant body of research there is little evidence that respite care, psychosocial interventions, group education and support impact significantly on depression, stress or coping skills in older carers.
- There is some evidence (based on mainly American research) to suggest that volunteering has a positive effect on older people's mental health.
- To date there is little research and consequently evidence to demonstrate the effectiveness of reminiscence, computer technology and lifelong learning in improving or maintaining mental health in later life.

Conclusion

In this chapter we have considered the main mental health issues for older people and types of interventions that may improve and maintain mental health. Because the population is ageing there is increased interest nationally and internationally in developing appropriate services and activities to promote and maintain mental well-being among older people. As we have seen, however, older people are not a homogeneous group and therefore their needs and expectations vary across age groups, cultures, ethnic groups and gender. What unfortunately often seems to happen is that older people are discriminated against twofold; first, because they are 'aged' and second because of who or what they are as a person. By considering the wider factors that impact on older people's mental health, the research evidence, examples of 'good practice' and the theoretical framework for mental health promotion, we should be able to develop effective, appropriate projects, services and activities that older people actually want to take part in.

References

Abrahamson, T.A., Trejo, L. and Lai, D.W.L. (2002) Culture and mental health: providing appropriate services for a diverse older population, *Mental Health and Mental Illness in Later Life*, Spring: 21–27.

Alpass, F.M. and Neville, S. (2003) Loneliness, health and depression in older males, *Aging and Mental Health*, 7(3): 212–16.

Antonelli, E., Rubini, V. and Fassone, C. (2000) The self-concept in institutionalized and non-institutionalized elderly people, *Journal of Environmental Psychology*, 20(2): 151–64.

Antonovsky, A. (1987) *Unravelling the Mystery of Health*. San Franscisco, CA: Jossey-Boss.

Arthur, S. (2002) *Money, Choice and Control: The Financial Circumstances of Early Retirement*. Bristol: Policy Press.

Bengtson, V.L., Burgess, E.O. and Parrott, T.M. (1997) Theory, explanation, and a third generation of theoretical development in social gerontology, *Journals Of Gerontology Series B: Psychological Sciences and Social Sciences*, 52(2): S72–S88.

Better Government for Older People (2005) *BGOP fundamentals*. Available online at www.bgop.org.uk/index.aspx?primarycat=2&secondarycat=4; accessed 13 November 2005.

Bostock, Y. and Millar, C. (2003) *Older People's Perceptions of the Factors that Affect Mental Well-being in Later Life*. Edinburgh: NHS Health Scotland.

Bowling, A. (1991) Social support and social networks: their relationship to the successful and unsuccessful survival of elderly people in the community. An analysis of concepts and a review of the evidence, *Family Practice*, 8(1): 68–83.

Brennan, P.F., Moore, S.M. and Smyth, K.A. (1995) The effects of a special computer network on caregivers of persons with Alzheimer's Disease, *Nursing Research*, 44(3): 166–72.

Cattan, M. (2002) *Supporting Older People to Overcome Social Isolation and Loneliness*. London: Help the Aged.

Cattan, M. (2009) Loneliness–interventions, in H. Reis and S. Sprecher (eds) *Encyclopedia of Human Relationships*. New York: Sage Publications.

Cattan, M. (2010) *Preventing Social Isolation and Loneliness among Older People*. Saarbrucken: Lambert Academic Publishing.

Cattan, M., Hughes, S., Giuntoli, G., Kime, N. and Fylan, F. (2010a) *The Needs of Frail Older People with Sight Loss*. London: Thomas Pocklington Trust.

Cattan, M., Kime, N. and Bagnall, A-M. (2010b) *Low-level Support for Socially Isolated Older People: An Evaluation of Telephone Befriending*. London: Help the Aged.

Cattan, M., Newell, C., Bond, J. and White, M. (2003) Alleviating social isolation and loneliness among older people, *International Journal of Mental Health Promotion*, 5(3): 20–30.

Cattan, M. and Tilford, S. (eds) (2006) *Mental Health Promotion: A Lifespan Approach*. Maidenhead: Open University Press.

Cattan, M., White, M., Bond, J. and Learmonth, A. (2005) Preventing social isolation and loneliness among older people: a systematic review of health promotion interventions, *Ageing and Society*, 25(1): 41–67.

Coleman, P. (1996) Psychological ageing, in J. Bond, P. Coleman and S. Peace (eds) *Ageing in Society: An Introduction to Social Gerontology* (pp. 68–96). London: Sage Publications.

Coleman, P.G. and O'Hanlon, A. (2004) *Ageing and Development*. London: Arnold.

Commission of the European Communities (2005) *Improving the Mental Health of the Population: Towards a Strategy on Mental Health for the European Union*. Brussels: European Union (EU).

Costello, J. and Kendrick, K. (2000) Grief and older people: the making or breaking of emotional bonds following partner loss in later life, *Journal of Advanced Nursing*, 32(6): 1374–82.

Crone, D., Smith, A. and Gough, B. (2005) 'I feel totally at one, totally alive and totally happy': a psycho-social explanation of the physical activity and mental health relationship, *Health Education Research*, 20(5): 600–11.

Daly, J. and Coffey, A. (2010) Staff perceptions of elder abuse, *Nursing Older People*, 22(4): 33–37.

Dean, J. and Goodlad, R. (1998) *Supporting Community Participation? The Role and Impact of Befriending*. Brighton: Rowntree Foundation.

Department of Health (DoH) (2009) *National Dementia Strategy*. London: Her Majesty's Stationery Office (HMSO).

Department of Health (DoH) (2010) *New Horizons. Confident Communities, Brighter Futures: A Framework for Developing Well-being*. London: DoH.

Dickenson, D., Johnson, M. and Samson Katz, J. (eds) (2000) *Death, Dying and Bereavement*. London: Sage Publications.

Dixon, J., Manthorpe, J., Biggs, S. et al. (2010) Defining elder mistreatment: reflections on the United Kingdom Study of abuse and neglect of older people, *Ageing & Society*, 30(4): 403–20.

Duggan, S., Deeny, P., Spelman, R. and Vitale C.T. (2010) Perceptions of older people on disaster response and preparedness, *International Journal of Older People Nursing*, 5: 71–76.

EUPHIX (2009) *Determinants of Health*. Available online at www.euphix.org/object_class/euph_determinants_of_health.html; accessed 18 July 2010.

European Union (EU) (2010) *Mental Health and Well-being in Older People: Making it Happen*. Madrid: EC/Spanish Ministry of Health and Social Affairs.

Evans, O., Singleton, N., Meltzer, H., Stewart, R. and Prince, M. (2003) *The Mental Health of Older People*. London: Office for National Statistics.

Fonda, S.J., Wallace, R.B. and Herzog, A.R. (2001) Changes in driving patterns and worsening depressive symptoms among older adults, *Journals of Gerontology: Social Sciences Series B*: 56B(6): S343–S51.

Forte, D. (2009) Relationships, in M. Cattan (ed.) *Mental Health and Well-being in Later Life*. Maidenhead: Open University Press.

Francis, J. and Allgar, V. (2005) *Things to Do, Places to Go: Promoting Mental Health and Well-being in Later Life. The Findings from a Call for Evidence of How to Promote Mental Health and Well-being in Later Life*. Leeds: Third Sector First, University of Leeds.

GfK Social Research (2010) *Survey of Carers in Households in England 2009/10*. London: NHS, The Information Centre.

Gilhooly, M., Hamilton, H., O'Neill, M. et al. (2005) Transport and ageing: extending quality of life via public and private transport, *ESRC Society Today*. Available online at www.esrcsocietytoday.ac.uk/ESRCInfoCentre/Plain_English_Summaries/envionment/mobility/index150.aspx; accessed 7 November 2005.

Giuntoli, G. and Cattan, M. (2010) *Defining Mental Well-being: Factors Affecting its Development in Later Life*. Leeds: Leeds Metropolitan University internal report.

Hammond, C. (2004) Impacts of lifelong learning upon emotional resilience, psychological and mental health: fieldwork evidence, *Oxford Review of Education*, 30(4): 551–68.

Hawkley, L.C., Thisted, R.A. and Cacioppo, J.T. (2009) Loneliness predicts reduced physical activity: cross-sectional and longitudinal analyses, *Health Psychology*, 28(3): 354–63.

Hayden, C. and Boaz, A. (2000) *Making a Difference Better Government for Older People Evaluation Report*. Available online at www.bettergovernmentforolderpeople.gov.uk/reference; accessed 2002.

Hays, T. and Minichiello, V. (2005) The contribution of music to quality of life in older people: an Australian qualitative study, *Ageing and Society*, 25: 261–78.

Helbostad, J.L., Sletvold, O. and Moe-Nilssen, R. (2004) Home training with and without additional group training in physically frail older people living at home: effect on health-related quality of life and ambulation, *Clinical Rehabilitation*, 18: 498–508.

HelpAge International (2002) *State of the World's Older People 2002*. London: HelpAge International.

HelpAge International (2005) *The Impact of the Indian Ocean Tsunami on Older People*. London: HelpAge International.

HelpAge International (2009) *Witness to Climate Change: Learning from Older People's Experience*. London: HelpAge International.

Herman, D.R., Solomons, N.W., Mendoza, I. and Qureshi, A.K. (2001) Self-rated health and its relationship to functional status and well-being in a group of elderly Guatemalan subjects, *Asia Pacific Journal of Clinical Nutrition*, 10(3): 176–82.

Hockey, J., Katz, J. and Small, N. (eds) (2001) *Grief, Mourning and Death Ritual*. Maidenhead: Open University Press.

Hopman-Rock, M. and Westhoff, M.H. (2002) Development and evaluation of 'aging well and healthily': a health education and exercise program for community living older adults, *Journal of Aging and Physical Activity*, 10: 363–80.

Johnson, C.S.J. (2005) Psychosocial correlates of nutritional risk in older adults, *Canadian Journal of Dietetic Practice and Research*, 66: 95–97.

Johnson, P. (2004) Long-term historical changes in the status of elders: the United Kingdom as an exemplar of advanced industrial economies, in P. Lloyd-Sherlock (ed.) *Living Longer: Ageing, Development and Social Protection*. London: Zed Books.

Jylhä, M. and Jokela, J. (1990) Individual experiences as cultural: a cross-cultural study on loneliness among the elderly, *Ageing and Society*, 10: 295–315.

Lopata, H.Z. (1980) Loneliness: forms and components, in R.S. Weiss (ed.) *The Experience of Emotional and Social Isolation*. Cambridge: MIT Press.

Marsden, G., Cattan, M., Jopson, A. and Woodward, C. (2010) Do transport planning tools reflect the needs of the older traveller? *Quality in Ageing and Older Adults*, 11(1): 16–24.

Matt, G.E. and Dean, A. (1993) Social support from friends and psychological distress among elderly persons: moderator effects of age, *Journal of Health and Social Behavior*, 34(3): 187–200.

Mein, G., Martikainen, P., Hemingway, H., Stansfield, S. and Marmot, M. (2003) Is retirement good or bad for mental and physical health functioning? Whitehall II longitudinal study of civil servants, *Journal of Epidemiology and Community Health*, 57: 46–49.

Mickus, M. and Owen, T. (2009) Coping, choice and control: pathways to positive psychological functioning and independence in later life, in M. Cattan (ed.) *Mental Health and Well-being in Later Life*. Maidenhead: Open University Press.

Milligan, C., Bingley, A. and Gatrell, A. (2005) *Cultivating Health: A Study of Health and Mental Well-being Amongst Older People in Northern England*. Lancaster: Lancaster University.

Moffatt, S. (2009) Work, retirment and money, in M. Cattan (ed.) *Mental Health and Well-being in Later Life* (pp. 64–83). Maidenhead: Open University Press.

Owen, T. (ed.) (2005) *Dying in Older Age, Reflections and Experiences from an Older Person's Perspective*. London: Help the Aged.

Paulson, S. (2005) The social benefits of belonging to a 'dance exercise' group for older people, *Generations Review*, 15(4): 37–41.

Penhale, B. and Kingston, P. (1997) Elder abuse, mental health and later life: steps towards an understanding, *Aging and Mental Health*, 1(4): 296–304.

Phillipson, C., Bernard, M., Phillips, J. and Ogg, J. (1998) The family and community life of older people: household composition and social networks in three urban areas, *Ageing and Society*, 18: 259–89.

Reinhardt, J.P. (1996) The importance of friendship and family support in adaptation to chronic vision impairment, *Journals of Gerontology Series B: Psychological Sciences and Social Sciences*, 51(5): 268–78.

Resnick, D.B. (2005) *Dying Declarations: Notes from a Hospice Volunteer*. Abingdon: Routledge.

Rook, K.S., Thuras, P.D. and Lewis, M.A. (1990) Social control, health risk taking, and psychological distress among the elderly, *Psychology and Aging*, 5(3): 327–34.

Ruuskanen, J.M. and Ruoppila, I. (1995) Physical activity and psychological well being among people aged 65 to 84 years, *Age and Ageing*, 24(4): 292–96.

Salkeld, G., Cameron, I.D., Cumming, R.G. et al. (2000) Quality of life related to fear of falling and hip fracture in older women: a time trade off study, *British Medical Journal*, 320: 341–46.

Satariano, W.A., Haight, T.J. and Tager, I.B. (2000) Reasons given by older people for limitation or avoidance of leisure time physical activity, *Journal of the American Geriatrics Society*, 48: 505–12.

Scaf-Klomp, W., Sanderman, R., Ormel, J. and Kempen, G.I.J.H. (2003) Depression in older people after fall-related injuries: a prospective study, *Age and Ageing*, 32: 88–94.

Seeman, T.E. (2000) Health promoting effects of friends and family on health outcomes in older adults, *American Journal of Health Promotion*, 14(6): 362–70.

Seymour, L. and Gale, E. (2004) *Literature and Policy Review for the Joint Inquiry into Mental Health and Well-being in Later Life*. London: Mentality.

Shyam, R. and Yadav, S. (2002) A study of depression, self-esteem and social support amongst institutionalized and non-institutionalized aged, *Journal of Personality & Clinical Studies*, 18(1–2): 79–86.

Sidell, M. (1996) Death, dying and bereavement, in J. Bond, P. Coleman and S. Peace (eds) *Ageing in Society: An Introduction to Social Gerontology*. London: Sage Publications.

Singleton, N., Aye Maung, N., Cowie, A., Sparks, J., Bumpstead, R. and Meltzer, H. (2002) *Mental Health of Carers*. London: Office for National Statistics.

Siren, A., Hakamies-Blomqvist, L. and Lindeman, M. (2004) Driving cessation and health in older women, *Journal of Applied Gerontology*, 23(1): 58–69.

Smith, J. and Baltes, P.B. (1997) Profiles of psychological functioning in the old and oldest old, *Psychology and Aging*, 12(3): 458–72.

Social Exclusion Unit (2006) *A Sure Start to Later Life: Ending Inequalities for Older People*. London: Office of the Deputy Prime Minister.

Soule, A., Babb, P., Evandrou, M. et al. (2005) *Focus on Older People*. London: National Statistics.

Sproston, K. and Nazroo, J. (eds) (2002) *Ethnic Minority Psychiatric Illness Rates in the Community (EMPIRIC)*. London: TSO.

Stathi, A., Fox, K. and McKenna, J. (2002) Physical activity and dimensions of subjective well-being in older adults, *Journal of Aging and Physical Activity*, 10(1): 76–92.

Third Sector First (2005) *'Thing to Do, Places to Go': Promoting Mental Health and Well-being in Later Life*. Leeds: Third Sector First.

Tijhuis, M.A.R., de Jong-Gierveld, J., Feskens, E.J.M. and Kromhout, D. (1999) Changes in and factors related to loneliness in older men: the Zutphen elderly study, *Age and Ageing*, 28: 491–95.

Tilford, S., Delaney, F. and Vogels, M. (1997) *Effectiveness of Mental Health Promotion Interventions: A Review*. London: Health Education Authority.

Tucker, J.S. (2002) Health-related social control within older adults' relationships, *Journals of Gerontology Series B: Psychological Sciences & Social Sciences*, 57B(5): P387–P95.

van Gool, C.H., Kempen, G.I.J., Pennix, B.W.J.H. et al. (2003) Relationship between changes in depressive symptoms and unhealthy lifestyles in late middle aged and older persons: results from the Longitudinal Aging Study Amsterdam, *Age & Ageing*, 32: 81–87.

van Tilburg, T., Gierveld, J.D., Lecchini, L. and Marsiglia, D. (1998) Social integration and loneliness: a comparative study among older adults in the Netherlands and Tuscany, Italy, *Journal of Social and Personal Relationships*, 15(6): 740–54.

Victor, C., Scambler, S.J., Bowling, A. and Bond, J. (2005) The prevalence and risk factors for loneliness in later life: a survey of older people in Great Britain, *Ageing & Society*, 25(3): 357–75.

Victor, C., Scambler, S. and Bond, J. (2009) *The Social World of Older People: Understanding Loneliness and Social Isolation in Later Life*. Maidenhead: Open University Press.

Victor, C.R. (1989) Inequalities in health in later life, *Age & Ageing*, 18(6): 387–91.

Wheeler, F.A., Gore, K.M. and Greenblatt, B. (1998) The beneficial effects of volunteering for older volunteers and the people they serve: a meta analysis, *International Journal of Ageing and Human Development*, 47(1): 69–79.

White, H., McConnell, E., Clipp, E. et al. (2002) A randomized controlled trial of the psychosocial impact of providing internet training and access to older adults, *Aging and Mental Health*, 6(3): 213–21.

Windle, G. (2009) What is mental health and mental well-being? in M. Cattan (ed.) *Mental Health and Well-being in Later Life*. Maidenhead: Open University Press.

Windle, G., Hughes, D., Link, P. et al. (2007) Public health interventions to promote mental well-being in people aged 65 and over: systematic review of effectiveness and cost-effectiveness, *Evidence Reviews*. Bangor, University of Wales. London: NICE.

World Health Organization (2002) *Active Ageing: A Policy Framework*. Geneva: WHO.

CHAPTER 17

Reflections and views from older people on health and social care

Ann Macfarlane

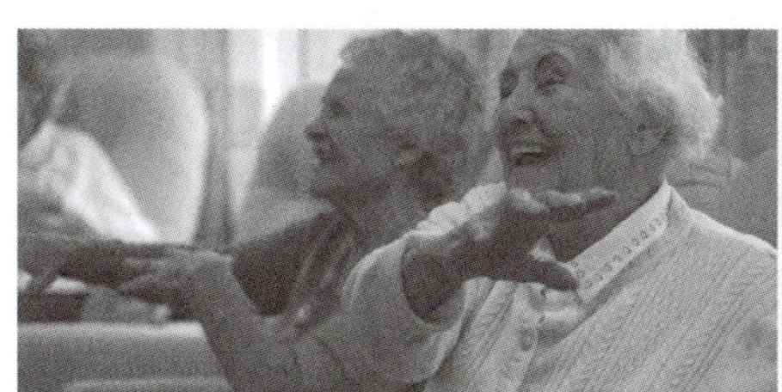
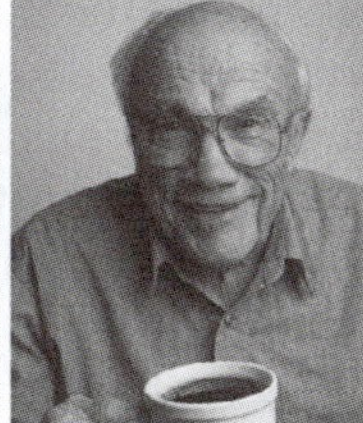
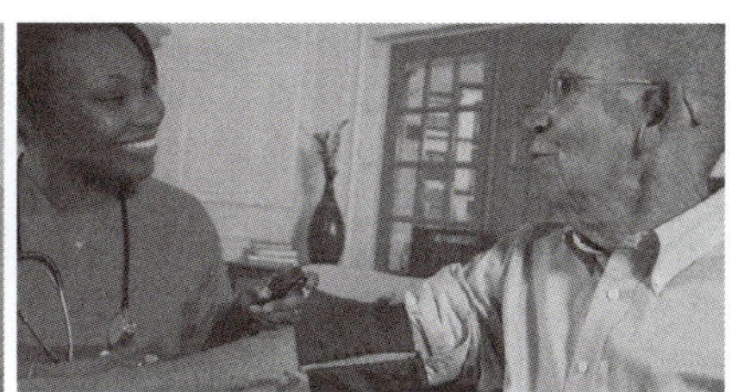

Learning objectives

At the end of this chapter, the reader will be able to:

- describe some direct personal experiences and observations of health and social care by older people in hospital, residential and hospice settings, and within a home environment
- identify the principles of independent living and older people
- identify what constitutes a good life for older people
- critique the importance of current legislation, personalization and co-production approaches
- identify the importance of discharge from hospital and good practice in health and social care issues for a return to maintaining health at home
- describe ways of working with older people with long-term conditions to manage in hospital and residential settings
- identify some solutions for health and social care professionals as they engage with older people in health care settings

Introduction

This chapter is written by an older woman who has been a disabled person for many years and experienced health care prior to and from the formation of legislation leading to the

1947 National Health Service Act. The chapter draws on the experiences of older people taking part in group sessions and the voices of many individual older people who want to be part of this book to support those planning, commissioning, delivering, monitoring and evaluating health and social care services. Other chapters also draw on the experiences of older people as it is their input that will help the nursing profession to continue to improve its practice and make health care provision for older people truly positive and empowering.

Introduction to some of the main causes of lack of confidence, self-esteem, dignity and self-worth that older people experience

Many older people, who experience hospitalization following traumatic experiences in the later stage in their lives, change from being an older person to a perpetual patient. Older people who have grown older with impairment and who already have many experiences of being in contact with the medical profession dread the thought of having to go back into institutionalized settings when they are ill. Once older people acquire the label of 'patient', and which is often retained, they remain in a world where much of the language is unintelligible and termed 'jargon', isolating them at a time when to have information and to be consulted is of vital importance. Many on admission to hospital or a residential setting are referred to as 'cases', treated as 'objects' and patronized. There is seldom acknowledgement of the status of older people, relating to what they did prior to becoming 'older', what they currently enjoy, how they spend time, and the roles and responsibilities they had and continue to have within family life and as citizens in wider society. Policies are designed to separate older people out and use language such as 'geriatric', 'dementia cases', 'frail elderly', 'vulnerable adults' and 'elderly mentally infirm' (EMI).

In practice, nurses and other medical practitioners become or remain remote, with practices and skills that focus on technical procedures. These can leave older people isolated from the very people who are employed to 'care' for them. Older people feel that current practices provide minimum human contact that results in touch from the use of rubber gloves, synthetic continence sheets and invasive procedures that include the insertion of catheters comprised of synthetic materials. There are many practices that leave older people (particularly those with high support needs) feeling undignified, not respected and less than human. These may relate to culture and behaviour, not understanding people's values, beliefs, religious needs and practices, the language older people speak and need to hear, and their basic human needs neglected through the progression of scientific research and treatment. Often procedures that keep older people alive are dehumanizing and sometimes treatments are continued long after they produce any health gains but are viewed as 'doing something'. Some intrusive treatments are prolonged to satisfy relatives who cannot bear to watch their older relative suffer and die and this is to the detriment of dignity and quality of life of the older person. It is also a fact that kind and caring practitioners find it difficult to sustain positive behaviour and practices in an institutional environment where negative ways of working have prevailed. There is no suggestion that older people should be 'written off' but rather that everything possible should be done to preserve dignity and quality care that results in well-being.

Scenario 17.1

Mavis, who has multiple long-term health conditions, one of them being a weak heart, says: 'Doctors and other professional people won't talk to each other and make decisions. Because of my weak heart, having an artificial leg and walking with a frame, and the fact that I have several steps leading down from my front door, makes it difficult for me to go outside. I have been told I can only go out in an ambulance with two attendants to keep hospital appointments. Therefore, I have no social life outside in the local community. I can no longer attend church, get my hair washed and styled as I have been used to, and I can't visit friends. I would like the doctors and other professional people supporting me to ask me what would assist me to become more independent and less isolated. This would immediately make me feel that people were interested in my well-being and give me confidence to believe that if action is taken I can become more in control of my life.'

- *Mavis is asking for the people supporting her to ask her what would assist her to become more independent and less isolated – ask this question of older people you are supporting at present and identify goals that they are suggesting themselves.*

Experiences of health and social care from older people themselves

Retired nurses who use health services have been heard to say, 'If only I knew when I was nursing what I know now . . .' By the time a retired nurse is in a position whereby they require nursing and social care input for themselves, this type of comment is far too late. People taking up a career in nursing and allied professions need to understand and apply principles of 'independent living'. Independent living is defined as having a voice, making choices and taking control. Principles should be embedded into policies and commissioning and integral to nursing standards. These principles should be addressed in basic, intermediate and advanced training in all health care courses as they apply to older people.

Key point

The principles of independent living that focus on older people having a voice and being listened to, making choices and taking control of their lives wherever and whenever possible, should be embedded into policies and commissioning and integral to nursing standards and practice.

The majority of older people are able to voice their opinions and make their wishes known. However, there are situations where, despite having capacity, older people (particularly if they have high support needs) have their wishes ignored or disregarded. Older people state that this can occur in their own home but is more likely to be evidenced on admission to an accident and emergency department or within a residential setting. They say that lying on a trolley, or in a hospital bed, makes it difficult to engage in conversation because they cannot hear or see or may feel afraid of making their wishes known. It is amazing how quickly one can feel dehumanized, especially once a person is deprived of their hearing aid, dentures, spectacles, personal clothing and jewellery. Often assumptions are made by professional people who have never been in contact with the older person before admission, which may lead to judgements being based solely on their medical condition and/or impairment. These assumptions can lead to inappropriate outcomes.

Many older people, who develop ill health, will have the experience of being admitted to a hospital bed to be nursed by strangers in an alien environment. They will often not be able to clearly see the people who come to them or understand what they say through the language used. They will not be able to hear sufficiently to know what is being said to them or about them as people stand at the end of the bed or walk away as they are speaking. They may have the courage to ask a question or request something, but they may not always get a response or one they can hear or interpret and this leads to a lack of appropriate support and can even add to or escalate their ill health.

Scenario 17.2

Phyllis, a single woman in her early 80s, had never been in hospital until one day, while alighting from a train at a main London Railway Station, she fell between the train and platform. She was admitted to a leading London hospital and was visited two days later by a friend. Phyllis was lying flat on her back awaiting an operation on her severely damaged femur. Her friend asked, 'What can I do to help you?' This fiercely independent and highly educated woman replied, 'Please tell the doctors who I am and ask them to send me someone with whom I can communicate. I don't know exactly what I have done to myself, I'm not sure what will happen next, and if I am going to be able to walk again. I'm frightened.'

- *What do you need to do to help Phyllis feel more informed about her situation and less frightened?*

Scenario 17.3

Mrs Carter called out when the drinks trolley came to the ward door, 'Please can I have some tea?' The domestic assistant brought a half cup of tea and placed it on the bed table far out of reach. 'Please can you give me my tea?' The domestic assistant was pushing the trolley down the corridor and did not hear the request. Mrs Carter called in vain for some time until a nurse came by and pushed the bed table near the bed but not quite near enough. In the struggle to reach the cup of tea Mrs Carter spilt it all over the bed and onto the floor. An agency nurse, who appeared to be asleep, eventually left his chair and came to the bedside and stared at the bedcovers. He eventually used a towel from the back of the locker to dry the floor. He left the ward with the wet bed sheet.

On return he threw back the bedcovers exposing Mrs Carter to other patients. Mrs Carter said, 'Please may I have more tea?' Without a word, the nurse left and some 10 minutes later came back with a cup of tea and placed it on the bed table, leaving it again just out of reach. He then went away again and finally came back with clean covers and a colleague to assist him. The curtains were pulled round the bed and the bed table with the tea on it was left to grow cold outside the curtains.

- *What could the nurse have done to ensure that Mrs Carter had a cup of tea in comfort?*
- *What effect did the nurse's action in this scenario have on Mrs Carter's sense of well-being and security in this ward?*
- *What would you do differently?*

These are some of the many scenarios that illustrate how any empathy, concern and care have gone from some members of the nursing profession to be replaced by a lack of understanding of what it is to be a human being in need of support. A recent report from The Patients Association 'Listening to Patients, Speak up for Change' (December 2010) reinforces the views and experiences of older people cited here.

Listening to older people in a group setting, many views were expressed on the experience of being in hospital. Older people said that nurses had treated them with kindness, courtesy, compassion and respect and they felt they had been listened to. One older person said that she was afraid she was going to die and she was desperate not to die alone but did not like to ask someone to stay with her. Older people said that despite their fears they welcomed staff with whom they were able to joke and be able to laugh. Several people said that they were treated as if, at 70 years old, their life was over. Everybody said how much they wanted staff to listen to their worries and views and not be dominated or dictated to. Group members said that often they did feel isolated and this was compounded if there were no other patients with whom they could communicate. They also stated that communication was a two-way process and it was important that they spoke up, if they were able to communicate verbally, and to make their wishes known. On the subject of receiving a diagnosis, especially one that might result in long-term treatment or death, they wanted nurses and other professional people to give them the time and understanding to express their fears, formulate questions and with opportunities to return to issues that they might not have thought of or found too difficult to articulate on receiving the diagnosis. There were many comments that focused on doctors and nurses giving mixed messages, resulting in confusion, annoyance and anger. These mixed messages were mainly about medication, date of discharge and support they might receive on leaving hospital.

Older people talked about how things had changed over the last few years. These included the proliferation of knowledge and information, particularly that found on web sites, and the openness of medical professionals that enabled people to have more choice and take risks in determining outcomes for well-being.

In terms of health and social care practitioners visiting older people at home, there were many positive views about the way people experienced respect, kindness and understanding but there was a request for more supervision. People who had had a negative experience felt that professional people coming into the home were left to work unsupervised. This resulted in poor practices, such as lack of cleanliness in hand-washing, leaving dirty dressings unprotected and disempowering language.

Support to help older people feel safe and in control

Older people talked about a nursing assessment that encompasses not only the immediate situation in which they find themselves but the longer term and that the initial assessment should come under regular review. They wanted health and social care professionals to have access to a brief life history set down in words, photographs and pictures that they themselves would provide. This would describe life lived prior to admission and include close family relationships, career paths, current hopes, their dreams and future goals. Older seriously ill people and perhaps moving to end-of-life care equally deserve to experience choice and control in their lives and there is an urgency to create a space in which the nurse and older person can talk sensitively and empathetically about hopes and dreams.

When life is coming towards an end, it demands a greater degree of urgency in listening to and understanding what would make a difference to older people. It is unlikely that the needs and wants of older people in a critical condition will be any greater than those in a less serious situation, but even more vital that a nurse or other professional practitioner respects the fact that the older person cannot keep hearing the phrase 'Wait a minute'. Hospices can perpetuate many of the institutional approaches and behaviours witnessed in hospital and residential settings. Within all training courses there is a need, therefore, to demedicalize much of the course content to reflect the importance of an 'independent living' approach.

The social model of disability and principles of independent living

The term 'independent living' comes from the Disabled Peoples' Movement. It came at a time when disabled people, particularly those with an academic background, debated and came to understand and write about the 'social model of disability'. The social model addresses the barriers that disabled people face in their daily lives, such as those presented in the built environment, within institutional structures and procedures, peoples' attitudes and behaviour, and lack of accessible, appropriate and timely information. The social model moves away from the notion that people's impairments are the problem, to an approach that addresses barriers that can be dismantled, improved or changed. The social model focuses on community and societal issues. Independent living concentrates on empowering people, giving them a voice, choice and control in their lives. Choice and control relate to all aspects of life, such as education, employment, housing, transport, medical care and personal assistance.

Key point

The social model of disability addresses the barriers that disabled people face in their daily lives, such as those presented in the built environment, within institutional structures and procedures, peoples' attitudes and behaviour, and lack of accessible, appropriate and timely information.

Independent living can make a huge difference to older people and their families, including:

- a wider range of options for housing and personal support in later life;
- greater awareness and take-up of personal social care and health budgets and direct payments amongst older disabled people;
- person-centred support planning to enable older disabled people to have a strong voice and influence over their own support and how to live life;

- innovative ways of enabling choice and control for older people in residential and nursing care settings and for older people with cognitive impairments, including those with dementia;
- opportunities for older disabled people to play a full part in family, community and civic life.

(Office of Disability Issues website)

The six principles of independent living that include older people

The following six principles should guide the planning, commissioning and provision of all support for older people at a strategic level. These principles encompass any situation in which older people find themselves.

- **Principle 1 seeks to increase the voice of older disabled people** in order for them to have choice and control.
- **Principle 2 ensures equal access for older people** over the services they may need or already receive.
- **Principle 3 enables older people to have choice and control** over the support they need to live their everyday lives, and this can include hospital and other institutional settings.
- **Principle 4 enables participation** in family, community and civic life and is an important goal for older people. All of the above principles should lead to this, and being in residential settings should not preclude this participation.
- **Principle 5 ensures that professional people working at a strategic level** have particular responsibility for making sure that policies and initiatives fit together in a strategic way – at national, regional and local levels.
- **Principle 6 promotes a new way of thinking** whereby at the broadest level, a different 'demographic dialogue' about older people is needed. This new way of thinking is one that reflects the realities, not just the fears, of population ageing and one that proactively plans for the changes ahead.

(Office of Disability Issues)

Applying independent living principles as they fit into the wider policy context for older people within a hospital, residential or hospice setting is crucial to achieving positive outcomes for older people.

Scenario 17.4

An older, long-term friend, Mrs Robson, who has severe diabetes and an above-knee left-leg amputation following gangrene, now has a prosthesis fitted to the left femur. A recent episode of ill health required hospitalization and stabilizing her diabetic condition took several weeks in an acute setting. She was transferred to a rehabilitation ward in a hospital close to her home and, after six weeks with some physiotherapy, she has made slow progress. The reasons that appear obvious to a layperson are not addressed by professional medical staff, including nurses. My friend, who was a senior social worker until retirement, and who has years of managing her diabetes, struggles to get her voice heard, and her views acknowledged

(*continued*)

and acted upon. Her meals are provided within a tight daily timetable that means her diabetes remains uncontrolled. Visiting times are rigid, she has no access to a radio, and she can only access TV programmes if she leaves her bed and goes to a day room which she is unable to do without assistance. Use of a mobile phone is refused and the wards have one landline phone to be shared between 40 people. She continues to require constant support to stand and walk from her bedside to the toilet, to the bathroom and to other day-time facilities. Due to a continual shortage of staff, my friend struggles with continence, with assessing and responding to her diabetic status, and has little intelligent stimulation. She has become totally institutionalized and it is difficult to envisage an outcome that will enable her to return home. Visitors to the hospital, such as those with mobility impairments, can only gain access to wards via a manually operated lift that is beyond the strength of all but those who can manually open and shut heavy doors.

Within a strictly controlled medical environment it is not difficult to see how changes in attitudes, the built environment, institutionalized procedures and approaches and access to information could greatly improve the quality of my friend's life and that of the people in the adjacent beds. To assist and hasten recovery, my friend needs access to family life, support to live in her own home and the right to access community life, including access to her general practitioner and other medical facilities and services. She also requires access to a personal budget that will enable her to achieve her goals and dreams. My friend states that the nursing staff, including occupational and physiotherapists and doctors, are kind, but they appear to have no knowledge of legislation and policies that could make a difference to her life and that of her family. This knowledge, put into practice, would make a significant difference to my friend's daily hospital routine and prepare her far more adequately for a return within her family.

- *How can you make sure you know about all the relevant legislation and policy needed to better support Mrs Robson?*
- *How can you work with other professions to ensure that Mrs Robson's needs are met to ensure a safe discharge to her own home?*

What constitutes a good life for older people?

Older people, including those with high support needs, tell us:

- meaningful relationships;
- personal identity and self-esteem;
- personalized support and care;
- personal authority and control;
- meaningful daily and community life;
- home and personal belongings.

(Older Peoples Programme, now the National Team for Inclusion)

While these keys to a good life were developed with older people, mainly in residential settings, it does not mean that they cannot be used to make a difference within medical environments. Older people tell us how much they would value nurses and other professional medical staff relating to them on a one-to-one basis – the need for personal identity and not being labelled a 'dementia sufferer', a 'stroke victim' and other negative terminology that hinders self-esteem and feeling good about self. Personalized support and care can improve health and well-being, particularly if nursing staff take care with helping older people to adequately undertake personal hygiene, with assistance where required, to dress, apply make-up, perfume, and have assistance with brushing hair and the toilet.

Personalization and co-production

'Personalization' means having the ability to design, provide and co-ordinate services that meet the needs of individual people who require support. 'Co-production' is about individuals, communities and organizations having the skills, knowledge and ability to work together, create opportunities and problem-solve. Co-production sounds simple but is a relatively new way of working and older people may need time to gain confidence, build trust and acquire a mutual understanding of policies and practices that will enable them to make decisions about how they want to live life, particularly after a crisis or illness where hospitalization has been a significant part of recovery. There are often forums for older people within local communities that have the ability to act as a reference group where local authorities, statutory community services and voluntary sector organizations can benefit from the input of these older peoples' groups. Organizations managed and controlled by disabled people, often called 'centres for independent living', have older people as members who work within the organizations. There is much expertise that older people can offer and this should be accessed to improve nursing practice.

A key part of personalization and co-production in the reform of public services is the promotion of voice, choice and control of older people, including those with high support needs. Nurses and other medical practitioners working with older people to deliver independent living will not only meet national and local targets that will achieve better outcomes for older people and their families, but it will make nursing older people much more rewarding. Older people will be given opportunities to say what makes life good for them and they will help to find the solutions to the difficulties they experience, and nurses and other medical staff will find their work more interesting. Working practices will enable older people to have and take more control and reach maximum health goals more quickly. Bad days will turn into good days and there will be a sense of achievement by the ill person, nurses and other medically trained practitioners who will leave their shift knowing they have made a difference to an older person's quality of life.

Key point

A key part of personalization and co-production in the reform of public services is the promotion of voice, choice and control of older people.

Many nurses say that they work in 'person-centred' ways and adopt 'person-centred' approaches. In practice this is not often the case and when nurses have the opportunity to think through their attitudes, behaviour, practices and the way in which they relate to older people, particularly those who are ill, they know this is not how they work. There is little evidence to suggest that older people are involved in their own health care, although work is being done with older people who have long-term conditions. An example of this has been focus groups where people with long-term conditions have been able to discuss together what works well for them in their own home environment. This shared knowledge and information can prove beneficial and lead to further health and practical gains. This work needs to be extended so greater numbers of older people benefit in terms of their health and well-being.

Older peoples' expectations are that they will receive treatment that will enable them to live long and healthy lives and do so in the comfort of their own homes. However, in the process of reaching optimum health, it is crucial that ill and disabled people also receive support, when required, from people dedicated to ensuring that basic nursing needs are met, and to a high standard. The nursing degree may result in nurses trained and qualified to carry out complex technical procedure but it continues to beg the question of who will be trained and available to provide basic personal hygiene, remove soiled bed linen and replace with clean sheets, and ensure older people experience good quality basic care that supports well-being. We know that in recent years many older people have died from lack of hydration and adequate nutrition. Further research has revealed that on average two older people a day die from thirst in hospital.

Discharge from hospital to living at home

Older people who are in hospital require accessible and timely information in formats that assist them to make appropriate choices and decisions for their future. This information exists and should be available well before discharge arrangements are made and activated. This information must be available in formats to enable those with different impairments to make choices and take control of their lives. Following an illness or trauma, older people state that they need time to make the best decisions and should not find their needs assessed without them being present and having decisions made for them by a professional medical team with the input of relatives. Many wanted close family involved but most of all they wanted to be present and to be the first to be informed about their illness or condition.

There are a variety of options in most communities, which should include going home as a priority. Older people need information on direct payments and personal and/or individual budgets that could support them in their own home. National organizations can provide information that enable older people to continue with local voluntary work or to return to their former paid employment or take on new challenges when they return to health Many older people who currently live in residential and nursing settings complain that they were taken straight from their hospital bed to a residential setting, often never having an opportunity to return to their home environment.

Scenario 17.5

Mrs Martin experienced a trauma resulting in a long hospital stay. Her illness became a series of long-term conditions and on assessment prior to discharge it was decided that she would be admitted to a nursing home while adaptations took place in her home. These were estimated to take six weeks. Mrs Martin stayed in the nursing home for almost a year and she never lost hope that she would return to her own home. She says: 'During that year I had to return to hospital several times and each time there was a delay in building works, adaptations and the delivery of equipment. Now I am in my own surroundings, I am so happy. I need five visits by nurses each day and I am still awaiting the equipment that will enable me to get in and out of the front door, but I have achieved my goal and many professional people and friends have supported me during the year long process.'

- *What can you do to ensure that you are as well informed as possible to support Mrs Martin and other older people through a lengthy period of repatriation to their own home?*

Because health workers often do not know the full extent of what help and support is available in the community, older people miss out on vital information that could make a significant difference to their quality of life and to decisions that may affect the rest of their lives, particularly in relation to their environment. It is well researched and documented that many older people reside in residential care or nursing home environments when returning home would have provided a far more appropriate outcome for them (Older People's Programme 2006). This is where 'person-centred' thinking, 'person-centred' approaches and co-production can make all the difference when decisions are taken that concern older people.

Many health and local authority older peoples' services work in partnership, using multidisciplinary teams, to work with older people to achieve positive outcomes. However, there continues to be an imbalance in the way in which all disciplines work, with a medical approach that continues to dominate. Health and social care practitioners are often compromised due to a perceived lack of time that can be spent with each older person. Initial additional time allocated to talking with and making plans with an older person could make a significant difference to the quality of their future life. Older people often know exactly what would improve their daily living. Time needs to be taken to observe, listen and act in ways that are truly 'person-centred' and these are skills that require rigorous practice and continuous application.

Organizations that can support older peoples' well-being

The social care Institute for Excellence (SCIE) provides TV online with a range of e-learning materials that enable health and social care practitioners to self-assess their knowledge and practices. Interactive programmes that are continually added to and updated, including information and best practice guides in paper format, provide a wealth of support and are easy to access. The website is also a source of information for the public, including patients. There is also a series of self-help booklets for people with long-term conditions produced by the Department of Health (DoH). The National Centre for Independent Living (NCIL) is another resource that supports older and disabled people. This organization supports a network of local centres for independent living managed and controlled by disabled people who advise on a range of issues that enhance the lives of older and disabled people, and can include assistance with acquiring direct payment and individual budgets. Age UK, together with other national organizations and local forums that support older people, offer a range of advice and practical services to remove or reduce difficulties older people experience.

How older disabled people manage within hospital and residential settings

To disabled older people, admission to hospital can bring feelings of fear. This fear specifically relates to how medical and nursing staff understand impairment. Disabled people who grow older often have an intimate knowledge of themselves in relation to their impairment. They have had to deal with all manner of situations at different stages of impairment, especially if the condition is one of deterioration. Many conditions, however, remain stable over many years and the person manages them on a day-to-day basis with or without assistance. To enter an unfamiliar environment can present barriers not experienced in a home setting. If a disabled older person enters a long-term residential setting, there may be more time for staff to familiarize themselves with the impairment and the barriers within the residential environment, but this may not be possible when a person is admitted to a hospital ward where the impairment is not the primary diagnosis.

To be in a system where individual needs are difficult to take into account presents huge fears for the disabled person. These fears may be around the fact that they cannot see their surroundings, cannot hear what is being said to them, may have intellectual impairment, may use mobility equipment, such as a walking frame or wheelchair, and may not be able to eat independently or manage the toilet without assistance. There are many issues that a disabled person may need help with and this demands *an accurate assessment of need*, excellent communication between practitioners and the disabled person themselves and the ability to get to know an individual's needs.

Disabled people themselves are likely to be able to communicate what they require and will probably know what is needed to assist in their recovery far better than the staff member, and it is this information and knowledge that staff need to understand and pass on to appropriate hospital personnel. Staff need to know the stress and insecurity experienced if a disabled person cannot access equipment that they need to function within a hospital environment. For an older person to have specific assistance ignored or denied is to deny that person their humanity and dignity and may heighten risk of that individual.

When an older person has been an active citizen and experiences a traumatic event that, besides the onset of illness, leaves them with residual impairment, then the fears may well be different. A person who becomes disabled when older is likely to have little or no knowledge of their rights and entitlements as a disabled person. They will require people who can give them timely and accurate information that will enable them to make choices and take as much control back into their lives as they would wish. This is particularly true of a person who may, at the time when discharge from hospital is being considered, need to make serious choices about their options around going home. Their home may not be so accessible to them and may require adaptations and equipment that would significantly delay discharge. This situation is likely to result in a temporary admission to a residential setting and, if managed proactively, could lead to discharge home when adaptations have been completed. However, it is known that institutionalization takes place very quickly and, without input from appropriately trained staff, it is likely the person will remain in a long-term environment. There can also be many inequalities that leave older disabled people angry and disempowered.

Scenario 17.6

Jack lived in a third-floor flat and had become more immobile over several years to the point where he could no longer access the stairs. There was no lift to his apartment. He also had severe diabetes that was affecting his eyesight. Jack's brother, George, two years older than Jack, lives in a neighbouring village governed by a different local council. George lives in a first floor flat, again with no lift and he, too, has deteriorating health. Jack's care manager insisted that Jack must consider entering a residential setting mainly on the grounds of his visual impairment. Jack was adamant that he wanted to stay put and asked for help with undertaking tasks such as someone to read and respond to his correspondence, a large dial watch, a large screen for his TV and for the chemist to sort out his medication so he could manage it better by himself. He also wanted more hours than allocated through an agency for housework and shopping. The care manager told Jack that his needs could not be adequately met and that he would be far safer if he was supported within a residential environment. Jack talked with George whose care manager had arranged for him to have a personal budget. George used the money to meet his needs which included having two personal assistants to assist him with bathing and dressing, preparing meals, some housework and laundry. He saved a little money each week until he had enough to get some help to go out to a football match.

Jack told his care manager about George and asked for his needs to be reassessed in the hope he could have a personal budget. However, his care manager was not well trained in how to provide Jack with a personal budget and she was far more concerned that the risk of Jack staying at home was too great. Eventually Jack was so worried about the future that he went into a residential setting where he has now been for eight years. When last visited Jack he was very angry: 'My capital will run out in four months and I don't know what will happen. George can't help me because he is struggling to pay his support charges. I wish I had taken George's advice and stuck out to stay in my own home but I felt I couldn't stand the strain of managing without appropriate help and I didn't have anyone else at the time to support me in considering all my options.'

- *What support did Jack need when he was living in his own home?*
- *How could you have better supported him?*

Some ideas and solutions that would make a difference when nursing ill and/or disabled older people

- Learn about the social model and independent living approaches.
- Observe, listen and act as appropriate and in a timely manner.
- Ensure practitioners receive appropriate and timely training in all aspects of health and social care and understand how this applies to positive outcomes for older people.
- Bring back the practice of the ward sister or nurse in charge visiting each older person at the beginning of every shift. This practice will pick up the concerns that people have

and that can often be dealt with quickly. Departmental matrons are being introduced in some hospital settings and it may be their responsibility to check on individual patients' welfare.

- Volunteers can bring huge gains to patient support and comfort. Such people could be strategically positioned within the hospital and residential environments to provide additional non-medical support, such as helping people to find and wear their hearing aids, spectacles and dentures and to gain access to facilities and services that would assist them to achieve independence. Volunteers could also be assigned to people whose needs may relate to someone talking with them and making notes for them to use with visitors or with medical and nursing practitioners so their needs could be met more effectively.
- Ensure that older people receive coherent messages about their condition and what is to happen. Current practices of being visited by different professional people who continually give confusing information leave older people bewildered.
- During the period when older people are in hospital, take time to find out about their lifestyle and their views about their discharge. Discuss issues in private rather than letting other people in the ward hear what is being said to and about the older person.
- Whenever possible ensure older people are able to dress appropriately and have their dignity preserved by enabling them to be clean, neat, have their hair brushed, have access to spectacles, contact lenses, their teeth and dentures cleaned and their feet washed and kept warm with footwear or blankets.
- Make a note of what assistance older people need, such as help with cutting food, reading a menu, making appointments and ensure this information is recorded in the notes. This is vital if an older person lacks regular visitors.
- Ask older people what they would like nearby so that they can access a drink, read the newspaper, do a crossword or make a telephone call.
- Make sure a call bell is left within reach.
- At out-patient appointments, come up to an older person and ask their name and find out other information, ensuring as much privacy as possible.
- Ensure disabled people are respected for what they know about their impairment and how to manage it. Ask them what would assist them during their hospital admission and remove barriers as appropriate.
- Allow time to provide up-to-date information about what options are available when assisting the older person to plan their own discharge.

Conclusion

It is the seemingly insignificant daily requirements of all of us that make a difference to our well-being in life and this is no different for older people, including older people who have high support needs. To have information in formats that are accessible and able to be understood is empowering and supports older people to make choices that will benefit them. Culturally sensitive support and an empathetic approach makes all the difference to older people who are ill and who may be far from home and relatives. The built environment has a major impact on a person's well-being and the availability of food that the person likes and is able to eat, particularly identifying and acknowledging cultural preferences, hot drinks and snacks as required, knowing where the toilet is situated and how help will be provided to access it, having items within reach, and the ability of someone to check with the older person that they have what they need before they are left alone really shows care and concern. These, and many other seemingly small things, contribute to positive outcomes that will greatly enhance well-being and quality of life. Older people who have been asked for their opinions on what they value most from health and social care professional people state that it is those who will listen, respect their opinions, give them time and empathy, and take action when required and where appropriate, who are the people they most value. Those are the people who make a difficult or painful experience more bearable. It does not seem much to ask but the rewards are great.

Key point

Older people who have been asked for their opinions on what they value most from health and social care professional people state that it is those who will listen, respect their opinions, give them time and empathy, and take action when required and where appropriate, who are the people they most value.

Acknowledgement

The chapter has been greatly enhanced by the input of individual older people who shared their stories and to the group of older people who generously shared their time and experiences at Age Concern, Kingston upon Thames.

Appendix 1: Further resources

There are many resources available to use to understand specific problems or services. It is, however, important to be aware of the agendas behind these resources that a range of positions might have been adopted and that it is useful to consider the background of resources so that they can be seen in this context. Some agencies might be involved in campaigns or canvassing, so this might not fit with the aims of your information-gathering. You may, however, choose to look at this information as part of the process of putting a picture together.

Sometimes this picture can be clarified by putting together a cross-section of presentations, comparing positions taken by organizations with known agendas. You can also look at the evidence used and its soundness – is this partisan or imbalanced?

You should also be aware of the way that organizations and information changes over time. Sometimes new information is found, and sometimes organizations fold up. This means that what you can find or get access to might only be available on the day that you find it!

It is also important to be aware of the importance of locality. Resources could be different in different places, or governed by different laws. You may, therefore, bear this in mind when looking for information – while the issue might be universal, for example good nutrition, the system for accessing this might be different in different places.

You may also need to be aware of the importance of the form in which information is provided. Some people may be adept at using computers; others may be good at reading or others comfortable with listening. For many people a range of different formats can be appropriate, but whatever the form, a careful thinking through the options may be needed. This may involve assessing preferences and continually monitoring them. In addition, thought may need to be given, not only to the format but also the tools that may be required. If someone has a visual impairment, for example, large book print may help, but the availability of this may need to be checked.

The following are examples of different resources which may be helpful to you.

General sites for nursing older people

Age UK

Information for older people and carers (www.ageuk.org.uk).

Alzheimer's Society

The Alzheimer's Society produces a number of leaflets to help those caring for someone with dementia (www.alzheimers.org.uk).

Arthritis Care

Arthritis Care produces many free publications on arthritis and related conditions as well as information on achieving optimum health for people with arthritis and how they can enjoy community life and undertake paid employment. Arthritis Care also campaigns on issues that affect the lives of those with arthritis (www.arthritiscare.org.uk).

British Geriatrics Society (BGS)

www.bgs.org.uk

National Development Team for inclusion (NDTi)

www.ndti.org.uk (this address includes the Older People's Programme plus the Older People's Programme 2006).

National Patient Safety Agency

www.npsa.nhs.uk

Office of Disability Issues

www.odi.dwp.org.uk

Royal College of Nursing

www.rcn.org.uk

Specialist sites

Aphasia Help

An aphasia-friendly website designed with support of people with aphasia (www.aphasiahelp.org/).

Association for Continence Advice (ACA)

A membership organization for health and social care professionals concerned with the progression of care for continence (www.aca.uk.com/index.php).

Bereavement Services Association (BSA)

The BSA provides a network for all those who provide bereavement support services, primarily within the NHS (www.bsauk.org/).

British Association for Parenteral and Enteral Nutrition (BAPEN)

www.bapen.org.uk/must_tool.html

British Dietetic Association

www.bda.uk.com/

CRUSE Bereavement Care

The charity CRUSE provides support and offers information, advice, education and training services with the aim to promote the well-being of bereaved people. Services are free to bereaved people (www.crusebereavementcare.org.uk/).

Department of Work and Pensions

Access to Work is a scheme that provides support to those who need it to undertake paid employment. The scheme is managed and financed by the DWP (www.dwp.gov.uk).

European Association of Palliative Care

www.eapcnet.org

Help the Hospices

A site for professionals, families and friends; includes information about carers' assessments, young carers, death and dying (www.helpthehospices.org.uk).

PromoCon

Provides a national service to improve the life for all people with bladder or bowel problems by offering product information, advice and practical solutions to both professionals and the general public (www.promocon.co.uk/aboutpromocon.shtml).

Royal National Institute for the Blind (RNIB)

The UK's leading charity offering information, support and advice to almost two million people with sight loss (www.rnib.org.uk).

Speakabaility

A useful website for people with aphasia and other communication difficulties (www.speakability.org.uk/).

The Bladder and Bowel Foundation

The UK's leading charity providing information and support for people with bladder and bowel control problems, their carers, families and health care professionals (www.bladderandbowelfoundation.org/).

The National Council for Palliative Care (NCPC)

The NCPC is the umbrella organization for all those who are involved in providing, commissioning and using palliative care and hospice services in England, Wales and Northern Ireland and promotes the extension and improvement of palliative care services for all people with life-threatening and life-limiting conditions (www.ncpc.org.uk).

Volunteering England

A UK charity offering information and advice to individuals and organizations on all aspects of undertaking voluntary work (www.volunteering England.org.uk).

Index

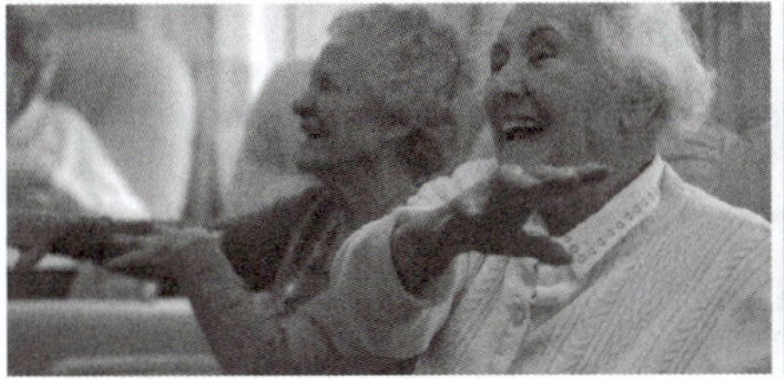
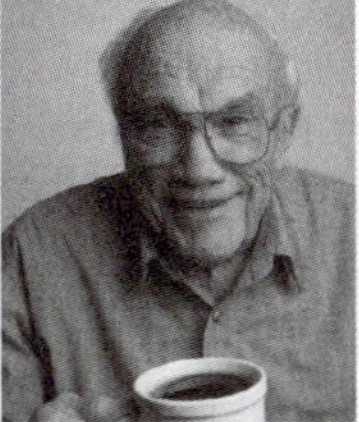
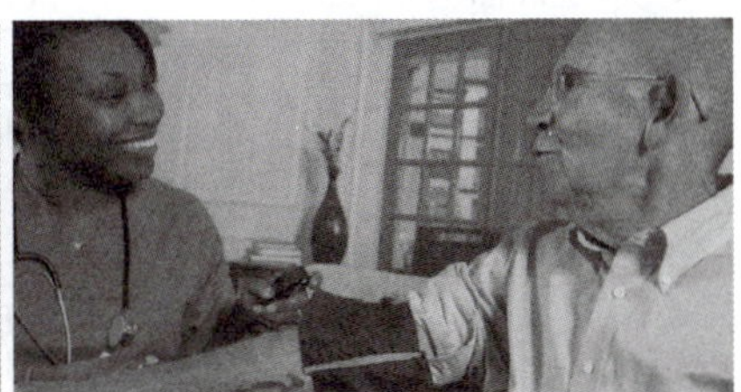

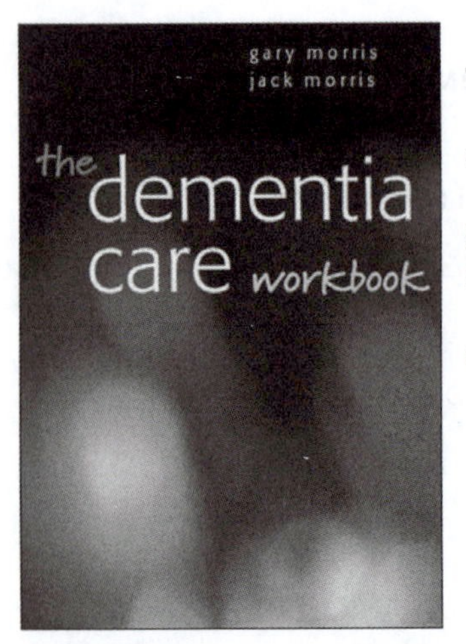

THE DEMENTIA CARE WORKBOOK

Gary Morris and Jack Morris

9780335234318 (Paperback)
2010

eBook also available

This excellent workbook builds upon the person-centred approach to dementia care, and gives students, practitioners and carers a new way of looking at dementia and the people who live with it. The authors reflect upon the reality of working within dementia care and the importance of working positively with others to achieve the best care possible.

The workbook is full of exercises and activities to try, all designed to help you engage, connect and empower the person with dementia as well their families/carers.

Key features include:

- Understanding how it feels to live with dementia.
- Recognising the issues and feelings involved for family carers or healthcare professionals
- Vignettes and examples of good and realistic practice throughout
- Encouraging you to examine your own practice and explore ways in which the care you give can be enhanced.

www.openup.co.uk

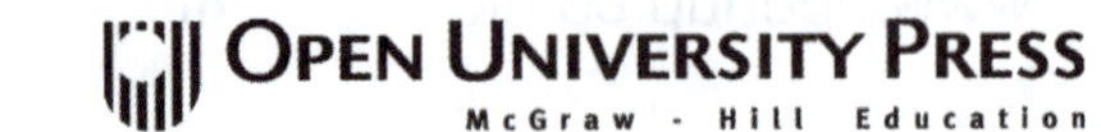